SHORT AND LONG TERM EFFECTS OF BREAST FEEDING ON CHILD HEALTH

ADVANCES IN EXPERIMENTAL MEDICINE AND BIOLOGY

SHORT AND LONG TERM EFFECTS OF BREAST FEEDING ON CHILD HEALTH

Edited by

Berthold Koletzko
University of Munich
Munich, Germany

Kim Fleischer Michaelsen
The Royal Veterinary and Agricultural University
Frederiksberg, Denmark

and

Olle Hernell
University of Umeå
Umeå, Sweden

Kluwer Academic / Plenum Publishers
New York, Boston, Dordrecht, London, Moscow

Library of Congress Cataloging-in-Publication Data

Short and long term effects of breast feeding on child health / edited by Berthold
Koletzko, Kim Fleischer Michaelsen, and Olle Hernell.
    p. cm. -- (Advances in experimental medicine and biology ; v. 478)
   "Proceedings of the 9th International Conference of the International Society for
Research in Human Milk and Lacation (ISRHML), held October 2-6, 1999, in Bavaria, Germany."
   Includes bibliographical references and index.
   ISBN 0-306-46405-5
   1. Breast feeding--Health aspects--Congresses. 2. Infants--Health and
hygiene--Congresses. 3. Infants--Nutrition--Congresses. I. Koletzko, B. (Berthold) II.
Michaelsen, Kim Fleischer. III. Hernell, Olle. IV. International Society for Research in
Human Milk and Lacation. International Conference. (9th : 1999 : Bavaria, Germany) V.
Series.

RJ216 .S4636 2000
613.2'69--dc21

                              00-034930

Proceedings of the 9th International Conference of the International Society for Research in Human Milk
and Lactation (ISRHML), held October 2–6, 1999, in Bavaria.

ISSN: 0065 2598

ISBN 0-306-46405-5

©2000 Kluwer Academic / Plenum Publishers, New York
233 Spring Street, New York, New York 10013

http://www.wkap.nl/

10 9 8 7 6 5 4 3 2 1

A C.I.P. record for this book is available from the Library of Congress

Preface

The quality of infant feeding is of major importance for child health, development, and well being. In addition to obvious short term effects of the diet on outcomes such as infant weight gain, results of research in recent years indicate a number of more subtle and complex effects on the quality of growth, tissue and organ development, functional outcomes, and behaviour. Moreover, there are strong indications for long-term effects of the early diet on health and body functions that extend for many years after the end of breast feeding, in some respects even well into adulthood. This phenomenon is often referred to as metabolic programming or metabolic imprinting. Breast feeding is the natural form of supplying food to the infant and is considered to be ideally adapted to the needs of both mother and child. Therefore, research on the physiological foundations and on the biological effects of breast feeding is a major priority in the health sciences.

The 9th International Conference of the International Society for Research in Human Milk and Lactation (ISRHML) was held at the Kloster Irsee Monastery near Munich, Germany from October 2 to 6, 1999 and focused on short and long term effects of breast feeding on child health. Scientists from 32 countries participated, of whom many are leading researchers in their fields. This book contains papers presented by the invited speakers of this conference, as well as short summaries of many of the presentations on original research results.

We are very grateful indeed to Ms. Frauke Lehner for her dedicated and meticulous editorial work on the contributions for this book. Moreover, we thank Ms. Karin Wandschura, Sandra Heussner, and Claudia Schäfer for their marvelous help in organising the conference. The conference and hence this book were only made possible by the generous financial support of the World Health Organisation, Geneva; the World Health Organization—Regional Office for Europe, Copenhagen; UNICEF, New York; the Danish International Development Agency (DANIDA), Copenhagen, Denmark; the Swedish International Development Cooperation Agency (SIDA), Stockholm; The Swedish National Food Administration, Uppsala, Sweden; The Swedish National Board of Health and Welfare, Stockholm, Sweden; and the Child Health Foundation—Stiftung Kindergesundheit, Munich. The contributions of these sponsors are greatly appreciated.

May this book contribute to enhancing knowledge of and support for breast feeding, as well as stimulate talented researchers to continue to strive for better understanding of the effects of infant feeding on child health.

München, December 1999

Berthold Koletzko, M.D.
Professor of Paediatrics
University of Munich, Germany
Olle Hernell, M.D.
Professor of Paediatrics
University of Umeå, Sweden
Kim Fleischer Michaelsen, M.D.
Professor of Paediatric Nutrition
Royal Agricultural and Veterinary University
Copenhagen, Denmark

Contents

Contents

Contents

1

BREASTFEEDING IN MODERN AND ANCIENT TIMES: FACTS, IDEAS, AND BELIEFS

Otmar Tönz
Schlösslihalde 26, CH-6006 Lucerne, Switzerland

1. INTRODUCTION

To receive nutrition out of the mother's body - after intrauterine parenteral nutrition has stopped and before individual, self-supporting and independent food procurement is possible: Suckling or Breastfeeding is the most natural way of providing nutrition to a newly born mammal, - is a wise and ingenious arrangement of nature. The intimate bond between mother and child is not suddenly disrupted with the cutting of the umbilical cord, and the infant continues to get warmth, protection and nutrition from the mother's body. In humans, breastfeeding has become a symbol of maternal devotion and infant security.

2. MYSTIFICATION OF BREASTFEEDING

Even though the act of breastfeeding seems self-evident and natural, cultural- and art history demonstrates that over the course of times people have always had great respect for this form of feeding and mothering an infant. The world's oldest existing bronze statuette, created by the Hethiters (Anatolia), shows a mother nursing her child. According to Greek

Short and Long Term Effects of Breast Feeding on Child Health
Edited by Berthold Koletzko *et al.*, Kluwer Academic/Plenum Publishers, 2000

1

mythology, the galaxies formed when milk (gr. γαλα) sprayed out from the breasts of Hera, the wife of Zeus, over the heavens. Old Egyptian Goddesses were often represented breastfeeding their sons. In Roman mythology, not even Bacchus was fed with wine but with the milk of the Nymphs.

In Christian art, Virgin Mary is shown many thousand-fold as "mother with child" or "Mater galaktotrophousa". The depiction of the breastfeeding Mary on the flight to Egypt is particularly popular. This scenery impressively radiates protection, rest, warmth and safety for the child in a harmful and threatening environment.

Another example of mystification of breastfeeding in the Middle age is the so called "Vision du Saint Bernhard de Clairveaux". The Holy Virgin Mary once appeared to Saint Bernhard, the founder of the Order of the Cistercians, while he was praying. She offered him her breast with the same milk with which she had nourished the Divine Infant. This vision, illustrated by many, more or less illustrious painters, occurred in the 12th Century. It may have been a symbol of spiritual inspiration or of the intimate bond between Heaven and Earth. How fortunate for Saint Bernhard that he did not live in our century: Sigmund Freud would have given a totally different interpretation of this daydream !

3.   UNUSUAL ASPECTS OF BREASTFEEDING

Over the course of the centuries, also in profane art, the breastfeeding mother was one of the most frequent motives in drawings, paintings, sculptures and even music (e.g. *F.Schubert* : Lied *"Vor meiner Wiege"*). Some of these paintings are rather peculiar, sometimes even of medical interest, as for instance *"la mujer barbuda"* (the bearded woman) by *Jusepe de Ribera* (1591-1652). He was a Spanish painter, born in Valencia, but working mostly in Naples, where he was therefore called "lo Spagnoletto" (Fig.1). Is it really possible that a woman with such a massive virilization can bear and nurse an infant? The painter describes important details in the legend next to the figures: Magdalena is a 52-year-old woman from the Abruzzes who has given birth to three children. She became severely virilized at the age of 37 and grew a full and abundant beard. The legend does not mention that she had another child thereafter. She was considered a great miracle of nature, and Ferdinand, the Vice King of Naples, ordered de Ribera to capture this extraordinary woman in a painting. But how could he show that this person really was a female, without undressing this poor and shy woman from the mountains? The solution of this dilemma: he laid an infant in her arms and thus gave a reason to uncover the breast as proof of her feminine nature. A very decent solution of a very delicate problem! It seems quite obvious that a 52-year-old woman who probably suffered from an androgen-producing tumour of the adrenal glands or ovaries would not be able to get pregnant and breastfeed her own infant. In fact, the baby is not sucking. So, de Ribera does not really deceive his spectators, except perhaps those who do not read his Latin explanations. On the other hand, based on observations of "relactating" grandmothers or even nursing men, she might have been able to breastfeed without having been pregnant

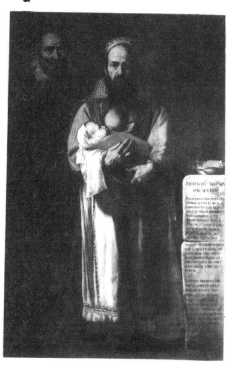

a

b

EN MAGNVM NATVRA MIRACVLVM MAGDALENA VENTVRA EX OPPIDO ACCVMVLI APVD SAMNITES VULGO EL ABRUZZO REGNI NEAPOLITANI ANNO- RUM 52 ET QVOD INSOLENS EST CVM ANNVM 37 AGERET COEPIT PUBES- CERE EOQVE BARBA DEMISSA AC PROLIXA EST UT POTIVS ALICUIUS MAGISTRI BARBATI ESSE VIDEATVR QVAM MULIERIS QVAE TRES FILIOS ANTE AMISERIT QVOS EX VIRO SVO FELICI DE AMICI QVEM ADESSE VIDES HABVERAT.

JOSEPHVS DE RIBERA HISPANVS CHRISTI CRVCE INSIGNITVS SVI TEM- PORIS ALTER APELLES IVSSV FERDI- NANDI DVCIS IN DEALCAEA NEAPOLI PROREGIS AD VIVUM MIRE DEPINXIT. ....KALEND. MART. MDCXXXI

Fig. 1.   a.) Jusepe de Ribera: La mujer barbuda (the bearded woman), Museo de Toledo, Spain.
b.) Latin legend next to figures.

Is there a fundamental reason why men should not be able to breastfeed? They have nipples, viable but admittedly rudimentary mammary glands, and they produce prolactin and also some estrogens. Even male new-borns can produce witch's milk in their enlarged breasts, and pubertal gynaecomastia - exceptionally even accompanied by galactorrhea - is a wide-spread phenomenon in young men. We know already from *Aristotle* that there are male animals, especially he-goats, who can nurse their young and who can be milked. Modern veterinary science confirms this phenomenon. Exactly 200 years ago, *Alexander von Humbolt,* one of the most famous scientists of his time, undertook a great research expedition to the equinoctial regions of the New Continent (South America) [1]. There he met *Francesco Lozano*, a man who had suckled his infant during 5 months. When the infant's mother became ill, the 32-year-old Lozano took the infant, pressed him to his breast, and the child started to suck at his nipple. He suddenly felt the accumulation of fluid in his breast gland and was able to feed the child. The son, exclusively nourished with his father's milk, throve excellently. *Humbolt* thereafter studied the scientific literature on this topic and found descriptions of similar cases, reported in earlier centuries. He mentioned also, that in old Russia, anatomists had occasionally found milk-producing glands in the male population. In the Talmud, there is another description of a father who nursed his son after his wife's death [2]. I suppose male breastfeeding is indeed possible in rare cases and under very special circumstances: it probably requires an extraordinary output of releasing hormones and estrogens, perhaps induced by intensive, mother-like feelings of fatherhood, maybe coupled with pre-existing hyperprolactinemia and enhanced responsiveness of the glandular tissues to hormonal and local stimuli by the sucking baby.

4.   FEEDING IN THE FIRST DAYS OF LIFE

The cultural – and scientific! –history of the past centuries was often surrounded by a haze of superstitious imaginations and beliefs. Until the middle of the 18th century, for instance, breastfeeding an infant during the first three days of life was not allowed: not only because children first had to be baptised in many regions, but also because colostrum was thought to be harmful to the infant and not compatible with meconium [3]. For this reason, different purges were in use to "remove the meconium from the stomach and intestines", while the mother's valuable first milk was withdrawn or even sucked off by whelps.

Table 1: Purges in common use for the new-born between 1500 and 1800, first reported by Paré in 1575 and last mentioned by Beaudeloque in 1790 (3)

Purge	Period of use						
Almond oil							
Almond oil & Syrup of roses							
Honey							
Butter							
Butter & Honey							
Sugar							
Almond oil & Sugar							
Sugared Wine							
Wine							
Butter & Sugar							
Syrup of roses / violets							
Pharmaceutical purges							
Others							
Rhubarb							
Sugared water							
	1500	1550	1600	1650	1700	1750	1800

The use of these purges resolved one problem which has remained a controversial topic until recent times: the problem of energy supply and fluid administration in the very first days of life before maternal lactogenesis is established. As shown in Tab. 1, there were many different fluids in use; some of them had a rather high caloric content, such as honey, butter, oils, red wine, sugar water etc.

The superstitious belief that colostrum and meconium were incompatible disappeared some two hundred years ago. Nevertheless, giving supplements during the first days of life – no longer as purges but as a supply of fluids and energy – was widely in use until our times. Results of different studies performed in the last decades, however, have shown that both are unnecessary, provided that maternal lactation be established by the third to fifth day after delivery. Yet in an older study at the Women's Hospital of Lucerne, years before UNICEF's rules were published, we have shown that only 5.6% of infants who later on were fully breastfed needed some milk supplements during the first days of life [4]. This number could probably even be lowered without causing any harm to the child [5]. This was in the eighties, when in many maternity hospitals more than 50% of newborns were supplemented with milk formula.

With regard to fluids, there still are some controversial ideas which I will not discuss in detail. UNICEF's "Ten Steps to Successful Breastfeeding" are undoubtedly valuable guidelines for hospitals; however, some recommendations lack a solid scientific basis, may go too far and do not respect different cultural and ethnic patterns in raising a child. This comment refers mainly to steps 6 and 9:

Give newborn infants no food or drinks other than breast milk unless medically indicated
Give no artificial teats or pacifiers to breastfeeding infants

Some comments on pacifiers or dummies (Step 9): nobody would have predicted 30 or 50 years ago that at the end of our century the pacifier would be object of a large number of scientific discussions and papers, some of which even had the honour to be published in the most celebrated journals like the Lancet and others [6-9]. In earlier decades, mostly hygienic and orthodontic aspects of pacifier use were discussed; now, there are new concerns and theses: dummy's use is said to affect intellectual development, to provoke nipple confusion and to shorten breastfeeding duration. The first thesis - that pacifier use has a negative influence on adult intelligence - remains a matter of belief, although this association has been evaluated using appropriate statistical methods [6]. The second concern - nipple confusion – was not confirmed by our own observations [10]; nevertheless, it may be wise not to introduce this ugly device before the infant is fully familiar with sucking at the nipples. Finally, the question whether pacifier use leads to shorter breastfeeding duration is a topic of ongoing discussions. I dare to summarise the respective studies as follows: when mothers are confident about nursing and motivated to breastfeed, the use of pacifiers will not affect breastfeeding duration. On the other hand, pacifiers may contribute to early termination of breastfeeding in situations where mothers are uncomfortable with breastfeeding and are using the pacifier as a weaning tool, trying to make the intervals between feedings longer and more regular, thus decreasing the total number of feedings [7].

After all, it is quite clear that a pacifier is not of vital importance, and we definitely do not advocate its general use. On the other hand, giving a pacifier to a crying baby is a custom of our people and cannot easily be eliminated. There is also no need to do so as long as it has not convincingly been demonstrated that it really hinders successful breastfeeding. Fortunately, many infants do not accept a pacifier even if mothers try to offer it repeatedly.

Step 6 of the UNICEF guidelines is no less controversial. Some retrospective studies show that children who have received milk supplements or even simple dextrose solutions during the first days of life may have a shorter breastfeeding duration. In these studies, however, cause and effect were probably confounded: infants of mothers with poor milk supply are more likely to be supplemented during the first days of life than infants from mothers with abundant milk production. The former will then probably be breastfed for a shorter time. This question can only be answered by a prospective study.

We therefore examined the influence of fluid supplements on breastfeeding in a prospective, randomised multicenter study [10]. About 600 mother-infant-pairs in 10 different Swiss maternity hospitals were randomly assigned to one of two groups: the conventional group where infants received a 10% sugar solution and if necessary an infant formula, both by bottle, or the UNICEF group where infants were nourished according to the UNICEF guidelines.

We did not find any difference in the sucking behaviour between the two groups during their hospital stay. There was also no significant difference in the duration and frequency of breastfeeding after 2, 4 and 6 months (methods and results of this study will be presented in more detail by Kind et al. in this issue).

In conclusion:

Avoiding artificial teats or pacifiers during the stay in the maternity ward had no influence on breastfeeding incidence and duration in mothers who are willing to breastfeed their infants. The pacifier may be an unpleasant civilisation phenomenon but it is not a civilisation disease.

Very few infants had to be supplemented with a formula.

It is an old habit - starting with the purges in the Middle Age mentioned above - to give additional fluids to infants in the first 2-4 days of their lives. In a strict sense, this is not an absolute necessity, and in countries with bad hygienic conditions it should be avoided. In our civilisation, however, I cannot see any substantial objections to giving supplements. The baby's water loss is up to 70 ml/kg/day, and a partial compensation will reduce the initial weight loss and decrease the incidence of thirst fever [11]. It is better to prevent than to treat dehydration and possible hypoglycaemia in infants at risk. Last but not least, giving supplements is an opportunity to quiet an infant who continues to cry after having sucked at the mother's not yet productive breasts. To simply prohibit fluid supplementation would be a rigid and puritanical approach and would not promote sensible, emotional mothering.

The argument that mankind survived during ten thousands of years without supplementary fluids in the first days of life is not valid. Firstly, the oldest testimonials suggest that newborns did in fact get some supplements [3], and secondly, the mortality rates in those times certainly have exceeded 5% in the first week of life. Even if nutritional problems were not always the cause of death in those infants, the strict imitation of such "natural patterns" does not meet today's safety demands.

5.   WEANING PROBLEMS

Another crucial question concerns an issue at the end of the breastfeeding period: for how long is exclusive breastfeeding adequate to satisfy the dietary needs of the young baby. When should we start to introduce supplementary foods, the so-called "Beikost"?

Based on data from 16 different studies, Margaret Neville [12] reported that the average daily milk intake in infants is about 800±200 ml/day at four to six months of life. Dewey showed in a cohort of small for date infants[13] that the milk production continues to increase slightly during the fifth and sixth months when they are exclusively breastfed, whereas it starts to decrease when Beikost is being introduced.

Interestingly, the amount of 800 ml/day does not amount to the whole milk production since on average about 13% of milk remains in the mammary gland [14]. Milk intake and production could therefore easily be enhanced if, for instance, a second baby would be nursed, or if the first infant would suck more vigorously. However, babies seem to be satisfied with this amount of milk, but they take in more calories, if semisolids in the form of vegetables, fruits or cereals are offered. For an average 6-month-old infant, 800 ml of milk equal about 540 kcal or 75 kcal/kg body weight. Using very sophisticated methods, Whitehead [15] reported that the energy requirement of such an infant is about 80-85 kcal/kg/day and increases slightly thereafter. In other words: after the fifth month of life, there is an inconsistency between need and supply of energy in the average breastfed infant, a discrepancy which continues to increase thereafter (Fig.2) [16].

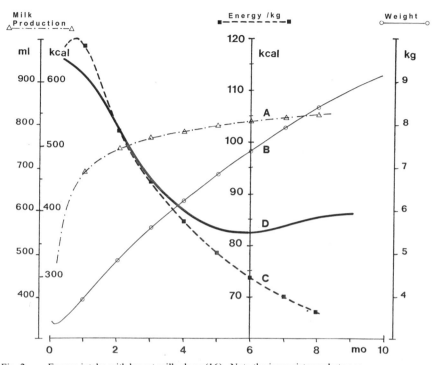

Fig. 2   Energy intake with breast milk alone (16). Note the inconsistency between requirement and supply after the fifth month.
A: milk production - energy intake (12); B: body weight; C: energy intake/ kg body weight (A/B); D: energy requirement/kg body weight (15).

The same is true for protein requirements. A 5½-month-old boy with a body weight of 7 kg, receiving 750 ml of milk would get exactly 1 g/kg/day of protein which surely would be insufficient at this age. Infants with a long breastfeeding duration are in fact smaller and weigh less, not only at 6 month but even at two or three years [17,18]. The difference in length, however, is minimal and merely of academic interest; however, it might be a sign of a transient sub-optimal nutrition. Since breastfed babies have the same head circumference as formula-fed infants, one could state that breastfed infants have more brain per kg body weight! Then again: the same brain power with a little bit more bone and muscle mass would certainly not be a disadvantage. The accepted time point for the introduction of supplementary foods remains the same as ever: not before the age of 4 months, and no later than 6 months of age. It should not be delayed until 6-8 months as some groups of uncritical breastfeeding proponents recommend. I also would like to emphasise that the first pap meals must not replace a meal from the breast, but should rather be offered as additional nourishment.

Concerning weight gain in breastfed infants, it is remarkable that breastfeeding obviously has an impact on the risk of overweight and obesity in later childhood, as has recently been shown in a study on more than 9'000 5- to 6-year-old children in Bavaria [19]. The prevalence of overweight and obesity was significantly lower in formerly breastfed children and a clear dose-response effect between breastfeeding duration and obesity was identified.

The time point for definite weaning can vary widely: it may be at 9 or 12 months, or even 2 or 3 years. In several traditional communities, breastfeeding for 2 years is felt to be physiological. Perhaps it is! Weaning after such a long time may not always be easy. If difficulties occur, I recommend the method of some African tribes described by Mathabane in "Kaffern-Boy": *"When my brother George was nearly two years old, our mother rubbed red pepper on her nipples and then put the child on her breasts. The hot spice burned on his lips and he cried awfully. This procedure was repeated four or fife times. After that, my little brother would no longer suck from those detestable, burning breasts and was thus weaned. Our father slaughtered a chicken and mother brewed beer, and some relatives were invited to appropriately celebrate the successful weaning. From this day on, little George was no longer a baby and he was allowed to sleep with the other children on the kitchen floor".*

In industrialised countries, breastfeeding duration is shorter, although it is much longer than it used to be some decades ago. A Swiss study performed by Conzelmann in 1994 (Fig.3), revealed breastfeeding rates of 80%, 60%, and 40% at 2, 4, and 6 months, respectively. In addition, there was a positive correlation between breastfeeding rates and socio-economic status [20]. Without any doubt, these rates are much higher than in earlier times.

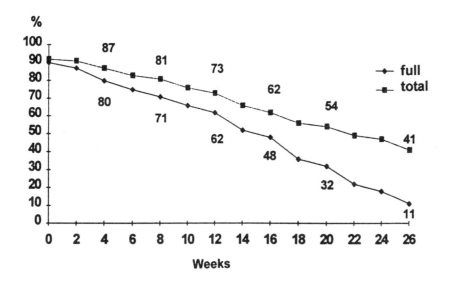

Fig 3.   Breastfeeding rates in Switzerland in 1994 (20).

6.   BREASTFEEDING IN EARLIER EPOCHS

We often assume that nearly all children were nursed by their mothers in earlier centuries. Unfortunately, this is merely an assumption or an idea but not a fact. Obviously, it is very difficult to know for sure what the situation was in earlier times. We have no statistics or medical descriptions from those times - infant feeding was not yet a topic of medical interest - and customs varied widely in different countries and over different time periods. In some regions mothers breastfed 80 or 90% of their infants, mainly the two or three first-born children of the family [21]; in other regions, like Bavaria, Tyrol, the Lausitz, Iceland, or cities, like Moscow, breastfeeding had nearly died out for several centuries [3].

Until the late 18th century, it was the social norm for upper and middle class mothers to employ wet-nurses rather than breastfeed their infants themselves. In the regions quoted above, however, infants were not breastfed at all. Particularly here in Southern Bavaria, they were fed almost exclusively with a flour pap, with or without addition of milk. It was already mentioned in 1524 that breastfeeding was rare in this region [22]. We have some indirect evidence that in many other countries the situation was not much better. For instance in Britain, there are gravestones from the 17th century with inscriptions like this : *"...she died... and left 8 children, 7 of them she nourished with her own breasts"* [3]. A clear indication that this was rather an exception. Other hints are given by the fact that doctors repeatedly wrote articles, proclamations and appeals to encourage women to breastfeed their infants themselves. A medical history study of the time period between 1750 and 1800 about the situation in England and France attests: *"All medical writers were doing their best to depopularize the almost universal use of pap as the sole means of bringing up infants by hand."* [23]

Without doubt, the most illustrious author of those times is Karl von Linné from Upsala, who, in 1752, wrote a booklet entitled: NUTRIX NOVERCA (The wet-nurse as a stepmother). In this article, he sharply criticises the bad habit of wet-nursing: *"We have scarcely been expelled from our mother's womb before we fall victims to a dangerous custom, which even denies us what nature has intended to give us, breast-milk, and this is highly imprudent; neither the whales nor the big lionesses or tigresses deny their new-borns their breastmilk"*. He also warns of one consequence of inhibited breastfeeding: breast cancer. *"Therefore, women of noble birth"* he says, *"more often have breast cancer than the farmers' women"*. With this, he anticipated a fact which was proven only some years ago for the pre-menopausal form of breast cancer [24].

I would like to point out that officially Linné did not write this book himself. It was a thesis of a young doctor named Frederick Lindberg who had to present this work "praeside Carolo Linnaeo" at the Faculty of Upsala. Nevertheless, we know that all of the 85 theses of his students were written by the master himself [25]!

The first useful statistics on breastfeeding actually come from Bavaria from the seventies of the last century [22]. The average breastfeeding duration in Schwaben, e.g., was 3½ weeks. In Munich, less than 10% of the babies were breastfed (Fig.5 a). In Niederbayern, even in 1905, 75% of all infants were never put to the breast [26], even though there had been a general rise in breastfeeding rates starting towards end of the 19th century.

7.   BREASTFEEDING AND MORTALITY

Actually, infant mortality rates in these regions of Southern Bavaria were much higher than in the Northern parts, the Frankenland, where the majority of babies were nursed by their mothers [27]. Mortality rate was 2.4 times higher in non-breastfed than in breastfed infants. After the first year, the formerly breastfed children were no longer at an advantage; on the contrary, they now had a higher mortality rate [22] (Tab.2). Evidently, infants who survived the critical first year without being breastfed represented a selection of very resistant and healthy children. This is in contrast to newer findings which indicate longer lasting protection after beastfeeding (see Hanson, L.Å., in this issue).

Table 2: Mortality rates in different provinces of Bavaria in 1882 (Bernheim [22])

	1st year		2nd - 5th year		6th - 10th year		Total 1st - 10th year
Oberbayern [1]	43.8		10.3		2.6		
Niederbayern [1]	44.5	44.0	10.8	9.8	3.4	2.9	56.7%
Schwaben [1]	43.6		8.7		2.7		
Pfalz [2]	27.6		15.2		3.6		
Oberfranken [2]	26.3	26.3	15.4	14.5	4.5	4.1	44.9%
Unterfranken [2]	25.0		13.0		4.1		

[1] Provinces with **low** breastfeeding rates
[2] Provinces with **high** breastfeeding rates

Nevertheless, the overall mortality rate was lower in breastfed infants. These lower mortality rates were associated with a lower number of infants in a family. The time interval between two children is much shorter after a new-born's or infant's death [26], and is longest after prolonged nursing [28]. Breastfeeding is a reliable contraceptive for 6-7 months [29]. Thus, the higher mortality rate was compensated by a higher birth rate in non-breastfeeding populations (Fig. 4). The *"life-wasting type"* describes a population with a low incidence of breastfeeding and high mortality and fertility rates, opposed to *"life-saving"* societies with a high incidence of breastfeeding and low mortality and fertility rates [30]. Both result in a demographic equilibrium, although the life-wasting way is certainly more troublesome and painful. It is astonishing that it was accepted by many people.

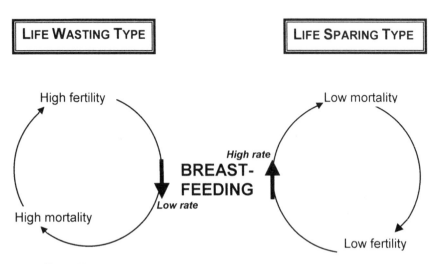

Fig. 4 Effects of breastfeeding activity on regulation of population size:
High breastfeeding rate – lower mortality – lower fertility – higher breastfeeding rate
Low breastfeeding rate – higher mortality – higher fertility – lower breastfeeding rate

There may be different reasons for his phenomenon. The most important one is perhaps a different mentality with regards to how a child was valued. Such a mentality is formed by a variety of traditional, religious, cultural and economic factors. The attitude to patiently endure and accept mortal blows of fate as God's providence was probably more prevalent in catholic communities (e.g. in Southern Bavaria). And then, of course, economic aspects may have played an important role as well: Often parents were not too unhappy when a baby - which was another hungry mouth to feed - went to heaven to pray there for the rest of the family [30].

8.   TWO "RENAISSANCES" OF BREASTFEEDING IN THE 20TH CENTURY

As already mentioned above, at the end of the 19th and the beginning of the 20th century, breastfeeding once again became popular in most European countries (Fig. 5 a + b). Common people now recognised that breastfed children throve better. The reduction of fertility associated with increased breastfeeding, on the other hand, lead to significantly smaller families. Mothers had more time to look after their infants and to nurse them themselves. The inverse correlation between breastfeeding rate and the number of children is obvious (Fig. 6) although there certainly are other contributing factors.

FIGURE 2. THE PERCENTAGE OF INFANTS EVER BREASTFED, MUNICH, 1869 - 1933.

FIGURE 1. THE PERCENTAGE OF INFANTS EVER BREASTFED, BADEN, 1873 - 1934.

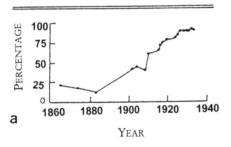

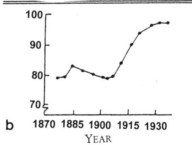

Fig. 5 The "first renaissance" of breastfeeding, starting at the end of the 19th century:
  a) Munich: low breastfeeding rate
  b) Baden: high breastfeeding rate

This first "renaissance" of breastfeeding lasted until the end of the thirties. Paediatricians and nurses supported the enthusiasm of young mothers. In St. Gallen - my birth place -, for instance, the breastfeeding rate rose from 58 to 97% between 1917 and 1934, whereas the birth rate fell from 27 to 15.5 per 1000 inhabitants between 1910 and 1935.

In 1940, in the middle of the 2nd World War, fertility again started to increase and culminated in an true baby boom in all European countries. This baby boom reached its peak in 1964. Curiously, in this children-loving atmosphere, the wings of breastfeeding enthusiasm began to become lame and the ardour for breastfeeding reached its nadir at the beginning of the seventies.

Since 1965, the birth rates in Europe have declined relentlessly until now. The fertility index, the number of children per woman in the reproductive age, was 2.7 in 1964 and has now reached 1.4 in Switzerland, 1.2 in Germany and 1.1 in Italy and Spain. A fertility index of 1.2 is less than 60% of the number necessary to maintain a stable reproduction. 1.2 signifies that only two generations from now - in about 2060 - the size of the population of the less than 20-year-olds will be less than 50% of its current, already insufficient size. We are living in a dying society.

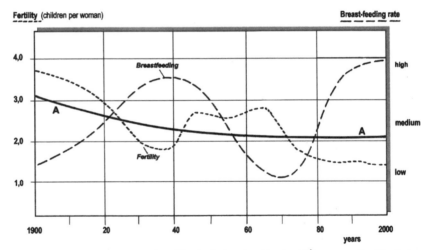

Fig. 6   Breastfeeding rates and fertility in Switzerland in the 20th century: Fertility index (children per woman in the reproductive age) and estimated breastfeeding rates (semi-quantitative), based on various sources. A : number of children per woman, required to maintain a stable reproduction.

Parallel to the marked decrease of our fertility, breastfeeding has experienced the "second renaissance". Concurrent with the lowest birth rates ever, we are confronted with the delightful fact of a very high breastfeeding frequency, which exactly mirrors the fertility rate (Fig.6).

The current boom started in the Scandinavian countries in 1973. Within 7 years, the breastfeeding rate in Sweden rose from 20 to over 80% in 2-month-old infants [31] (Fig. 7). In Central Europe, a less impressive wave followed two or three years later. The WHO reacted with the publication of the "International Code of Marketing of Breast-milk Substitutes" in 1981, the "Ten Steps" 1989 and UNICEF's "Baby friendly Hospital Initiative" 2 years later. UNICEF did not stand at the beginning of this development but rather jumped onto a running train and immediately proceeded to the conductor's cab!

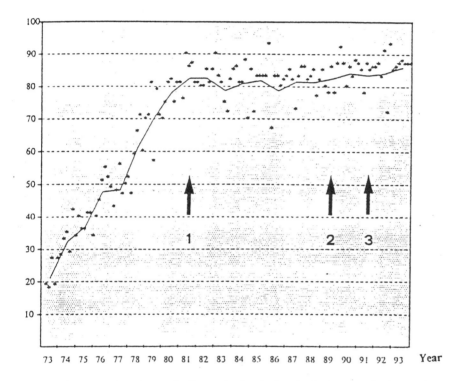

Fig. 7   The "second renaissance" of breastfeeding in Sweden in the seventies (31) and activities of WHO/UNICEF that followed:
1) International code of marketing of breast milk substitutes
2) Ten steps to successful breastfeeding
3) Baby-friendly hospital initiative

A new, not yet published European study from 12 different countries (1991-93), reveals a rather satisfactory breastfeeding activity : 67% at two, 42% at four and 27% at six months of age (F.Haschke, by courtesy [19]). However, there are large differences between the Nordic countries which have high breastfeeding rates, and England, France and the Latin nations which lower breastfeeding activities.

Manifold factors have lead to higher motivation to breastfeed: fewer children, more time, more money, but also more fears of synthetic, chemically produced foods, an increased scepticism regarding purely technical ways of thinking and the "back to nature" movement. New knowledge about the "womanly art of breastfeeding" was introduced in the last decades, not by paediatricians or obstetricians but rather through the initiative of active women working for La Leche League or as Lactation Consultants: early skin-to-skin contact immediately after birth, the first sucking in the first hour after delivery, rooming-in, correct positioning of the infant, proper handling of the breast - no longer the so-called cigarette-grasp, depicted in so many paintings, but the hand-holding used in old Egypt (Fig. 8a+b) – and, finally, feeding on demand.

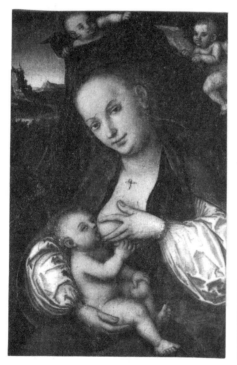 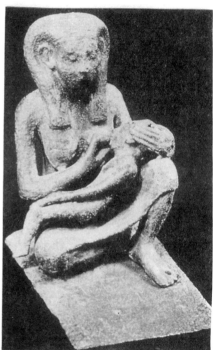

Fig. 8 Methods of holding the breast during nursing:
     a) so-called "Cigarette grasp" (no more recommended). Lukas Cranach d.Ä. (1472-
       1553), Monastery of Capuchins, Innsbruck, Austria
     b) so called "C-grasp", Egypt, Median Empire (1900 B.C.)

A final comment to this last point: paediatricians of the first generations recommended scheduled feeding: 5 feedings a day and none in the night [32]. This schedule was derived from the experience of wet-nursing in hospitals. Not only the rigid timetable 6-10-2-6-10 o'clock was wrong, even "wronger" was the total number of meals. Even highly motivated mothers suffered from the "insufficient milk syndrome" after a few weeks of nursing their infants according to this rigid feeding schedule. The recently published European Growth Study revealed that when feeding occurs on demand the number of feedings is significantly higher (Tab.3).

Table 3: Mean number of breastfeedings in 24 h (33) from the Euro-Growth Study 1991-93 (12 countries)

Age (mo)	feedings/24 h		(n)
1	**7.1**		(1152)
	4	*0.7%*	
	5	*7.6 %*	
	6	*31.1 %*	
	7	*25.7 %*	
	8	*25.3 %*	
	9+	*9.5 %*	
2	**6.6**		(873)
4	**6.2**		(487)
6	**5.8**		(254)

In the first two months of life, more than 80% of infants took 6 to 8 meals in a 24-hour-period (also at night!) and only 8% were satisfied with the 5 feedings [33] once recommended by the great-grandfathers of paediatrics.

All these factors taken together have led to the present situation of widespread, self-evident and natural breastfeeding.

My final question: is today's delightfully high breastfeeding rate really indicative of a vital and healthy society, or is it perhaps the contrary, a symptom of a morbid population? This question confuses me and even makes me sad. It reminds me of the phenomenon of forcefully blossoming trees in a dying forest. What should we do? It certainly would not be wise to discourage breastfeeding (we would be treating a symptom rather than the cause of the problem). On the contrary, breastfeeding offers so many advantages to both mother and infant that we should support it by all means.

REFERENCES

1. Von Humbolt, Alexander : Reise in die Aequinoctial-Gegenden des neuen Kontinents 1799-1805. Kap.VI, Cotta, Stuttgart
2. Rohn, R D 1984: Galactorrhea in the adolescent. J Adolesc Health Care, **5**: 37-49
3. Fildes, V A 1986: Breasts, bottles and babies. A history of infant feeding. University Press, Edinburgh
4. Tönz, O, Schubiger G 1990 : Ernährung in den ersten Lebenstagen: Wieviele Kinder brauchen eine Zusatznahrung Schweiz Med Wschr :**120** : 1487-92
5. Kind C, Drack G, Lorenz U , 1994 : Avoiding early formula supplementation in breast-fed newborns: effects of a change in nursing policy. Pädiatr Paedol **29**: 51-56
6. Gale, C R, Martyn C N 1996 : Breastfeeding, dummy use and adult intelligence. Lancet **347** : 1072-75
7. Victora C G, Behague D P, Barros F C, Olinto M T A, Weiderpass E 1997 : Pacifier use and short breastfeeding duration: Cause, consequence or coincidence. Pediatrics **99**: 445-53
8. Righard L, Alade M O 1997 : Breastfeeding and the use of pacifiers. Birth **24**: 116-20
9. Howard R C, Howard F M, Lanphear B et al. 1999 : The effects of early pacifier use on breastfeeding duration. Pediatrics **103(3)** : e33
10. Schubiger G, Schwarz U, Tönz O 1997 : UNICEF/WHO baby-friendly hospital initiative: does the use of bottles and pacifiers in the neonatal nursery prevent successful breastfeeding ? Eur J Pediatr **156**: 874-77
11. Dahms B B, Krauss A N, Gartner L M et al. 1973: Breast feeding and serum bilirubin values during the first 4 days of life. J Pediatr **83**: 1049-54
12. Neville M C, Keller R, Seacat J et al. 1988 : Studies in human lactation: milk volumes in lactating women during the onset of lactation. Amer J Clin Nutr **48**: 1375-86
13. Dewey K G, Cohen R J, Brown K H, Rivera L L 1999 : Age of introduction of complementary foods and growth of term, low-birth-weight, breast-fed infants: a randomised intervention study in Honduras. Amer J Clin Nutr **69**: 679-86
14. Dewey K G, Heinig M J, Nommsen L A, Lonnerdal B 1991 : Maternal versus infant factors related to breast milk intake and residual milk volume: the DARLING study. Pediatrics **87**: 829-37
15. Whitehead R G 1995 : For how long is exclusive breastfeeding adequate to satisfy the dietary energy needs of the average young baby. Pediatr Res **37**: 239-43
16. Tönz O 1996 : Von der Mamma zur Pappa. Monatsschr Kinderheilk **144(2)**: S150-55
17. Dewey K G, Peerson J M, Brown K H et al. 1995 : Growth of breastfed infants deviates from current reference data: a pooled analysis of US, Canadian, and European data sets. Pediatrics **96**: 495-503
18. Von Kries R, Koletzko B, Sauerwald T et al 1999 : Breast feeding and obesity: cross sectional study. Brit Med J **319**: 147-50
19. Haschke F, van t'Hof M A and the Euro-Growth Study Group : Euro-Growth references for breastfed boys and girls: The influence of breast feeding and solids on growth until 36 months of age. J Ped Gastroenterol Nutr (in press)
20. Conzelmann-Auer C, Ackermann-Liebrich U 1995 : Frequency and duration of breastfeeding in Switzerland. Soz- Präventivmed **40**: 396-98

21. Kintner H J 1985 : Trends and regional differences in breastfeeding in Germany from 1871 to 1937. J Fam Hist **10**: 163-85

22. Bernheim H 1888 : Die Intensitätsschwankungen der Sterblichkeit in Bayern und Sachsen und deren Factoren. Z Hyg **4**: 525-81

23. Bracken F J 1956 : The history of artificial feeding of infants. Maryland State Med **5**: 40-54

24. Newcomb P A , Storer B E, Longnecker M P et al. 1994 : Lactation and a reduced risk of premenopausal breast cancer. New Engl J Med **330**: 81-87

25. Fredbärj T 1957 : Linné as pediatrician. Act paediatr **46**: 215-31

26. Knodel J, van de Walle E 1967 : Breast feeding, fertility and infants mortality: an analysis of some early German data. Popul Stud **21**: 109-131

27. Knodel J 1977 : Breast feeding and population growth. Science **198**: 1111-15

28. Knodel J 1977 : Infant mortality and fertility in three Bavarian villages: an analysis of family histories from the 19th century. Popul Stud **22**: 297-318

29. Kennedy K I, Kotelchuck M, Visness C M et al 1998 : Users' understanding of the lactational amenorrhea method and the occurrence of pregnancy. J Hum Lact **14**: 209-18

30. Imhof A E 1981 : Unterschiedliche Säuglingssterblichkeit in Deutschland, 18.-20. Jahrhundert – Warum ? Z Bevölkerungswissensch **7**: 343-84

31. Zetterström R 1994 : Trends in research on infant nutrition, past present and future. Acta paediatr Suppl **402**: 1-3

32. Manz F, Manz I, Lennert T 1996 : Zur Geschichte der ärztlichen Stillempfehlungen in Deutschland. Monatsschr Kinderheilk **145** : 572-87

33. Manz F, van't Hof M A, Haschke F 1999 : The mother-infant relationship: who controls breastfeeding frequency? Lancet **353**: 1152

2

BEER AND BREASTFEEDING

Berthold Koletzko, Frauke Lehner
Div. Metabolic Diseases and Nutrition, Dr. von Haunersches Kinderspital, University of Munich, Germany

Key words: Beer, lactogenesis, prolactin

Abstract: Traditional wisdom claims that moderate beer consumption may be beneficial for initiation of breastfeeding and enhancement of breastfeeding success. Here we review the question whether or not there is any scientific basis for this popular belief. There are clear indications that beer can stimulate prolactin secretion which may enhance lactogenesis both in non-lactating humans and in experimental animals. The component in beer responsible for the effect on prolactin secretion is not the alcohol content but apparently a polysaccharide from barley, which explains that the effect on prolactin can also be induced by non-alcoholic beer. No systematic studies are available to evaluate the clinical effects of beer on induction of lactogenesis, and short term studies have shown a reduced breast milk intake by infants after moderate alcohol consumption of their mothers. It is conceivable that relaxing effects of both alcohol and components of hop might also have beneficial effects on lactogenesis is some women, but there is no hard evidence for causal effects. It appears prudent not to generally advocate the regular use of alcoholic drinks during lactation but to rather refer mothers to non-alcoholic beer, even though no adverse effects of an occasional alcoholic drink during lactation have been documented.

Traditional wisdom not only in Bavaria, but also in many other areas of the world claims that moderate consumption of beer may be beneficial for initiation of breastfeeding and enhancement of breastfeeding success [1]. During the early part of the 20th century, beer companies marketed low alcoholic beers or "tonics" as a means for women to stimulate appetite,

Short and Long Term Effects of Breast Feeding on Child Health
Edited by Berthold Koletzko *et al.*, Kluwer Academic/Plenum Publishers, 2000

increase their strength and enhance milk production [2]. Also in more recent years, beer has been discussed as a beverage with possible special effects on lactation [3-5]. At a conference discussing breastfeeding in a Baroque monastery with an active monastery brewery (Irseer Klosterbräu), located close to the world's beer capital Munich, it seems appropriate to briefly review the question whether or not there is any scientific basis for the popular belief that beer consumption has effect on the initiation of breastfeeding.

Some have proposed that beer drinking may facilitate the initiation of breastfeeding by a soothing effect [4,6]. Several authors have discussed effects on the secretion of the hormone prolactin by the adenohypophysis. Prolactin, in concert with the gradual fall in progesterone levels during the postpartum period, effectively stimulates lactogenesis during the first days after child birth [5,7]. The effects of alcohol consumption on the secretion of prolactin is controversial [8], but beer indeed seems to have a stimulating effect [9]. De Rosa and coworkers [10] studied 11 female volunteers aged 18-36 years during the early follicular phase of the menstrual cycle. At three times with an interval of 48 hours, the subjects were given 1 litre of one of three fluids under standard conditions. After 12 hours of fasting and fluid deprivation, and at least 1 hour of bed rest, the subjects consumed within 15 minutes 1 litre either of beer (6 % ethanol), sparkling water or sparkling water with 6 % alcohol. Prolactin was measured from blood samples obtained at 0, 30, 60, 90 and 120 minutes. Peak values were obtained at 30 minutes in all three groups, but the prolactin increase was significantly larger after beer (27.1 ± 13.7 ng/ml) than after water (12.6 ± 4.1 ng/ml) or water with alcohol (12.0 ± 2.2 ng/ml) ($p < 0.05$). An induction of prolactin secretion by beer consumption was also reported by Carlson et al [11]. Five healthy men aged 31-47 years and seven healthy, non-lactating women aged 22-46 years were studied in the late morning after their usual breakfast. After collection of 3 baseline samples, the subjects consumed 800 ml of beer with 4.5 % alcohol in 30-45 minutes, and blood samples were collected at 15 minute intervals for 2.5 hours. In the male subjects, serum prolactin levels increased after beer consumption from 7.0 ± 1.5 ng/ml ($M \pm SE$) to 12.0 ± 2.1 ng/ml ($p < 0.025$). In females there was an increase from 9.6 ± 1.8 ng/ml to a peak of 22.6 ± 2.6 ng/ml ($p < 0.005$). A similar response was observed in one woman who drank nonalcoholic beer. Pretreatment of the women in the study with naloxone had no effect on prolactin secretion. In contrast to beer, there was no prolactin response in female volunteers after oral ingestion of a hot cacoa drink or a an aqueous solution of D,L-salisonol, a tetrathydoisoquinolone component of beer and some other alcoholic beverages which had been proposed as a potential responsible agent [12]. These two studies as well as other data [13-16] demonstrate that neither ethanol alone nor a simple volume stimulus induce a rise of serum prolactin, whereas beer drinking can induce an acute increase of prolactin secretion in non-lactating humans.

A similar effect of beer on prolactin secretion was also reported in animal experiments. A study aimed primarily at investigating a potential relationship between beer intake and development of mammary adenocarcinoma [17] investigated female C_3H/St mice that were infected with a b-type RNA virus (Bittner particle) to induce mammary adenocarcinomas. The animals were either given water or decarbonated light beer (Budweiser) as the sole liquid. While there was no difference in tumor prevalence or tumor growth, beer drinking mice tended to have higher serum prolactin levels at 49 days after weaning (65 ± 35 ng/ml) than controls (53 ± 23 ng/ml; n.s.). Similarly, intravenous injection of an aqueous beer extract induced a marked increase of prolactin secretion in ewes [18].

Sawagado and Houdebine from the Laboratoire de Physiologie de la Lactation at Jouy-en-Josas, France, attempted to further characterise the lactogenic compound in beer [18]. Mature virgin Wistar rats aged 14 weeks were given orally for 4 days lyophilised beer powder produced from Pelfort ordinary stout, or aqueous barley extracts. Measurements of beta-casein contents in rat mammary gland by radioimmunoassay demonstrated a marked beta-casein accumulation with both beer and barley administration, which could be prevented by the simultaneous administration of the dopaminergic drug CB 154. Thus, it appeared that the effect on casein accumulation was mediated by prolactin. Further studies in ewe showed that beer powder, barley extract and a crude malt extract, but not hop extract triggered a prolactin response, which suggested that the lactogenic principle in beer does not derive from hop but from beer barley and malt. The authors also found that maltose, which is abundantly found in barley, was unable to stimulate a prolactin response.

In order to identify the class of molecules to which the lactogenic compound or compounds belong, Sawagado and Houdebine went on and treated beer, barley and malt extracts with various solvents [18]. It turned out that the active compound in beer is insolubilized in 50 % ethanol. After resuspension in water and extraction with chloroform, the active compound was detected in the water phase. Thus, the authors concluded that the active molecule is neither a protein not a lipid but rather a polysaccharide. It turned out that more alcohol was required to precipitate the lactogenic activity from beer than from barley and malt suggests that the active polysaccharides might be partly cleaved into smaller molecules during the fermentation process.

In further studies, the authors found that several other plants also contain lactogenic compounds, including cotton seed, Europhorbia hirta and Accacia nilotica. Thus, in addition to beer some other plants or plant extracts might be utilisable for enhancing lactogenesis.

In an electronic literature search, we did not find any controlled studies that investigated the possible clinical effects of beer consumption on lactogenesis and breastfeeding success. Indeed, it seems rather difficult to realise such a controlled study due to both ethical and practical limitations. However, studies are available that investigated the effects of alcoholic drinks on the short-term behaviour of breastfed infants.

Menella and Beauchamp studied a group of 12 lactating women in a study with a cross-over design [19]. On two consecutive days, they consumed either beer with 4.5 % alcohol providing an alcohol intake of 0.3 g/kg, or an equal volume of non-alcoholic beer. Following alcoholic beer consumption, the odor of expressed milk was altered and infants drank less milk (149.5±13.1 ml vs. 193.1±18.4 ml, p<0.05) than after maternal consumption of non-alcoholic beer. In contrast to the alteration of drinking behaviour, there was no significant difference in maternal perception of their infant's behaviour or their own lactational performance. A similar effect on infant feeding was observed in another study on 12 mother-infant pairs after maternal consumption of either orange juice or orange juice with a small amount of alcohol (0.3 g/kg) [20]. When the mothers had consumed alcohol, their infants sucked more frequently during the minute of feeding (67.0±6.5 vs. 58.4±5.9 sucks/minute, p<0.05), but consumed significantly less breast milk milk (120.4±9.5 ml vs. 156.4±8.2 ml, p<0.001). Both these studies could not provide information on potential longer-term effects of maternal alcohol intake on breastfeeding.

In addition to these short-term observations, concern arises with regard to early alcohol exposure of the breastfed infant in view of the proposed potential long-term effects of early flavour experience on later preferences for foods and drinks [21]. It has been considered that exposure to significant amounts of alcohol during early life might enhance later alcohol consumption. Moreover, the possible pharmacological effects of alcohol in young infants let lead us to consider a regular alcohol intake of breastfeeding women undesirable [22,23], even though modest consumption has not been associated with adverse effects [5].

In conclusion, there are clear indications that beer can stimulate prolactin secretion which may enhance lactogenesis. The active principle responsible for the effect of beer on prolactin is not the alcohol content but apparently a polysaccharide from barley, which explains that the effect on prolactin can also be induced by non-alcoholic beer. However, no systematic studies are available to evaluate the clinical effects of beer on induction of lactogenesis, and short term studies have shown a reduced breast milk intake by infants after moderate alcohol consumption of their mothers. It is conceivable that relaxing effects of both alcohol and components of hop might also have beneficial effects on lactogenesis is some women, but no hard evidence of causal effects is available. It appears prudent not to generally advocate the regular use of alcoholic drinks during lactation but to rather refer mothers to non-alcoholic beer, although no adverse effects of an occasional drink during lactation have been documented.

REFERENCES

1. Routh CHF. Infant feeding and its influence on later life. New York: William Wood and Company; 1879.

2. Krebs R. Making friends is our business - 100 years of Anheuser Busch. St. Louis: Anheuser-Busch Inc.; 1953.

3. Visser W. [Nutrition during pregnancy and breast feeding. Drink dark beer and eat for two?]. TVZ. 1992;(5):170-3.

4. Falkner F. Beer and the breast-feeding mom, questions and answers. J.Am.Med.Ass. 1987;258:2126

5. Lawrence RA. Breastfeeding. A guide for the medical profession. 4 ed. St. Louis: Mosby Year Book Inc.; 1994.

6. Grossman ER. Beer, breast-feeding, and the wisdom of old wives [letter]. J.Am.Med.Ass. 1988;259(7):1016

7. Neville MC. Jensen RG, editors.Handbook of milk composition. San Diego: Academic Press; 1995;Lactogenesis in Women: a cascade of events revealed by milk composition. p. 87-98.

8. Toro G, Koloday RC, Jacobs LS, Masters WH, Daughaday WH. Failure of alcohol to alter pituary and target organ hormone levels. Clin.Res. 1973;21:205

9. Marks V, Wright JW. Endocrinological and metabolic effects of alcohol. Proc.R.Soc.Med. 1977;70(5):337-44.

10. De RG, Corsello SM, Ruffilli MP, Della CS, Pasargiklian E. Prolactin secretion after beer [letter]. Lancet 1981;2(8252):934

11. Carlson HE, Wasser HL, Reidelberger RD. Beer-induced prolactin secretion: a clinical and laboratory study of the role of salsolinol. J Clin Endocrinol.Metab. 1985;60(4):673-7.

12. Duncan MW, Smythe GA. Salsolinol and dopamine in alcoholic beverages [letter]. Lancet 1982;1(8277):904-5.

13. Earll JM, Gaunt K, Earll LA, Djuh YY. Effect of ethyl alcohol on Ionic calcium and prolactin in man. Aviat.Space.Environ.Med. 1976;47(8):808-10.

14. Wartofsky L, Dimond RC, Noel GL, Adler RA, Frantz AG, Earll JM. Effect of an oral water load on serum TSH in normal subjects, and on TSH and prolactin response to thyrotropin-releasing hormone (TRH) in patients with primary hypothyroidism. J Clin Endocrinol.Metab. 1975;41(4):784-7.

15. Ylikahri RH, Huttunen MO, Harkonen M, Leino T, Helenius T, Liewendahl K, Karonen SL. Acute effects of alcohol on anterior pituitary secretion of the tropic hormones. J Clin Endocrinol.Metab. 1978;46(5):715-20.

16. Ylikahri RH, Huttunen MO, Harkonen M. Letter: Effect of alcohol on anterior-pituitary secretion of trophic hormones. Lancet 1976;1(7973):1353

17.   Schrauzer GN, Hamm D, Kuehn K, Nakonecny G. Effects of long term exposure to beer on the genesis and development of spontaneous mammary adenocarcinoma and prolactin levels in female virgin C3H/St mice. J Am Coll.Nutr 1982;1(3):285-91.

18.   Sawagado L, Houdebine LM. Identification of the lactogenic compound present in beer. Ann.Biol.Clin Paris. 1988;46(2):129-34.

19.   Mennella JA, Beauchamp GK. Beer, breast feeding, and folklore. Dev Psychobiol. 1993;26(8):459-66.

20.   Mennella JA, Beauchamp GK. The transfer of alcohol to human milk. Effects on flavor and the infant's behavior [see comments]. N.Engl.J Med. 1991;325(14):981-5.

21.   Mennella JA, Beauchamp GK. Early flavor experiences: research update. Nutr Rev. 1998;56(7):205-11.

22.   Koletzko B. Alkoholgehalt in Medikamenten für Kinder. Med.Monatschr.f.Pharmazeuten 1995;18:194-5.

23.   Koletzko B (editor). Kinderheilkunde. 11 ed. Berlin: Springer Verlag; 1999.

3

DOES BREAST-FEEDING PROTECT AGAINST CHILDHOOD OBESITY?

[1]R. von Kries, B. [2]Koletzko, [2]T. Sauerwald, and [2]E. von Mutius

[1]*Institute for Social Paediatrics and Adolescent Medincine, Munich;* [2]*Dr. von Haunersches Kinderspital, Munich*

Key words: breast-feeding, overweight, obesity , prevention

Abstract: The impact of breast-feeding on overweight and obesity in children at school entry was assessed in a cross sectional study in Bavaria in 1997. The school entry health examination enrolled 134577 children. Data on early feeding were collected in two rural districts (eligible population n=13.345). The analyses were confined to 5 or 6 year old children with German nationality. The main outcome measures were overweight (BMI>90th percentile for all German children seen at the 1997 school entry health examination in Bavaria) and obesity (BMI>97th percentile). Information on breast-feeding was available for 9206 children of whom 56% had been breast-fed for any length of time. In non breast-fed children the upper tail of the BMI distribution was enlarged as compared to the breast-fed children whereas the median was almost identical. The prevalence of obesity in children who had never been breast-fed was 4.5% as compared to 2.8% in ever breast-fed children. A clear dose response effect for the duration of breast-feeding on the prevalence of obesity was found: 3.8%, 2.3%, 1.7% and 0.8% for exclusive breast-feeding for up to 2, 3 to 5, 6 to 12 and more than 12 months, respectively. The results for overweight were very similar. The protective effect of beast feeding on overweight and obesity could not be explained by differences in social class or lifestyle. The adjusted odds ratios of breast-feeding for any length of time was 0.71 (95% CI 0.56-0.90) for obesity and 0.77 (95%CI 0.66-0.88) for overweight. This data set did not allow to adjust for maternal weight, an important risk factor for obesity in children. Maternal overweight, however, could not explain the effect of breast-feeding on overweight and obesity in a similar study. The reduction in the risk for overweight and obesity is therefore more likely to be related to the properties of human milk than to factors associated with breast-feeding. The potential relevance of different components of human milk for the observed reduction in the risk for overweight and obesity is discussed. The preventive effect of breast-feeding on overweight and obesity is an important additional argument for the promotion of breast-feeding in industrialised countries.

1.   INTRODUCTION

In industrialised countries overweight is the most frequent nutritional disorder in children and adolescents, with a continuing increase of its prevalence [1, 2]. Overweight children have a high risk for overweight in adulthood [3-5] and for health disturbances such as arterial hypertension, dyslipidaemia, coronary heart disease, gout and others [6]. Since therapeutic interventions in obese children aiming at weight loss are costly and have less than satisfactory long-term success rates[7], identification of strategies for effective prevention of obesity is particularly attractive.

We have recently addressed the question whether prolonged breast-feeding might have long-term programming effects on the prevalence of overweight and obesity in children at school entry [8]. In this study, carried out in Bavaria, the risk for overweight and obesity decreased by duration of exclusive breast-feeding.

The aim of this article is
-    to summarize the results of the Bavarian study [8]
-    to discuss whether the apparently reduced risk for overweight and obesity in breast-fed children can be attributed to the properties of human milk
-    to give further details on the lower prevalence of overweight/obesity in breast-fed children in Bavaria
-    to stimulate the discussion as to which components of human milk might be instrumental in reducing the risk for obesity in breast-fed children

2.   STUDY DESIGN AND MAIN RESULTS OF THE BAVARIAN STUDY

2.1   Study design and setting

The study was part of the bavarian school entry health examinations 1997 enrolling 134,577 children (figure 1). From February 1997 to August 1997 13.345 children examined in two rural Bavarian regions (Oberpfalz and Niederbayern) and their parents were given a questionnaire on risk factors for atopic diseases. The overall response rate by the parents was 76.2%. The total number of completed questionnaires was 10.163. These data were linked with data on length and weight measured as part of the routine health examination. The BMI was calculated as weight / length^2 . The analysis was confined to the 5 year old (n=1975) and 6 year old (n=7382) German children leaving 9357 questionnaires for the analyses. The age and sex specific distribution of the BMI in all German children investigated during the 1997 school health examination in Bavaria was used as the reference to define overweight (BMI>90th percentile) and obesity (BMI>97th percentile).

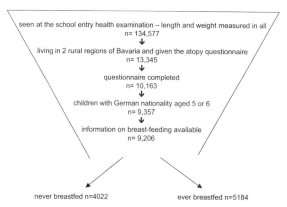

Figure 1: Overweight and Obesity in Bavarian Children at school entry in 1997

The main exposure was exclusive breastfeeding and its duration. The question on breastfeeding was: „Was your child breastfed". If the answer was yes the further question was: "For how long was your child exclusively breastfed". The categories offered to answer this question were: for not more than 2 months, 3 to 5 months, 6 to 12 months and for more than a year.

In order to identify covariables potentially associated with breastfeeding several additional items were considered. These regarded housing characteristics and lifestyle (e.g. the age of the house, child's own bedroom, maternal smoking in pregnancy, spare time spent outside in summer and winter), questions on the child's health (e.g. prematurity, low birth weight,) and questions on diet (time of introduction of solid food, consumption of own cooked food or industrial ready-to-meal products, food bought in health food shops) and explorative questions (never, less than once weekly, once or twice, 3 - 6 times weekly or daily) on the consumption of selected dietary items (milk products, fish, meat, fat, carbohydydates). The highest education of either parent was used as a marker for social class.

2.2   Main results

There was a progressive reduction of the prevalence of overweight and even more pronounced of obesity in children at school entry by duration of breastfeeding (figure 2). Several indicators of social class and lifestyle differed significantly between breastfed and not breastfed children. Many of these were also associated with overweight or obesity. High parental education, prematurity and low birth weight reduced the risk of overweight and obesity, whereas maternal smoking during pregnancy increased the risk. Full fat milk products (milk, quark or yogurt, whipped cream) and sweet deserts may be avoided by overweight children suggesting a spurious "protective" effect of these products as compared to a "risk" associated with the consumption of the low fat version of these products. There was also an apparent reduction of the risk for overweight and obesity associated with a high consumption of butter and breakfast cereals [8].

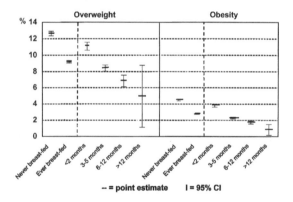

Figure 2: Overweight (BMI>90th percentile) and obesity (BMI>97th percentile). Prevalence in german children aged 5 or 6: relation to breast-feeding

Parental education was the only factor accounting for a > 10% shift of the odds ratio for breastfeeding and overweight and obesity towards unity. Other factors which remained significantly associated with overweight/obesity in the final logistic regression model were high parental education, maternal smoking in pregnancy, low birth weight, having an own bedroom and frequent consumption of butter (table 1). The adjusted odds ratios by duration of breastfeeding are shown in table 2. Being ever breast-fed reduced the risk of overweight by more than 20% and breastfeeding for six months or

Table 1: Independent risk factors for overweight and obestity: final logistic regression model

	Overweight		Obesity	
	OR	95% CI	OR	95% CI
Breastfeeding	0.79	0.68 – 0.93	0.75	0.57 – 0.98
High parental education	0.81	0.70 – 0.95	0.75	0.58 – 0.98
Maternal smoking In pregnancy	1.52	1.18 – 1.95	1.85	1.26 – 2.71
Birthweight < 2500 g	0.68	0.53 – 0.88	0.81	0.54 – 1.20
Own bedroom	1.24	1.05 – 1.46	1.20	0.91 – 1.59
Butter>= 3x/ week	0.72	0.62 – 0.84	0.69	0.54 – 0.90

Table 2: Impact of the duration of breast-feeding on overweight and obestiy in German children aged 5 or 6: OR's adjusted for parental education, maternal smoking in pregnancy, low birth weight, own bedroom and frequent consumption of butter

		Overweight		Obesity	
		OR	95%CI	OR	95%CI
Breast-fed for					
<2 months	(n=2,084)	0.89	0.73-1.07	0.90	0.65-1.24
3-5 months	(n=2,052)	0.87	0.72-1.05	0.65	0.44-0.95
6-12 months	(n=863)	0.67	0.49-0.91	0.57	0.33-0.99
>12 months	(n=121)	0.43	0.17-1.07	0.28	0.04-2.04
Ever breast-fed	(n=5,184)	0.79	0.68-0.93	0.75	0.57-0.98

more reduced the risk by over 35 %. Even more pronounced effects were observed regarding obesity (25% and 43% respectively).

3. CAN THE APPARENTLY REDUCED RISK FOR OVERWEIGHT AND OBESITY IN BREAST-FED CHILDREN CAN BE ATTRIBUTED TO THE PROPERTIES OF HUMAN MILK?

With all cross sectional studies there is a risk of recall/information bias. Some misclassification regarding the duration of breastfeeding is likely, if mothers have to remember details of the child's earlier feeding. This misclassification, however, is unlikely to be related to the outcome because the overt aim of the study was the search for risk factors of atopic diseases. Selection bias is also unlikely: the return rate of the questionnaires was high and unrelated to the outcome measure [8]. Random misclassification of the measurement of length and weight is likely, as it is difficult to ensure that all persons involved in the measurement in more than 10 different public health offices use exactly the same equipment in exactly the same way. This misclassification, however, is unlikely to be dependent on breastfeeding, as this information was not known to the persons involved in the measurement.

Breastfeeding was associated with a number of lifestyle and dietary factors documented as part of the study. With the exception of parental education none of these was a confounder of the association of breastfeeding and overweight/obesity. High parental education in breastfed children, however, only partially explained the association of breastfeeding and overweight/obesity.

Information on important risk factors for overweight, which might be confounders of the presumed protection by breastfeeding, could not be optimally assessed:
lifestyle and social class
-   Parental education may not be the optimal indicator of social class, but additional information is difficult to obtain in Germany because a potential impact of social class on health is not perceived by the German population.
-   Physical activity is certainly an important risk factor for overweight/obesity. As the questionnaire had not been originally designed for this purpose these questions were limited to "time for playing outdoors", which - though associated with breastfeeding - was not associated with overweight/obesity and was not a confounder.
-   Diet is another important lifestyle factor associated with the risk for adiposity – the questions were confined to a semi-quantitative assessment of the present diet. Many overweight children, however, might have changed diet to reduce their weight.
Genetic risk factors for overweight/obesity
-   Parents' weight is an important indicator of the genetic risk for overweight/obesity [9-11] and maternal overweight appears to be associated with a short duration of or no breastfeeding [12]. A positive family history of adiposity was not a confounder of the association between breastfeeding and overweight/obesity in a previous study [9].

In our cohort study on this issue presented at this meeting by Dr. Bergmann prolonged breastfeeding was less common in overweight mothers but maternal overweight was not a confounder of the association of breastfeeding and overweight/obesity.

A strong argument against a role for lifestyle factors associated with breast-feeding to explain the observed protective effect comes from a study on Canadian adolescents born in the 1960ties [9]. In this study a similar dose related, protective effect of breast feeding on the later prevalence of overweight/obesity was found. If this dose dependent protective effect were caused by lifestyle factors associated with breastfeeding similar confounding factors should have to have been operative during the different time periods in different societies. In Kramer's study only 18.5% of the children had been breastfed as compared to 56% our study suggesting other mothers might have chosen to breastfeed their children in the nineties in Bavaria than in the sixties in Canada. The lifestyle in the early sixties in Canada was almost certainly different from that in Bavaria in the early nineties. Although it is difficult to rule out that unknown factors associated with the lifestyle of families of breastfed children might be causative for the apparent protective effect of breastfeeding this does not appear likely.

4. FURTHER DETAILS ON THE "LOWER PREVALENCE OF OVERWEIGHT/ OBESITY IN BREAST-FED CHILDREN" IN BAVARIA

The age and sex specific distribution of the BMI in all German children investigated during the 1997 school health examination in Bavaria was used as the reference to define overweight (BMI>90th percentile) and obesity (BMI>97th percentile). The 90th and 97th percentile in Bavaria are considerably higher than the widely used French reference values [13] (table 3). This means that most children defined as overweight according to the Bavarian percentiles would have BMI values above the 95th percentile of the French reference values.

The lower prevalence of overweight/ obesity in breast-fed children in Bavaria does not reflect a shift in the entire distribution of the BMI's in breast-fed children as compared to those on formula. There is no shift of the mean but the upper tail of the distribution is "fatter" in non breast-fed children (figure 3). This has implications for further studies: These findings might not be reproduced, if only means and their 95% confidence intervals are considered. The biological model to explain the observed protective effect on overweight and obesity should match a shift in the "upper tail".

Table 3: BMI: 90th percentile and 97th percentile for German children in
Bavaria 1997: compared to reference values by Rolland-Cachera et al. 1991.

age in years	Gender	90th percentile		97th percentile	
		Bavaria	Rolland-Cachera	Bavaria	Rolland-Cachera
5	male	17.24	17.07	19.22	17.89
6	male	17.53	17.18	19.77	18.08
5	female	17.39	16.81	19.39	17.68
6	female	17.70	16.91	19.93	17.83

As the study was cross sectional we do not have data on the BMI during
the first five years of life in these children. The data of our cohort study on
this issue presented at the meeting by Dr. Bergmann suggest, that the
protective effect of breastfeeding emerges only after the 4th year of life.

5. WHICH COMPONENTS OF HUMAN MILK MIGHT BE INSTRUMENTAL IN REDUCING THE RISK FOR OBESITY IN BREAST-FED CHILDREN?

The components of human milk feeding accounting for a lower risk for
overweight/obesity in breast-fed infants might be related to the hormonal
response, bioactive factors present in human milk, a lower caloric intake
and/or a lower protein intake, all of which might potentially have long-term
effects [14].

Lucas et al [15, 16] reported significantly higher plasma insulin
concentrations in bottle than breast fed infants, which would be expected to
stimulate fat deposition and thus might affect early development of
adipocytes. Human milk also contains bioactive factors that may modulate
tissue growth and development. Breast milk contains both epidermal growth
factor and tumor necrosis factor alpha, both of which are known to inhibit
adipocyte differentiation in vitro [17-19].

Moreover, nutrient intakes of breast and bottle fed infants differ between
breast and formula fed babies [20]. Recent data indicate that the metabolisable
energy and protein intakes of breast-fed are considerably lower than
previously assumed and significantly below those found in populations of

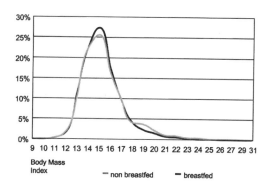

Figure 3: Distribution of the BMI in breastfed and non breastfed German children aged 5 and 6 in two rural Bavarian regions

formula-fed infants [21, 22]. These early differences in macronutrient supply might have long term effects on substrate metabolism. In longitudinal follow-up studies, Rolland-Cachera and coworkers [23-25] observed a significant relationship between the dietary protein intake at the age of 10 months with later BMI and body fat distribution. The authors proposed that a high protein intake in early childhood might predispose to an increased risk of obesity at a later age. Indeed, in animal studies the early protein availability during fetal and postnatal development was found have long-term metabolic programming effects on glucose metabolism and body composition in adult life [26-28].

6.   CONCLUSIONS

- ◆ Based on the data of this cross sectional study enrolling almost 10,000 children there is strong evidence that breast-fed children are less likely to be overweight or obese at school entry than formula fed children.
- ◆ This effect reflects "fattening" of the upper tail of the BMI distribution for non breast-fed children but is not due to a shift of the mean.

♦ There is some evidence that the reduced risk of overweight/obesity in breast-fed children is related to the properties of human milk and not to different genetics or lifestyle factors in these children. Further research for confirmation of this statement is needed, however.

♦ The causal factor in human milk, accounting for its protective effect against overweight awaits identification.

REFERENCES

1. Freedman DS, Srinivasan SR, Valdez RA, Williamson DF, Berenson GS. Secular increases in relative weight and adiposity among children over two decades: the Bogalusa Heart Study. Pediatrics 1997;99:420-6

2. Ogden CL, Troiano RP, Briefel RR, Kuczmarski RJ, Flegal KM, Johnson CL. Prevalence of overweight among preschool children in the United States, 1971 through 1994. Pediatrics 1997;99:E1

3. Charney E, Goodman HC, McBride M, Lyon B, Pratt R. Childhood antecedents of adult obesity. Do chubby infants become obese adults? N Engl J Med 1976;295:6-9

4. Stark O, Atkins E, Wolff OH, Douglas JW. Longitudinal study of obesity in the National Survey of Health and Development. Br Med J (Clin Res Ed) 1981;283:13-7

5. Abraham S, Collins G, Nordsieck M. Relationship of childhood weight status to morbidity in adults. HSMHA Health Rep 1971;86:273-84

6. Power C, Lake JK, Cole TJ. Measurement and long-term health risks of child and adolescent fatness. Int J Obes Relat Metab Disord 1997;21:507-26

7. Canadian.Task.Force. Periodic health examination, 1994 update: 1. Obesity in childhood. Canadian Task Force on the Periodic Health Examination. Cmaj 1994;150:871-9

8. von Kries RK, B. Sauerwald,T. von Mutius, E. Barnert, D. Grunert, V. von Voss, H. Breast feeding and obesity: cross sectional study. BMJ 1999;319:147-150

9. Kramer MS. Do breast-feeding and delayed introduction of solid foods protect against subsequent obesity? J Pediatr 1981;98:883-7

10. Poskitt EM, Cole TJ. Nature, nurture, and childhood overweight. Br Med J 1978;1:603-5

11. Zive MM, McKay H, Frank-Spohrer GC, Broyles SL, Nelson JA, Nader PR. Infant-feeding practices and adiposity in 4-y-old Anglo- and Mexican- Americans. Am J Clin Nutr 1992;55:1104-8

12. Hilson JA, Rasmussen KM, Kjolhede CL. Maternal obesity and breast-feeding success in a rural population of white women [published erratum appears in Am J Clin Nutr 1998 Mar;67(3):494]. Am J Clin Nutr 1997;66:1371-8

13. Rolland-Cachera MF, Cole TJ, Sempe M, Tichet J, Rossignol C, Charraud A. Body Mass Index variations: centiles from birth to 87 years. Eur J Clin Nutr 1991;45:13-21

14. Hamosh M. Does infant nutrition affect adiposity and cholesterol levels in the adult? J Pediatr Gastroenterol Nutr 1988;7:10-6

15. Lucas A, Sarson DL, Blackburn AM, Adrian TE, Aynsley-Green A, Bloom SR. Breast vs bottle: endocrine responses are different with formula feeding. Lancet 1980;1:1267-9

16. Lucas A, Boyes S, Bloom SR, Aynsley-Green A. Metabolic and endocrine responses to a milk feed in six-day-old term infants: differences between breast and cow's milk formula feeding. Acta Paediatr Scand 1981;70:195-200

17. Koldovsky O. Hormones in milk. Vitam Horm 1995;50:77-149

18. Hauner H, Rohrig K, Petruschke T. Effects of epidermal growth factor (EGF), platelet-derived growth factor (PDGF) and fibroblast growth factor (FGF) on human adipocyte development and function. Eur J Clin Invest 1995;25:90-6

19. Petruschke T, Rohrig K, Hauner H. Transforming growth factor beta (TGF-beta) inhibits the differentiation of human adipocyte precursor cells in primary culture. Int J Obes Relat Metab Disord 1994;18:532-6

20. Dewey KG, Lonnerdal B. Milk and nutrient intake of breast-fed infants from 1 to 6 months: relation to growth and fatness. J Pediatr Gastroenterol Nutr 1983;2:497-506

21. Whitehead RG. For how long is exclusive breast-feeding adequate to satisfy the dietary energy needs of the average young baby? Pediatr Res 1995;37:239-43

22. Heinig MJ, Nommsen LA, Peerson JM, Lonnerdal B, Dewey KG. Energy and protein intakes of breast-fed and formula-fed infants during the first year of life and their association with growth velocity: the DARLING Study. Am J Clin Nutr 1993;58:152-61

23. Rolland-Cachera MF, Deheeger M, Akrout M, Bellisle F. Influence of macronutrients on adiposity development: a follow up study of nutrition and growth from 10 months to 8 years of age. Int J Obes Relat Metab Disord 1995;19:573-8

24. Rolland-Cachera MF, Deheeger M, Bellisle F. Nutrient balance and android body fat distribution: why not a role for protein? [letter; comment]. Am J Clin Nutr 1996;64:663-4

25. Deheeger M, Akrout M, Bellisle F, Rossignol C, Rolland-Cachera MF. Individual patterns of food intake development in children: a 10 months to 8 years of age follow-up study of nutrition and growth. Physiol Behav 1996;59:403-7

26. Burns SP, Desai M, Cohen RD, et al. Gluconeogenesis, glucose handling, and structural changes in livers of the adult offspring of rats partially deprived of protein during pregnancy and lactation. J Clin Invest 1997;100:1768-74

27. Desai M, Byrne CD, Zhang J, Petry CJ, Lucas A, Hales CN. Programming of hepatic insulin-sensitive enzymes in offspring of rat dams fed a protein-restricted diet. Am J Physiol 1997;272:G1083-90

28. Desai M, Hales CN. Role of fetal and infant growth in programming metabolism in later life. Biol Rev Camb Philos Soc 1997;72:329-48

4

NUTRIENTS, GROWTH, AND THE DEVELOPMENT OF PROGRAMMED METABOLIC FUNCTION

Alan A Jackson

Institute of Human Nutrition, Fetal Origins of Adult Disease Division, University of Southampton, UK

Key words: fetus, infant, child, growth, protein, amino acids, lipids, metabolic capacity

Abstract: For each individual, the genetic endowment at conception sets the limits on the capacity or metabolic function. The extent to which this capacity is achieved or constrained is determined by the environmental experience. The consequences of these experiences tend to be cumulative throughout life and express themselves phenotypically as achieved growth and body composition, hormonal status and the metabolic capacity for one or other function. At any time later in life the response to an environmental challenge, such as stress, infection or excess body weight is determined by an interaction amongst these factors. When the metabolic capacity to cope is exceeded, the limitation in function is exposed and expresses itself as overt disease. During early life and development the embryo, fetus and infant are relatively plastic in terms of metabolic function. The effect of any adverse environmental exposure is likely to be more marked than at later ages and the influence is more likely to exert a fundamental effect on the development of metabolic capacity. This has been characterised as "programming" and has come to be known as "the Barker hypothesis" or "the fetal origins hypothesis". Barker has shown that the size and shape of the infant at birth has considerable statistical power to predict the risk of chronic disease in later life. These relationships are graded and operate across a range of birth weight, which would generally be considered to be normal, and are not simply a feature of the extreme of growth retardation. The first evidence showed strong relations between birth weight and heart disease, the risk factors for heart disease, diabetes and hypertension, and the intermediary markers for heart disease, blood cholesterol and fibrinogen. Strong associations have also been found for bone disease, allergic disease and some aspects of brain function. In experimental studies in animals it is possible to reproduce all of the metabolic features predicted from this hypothesis by moderating the consumption of food, or its pattern during pregnancy, and determining metabolic behaviour in the offspring. It has been shown that aspects of maternal diet exert an influence on fetal growth, especially the dietary intake of carbohydrate, protein and some micronutrients. However, these relationships are less strong than might have been predicted, especially when compared with the associations which can be drawn with maternal shape, size and metabolic capacity. Maternal height, weight and body composition relate to the metabolic capacity of the mother and her ability to provide an environment in which the delivery of nutrients to the fetus is optimal. Current evidence suggests that the size of the mothers determines her ability to support protein synthesis, and that maternal protein synthesis, especially visceral protein synthesis, is very closely related to fetal growth and development. It is not clear the extent to which the effect of an adverse environment in utero can be reversed by improved conditions postnatally, but some care is needed in exploring this area, as the evidence suggests that "catch-up" growth imposes its own metabolic stress and may in itself exert a harmful effect.

1.   DEVELOPMENT OF METABOLIC CAPACITY, VULNERABILITY, PLASTICITY

The processes, which underlie normal growth and development from conception to birth take place as structured changes which proceed in an orderly fashion and at a defined rate. The integration of this process in time and space is critical for a successful outcome, and each succeeding period in the process is to an extent determined by the success of all the prior components of the process. Therefore length, weight and body composition at birth reflect the integration of this complexity, and the functionally capacity of individual organs and tissues will be determined by the extent and nature of these interactions. Thus at any point in time, metabolic function is determined by past experience and will in turn shape and modulate function in the future[1].

The developing fetus is extremely plastic and the opportunity exists for it to be substantially moulded by its environment. For this reason the mother seeks to maintain an environment which is characterised by constancy, to protect development and limit the potential perturbations experienced by the fetus. With time the plasticity declines, function and metabolic capacity become more set. A normal part of growth is the development of a reserve capacity for most metabolic functions and processes, which provides a buffer against change and gives the individual the ability to cope with a wider range of environmental perturbations without obvious upset[2]. The evidence suggests that although the upper limit of aspects of this metabolic capacity may be genetically determined, the achieved metabolic capacity may be determined by environmental effects which operate during fetal and early life, making these programmed functions[3]. Programming is a term which characterises the general ability of the phenotype of the organism to be moulded by environmental experiences. It embraces the idea of critical environmental stimuli operating at defined sensitive periods during development, having the ability to induce long-lasting changes in form, function or behaviour of an individual. The environmental change which underlies the response might be characterised by functions as diverse as effect of temperature of incubation on gender of crocodiles to fixation and parenting in geese[4-5]. The ability of an organism to respond effectively to variation in the environment has clear survival value for individuals and the species.

For the human, birth marks a point along the development of these processes, where without entire independence the newborn has sufficient robustness to withstand a range of environmental perturbation. Achieved size is a crude marker for metabolic capacity; in general the metabolic machinery or the enzymic capacity of a larger liver is greater than that of a smaller liver, and a larger muscle mass has a greater capacity to remove glucose from the circulation at a faster rate. Thus, in many ways, size at birth may reflect, or act as an indirect marker for metabolic capacity, and achieved growth will to some extent be a reflection of this size and hence capacity[1]. Metabolic disorders supervene when the available capacity is not adequate for the demand imposed, and hence individuals with less capacity are more susceptible to the same environmental challenge. Ageing represents the loss of capacity and those who achieve a lower overall capacity are more likely to hit the critical, minimum level for normal function, at an earlier age, and therefore more likely to be younger when they first manifest diseases associated with ageing[3].

2.   INFANT-CHILDHOOD-PUBERTY MODEL OF GROWTH

Growth represents the formation of new tissue, which means that sufficient energy needs to be available to enable the net deposition of protein and water as new tissue[6]. At all stages of life and development the potential for growth is determined by the genetic makeup of the individual. However, the phenotypic expression of this potential is determined by a number of factors, amongst which the interaction of the available energy and nutrients, with the modulating influence of the hormonal milieu is of special and most critical importance[7]. The relative importance of nutrients and hormones is not constant, but changes at different stages of development, so that for any one period the major drive towards net tissue deposition is likely to vary from any other stage. Three major phases of growth have been identified by Karlberg, based upon the relative importance of the balance of substrate and hormones at the different stages: fetal-infant; childhood; and pubertal[8]. Thus, it is suggested that although the overall pattern of growth during early life may approximate a smoothed curve, this might in reality comprise the sum of three independent curves, for each of the three separate periods. The dominant driver for the fetal-infant period is the availability of substrate. Hormonal factors are required, but the normal process is limited by the availability of energy, substrate and cofactors, with the growth trajectory during infancy representing an extension of the fetal growth pattern or trajectory. This period may extend up to the second half of the first year. The childhood phase of growth commences at some time between 6 and 18 months of age and last up to 10 to 12 years. The main driver for this part of the process appears to be the growth hormone axis. The timing of the end of the infant period and the start of the childhood period may be critical in determining the extent of stunting in later life. The pubertal phase of growth is primarily driven by sex steroids, and therefore is gender specific. It begins at some time between 8 to 10 years and continues until full maturity is achieved. At all ages and all stages, the quantity and quality of nutrients available will exert an influence on the process and patterning of growth, but an early insult will have a more marked effect for the same level of change. It appears that the transition periods may be the most critical for adverse influences, for example the increased likelihood of stunting if the transition from infant to childhood periods is delayed.

3.   ROLE OF ENERGY AND NUTRIENTS

The rate of growth is critically dependent upon the availability of sufficient energy, although it may be constrained by the limited availability of one or other nutrient. Although the data are not sufficiently clear, it is likely that the quality of growth (the pattern and composition of tissues being deposited) is importantly influenced by the pattern of macronutrients available as sources of energy. It appears that for the late fetus there is an exceptional dependence upon glucose and amino acids as energy substrates, with very little utilization of lipids. However, up to one half of the weight gained by the fetus during the third trimester may be associated with adipose tissue, and as much as 40% of the variation in birth weight might be due to differences in fat mass. The sources of energy for the late fetus are unusually dependent upon the oxidation of glucose and amino acids and we have insufficient understanding of the factors which modulate the availability and utilisation of macronutrients of the human fetus during this time.

4.   AMINO ACID METABOLISM: ESSENTIAL AND NON-ESSENTIAL

Amino acids are utilised as the building blocks for protein synthesis, as well as for the formation of a diverse range of complex molecules of fundamental importance to metabolism. In nutrition, the amino acids have classically been divided into two groups; those that need to be provided preformed in the diet, essential amino acids, and those which can be synthesised in adequate amounts by the host, non-essential amino acids[9,10]. Even for adults, this division is less sharp than previously recognised, but for the fetus all amino acids have to be provided preformed either from the mother or from the placenta until the pathways for *de novo* formation are adequately developed and mature. The time and pace of this maturation varies, with some pathways not achieving significant or adequate function until after birth, for example the ability to synthesise adequate amounts of cysteine and taurine. The pattern of amino acids required by the developing fetus is very different to that found in dietary protein, the "goodness of fit" is poor. Therefore there must be considerable modification to produce an appropriate pattern, either by maternal metabolism or placental formation. The accumulation during late gestation by the fetus of non-essential amino acids is far greater than the accumulation of essential amino acids. Amongst the essential amino acids there is a particular demand for amino acids which are synthesised in large amounts by the placenta: glycine and glutamine[11]. Therefore, it is important for fetal growth that the capacity for these metabolic interconversions is adequate and achieved by the appropriate stage of development. For example, about 90% of the fetal need for glycine appears to be dependent upon placental formation through a metabolic pathway which is dependent upon folate[12]. Thus it might be expected that impairment of folate status would result in a shortfall in the availability of glycine to the fetus. Given the critical role played by glycine in intermediary metabolism, and the heavy demand on glycine for the formation of structural proteins such as collagen, it would be expected that a marginal folate status might result both in a limitation in skeletal development and in the functional capacity of intermediary metabolism.

5.   FETAL ORIGINS OF ADULT DISEASE

Until recently it was generally considered that the chronic non-communicable diseases of adulthood, heart disease, hypertension, diabetes and cancer, were caused by a genetic predisposition acting with lifestyle factors such as smoking, diet and activity. Over the last decade it has become clear that other factors may play a substantial role, and in particular programming of the metabolic capacity during early life may be especially important. The first evidence for this proposition came form a series of epidemiological studies carried out by Barker and his colleagues which suggested that growth during early life potentially represents a major risk factor for the later development of ischaemic heart disease[4;13]. The proposition is that early nutritional exposure programmes future metabolic competence and behaviour by imprinting a change upon genomic expression. The first evidence came from ecological studies which showed that geographical differences in death from ischaemic heart disease in England and Wales were related to differences in infant mortality 70 years ago[14], suggesting that growth and development in the perinatal period may be related to an important risk factor for heart disease. In retrospective cohort studies of men and women born in Hertfordshire between 1911-1930 and Sheffield between 1907 and 1924, it was shown that those with the lowest weight at birth and 1 year had the highest death rates for heart disease, and thus for example in Hertfordshire men the standard mortality rate was 111 for those less than 18 lbs at 1 year compared with 42 in those weighing over 27 lbs at one year[15-16]. Early growth relates directly to current clinical evidence of coronary vascular disease[17], and also to risk factors (such as hypertension, diabetes or obesity)[4;13], and intermediary markers (such as blood lipids and clotting factors), for ischaemic heart disease[18-20]. The general nature of these observations has been replicated in many studies throughout the world, and the weight of evidence is such that it can be stated with reasonable confidence that the pace and pattern of early growth represents a major risk factor for the development of disease during later life. However, this statement it too bald for the more fundamental implication carried by the relationships which have been characterised. Thus although disease or death has been used as a sharp end point to characterise the clinical importance of the relationships, the metabolic basis for the pathological changes is evident from much earlier in life. Thus for example, in studies carried out in children in England, India, Jamaica and elsewhere, the metabolic differences which underlies the risk of disease are already evident, from as early as 3 or 4 years of age[21]. Thus programmed metabolic changes contribute to the determination of the capacity for metabolic function during the entire life of an individual. The metabolic function of an adult, represents the cumulative experience of their environmental exposure throughout their entire life experience. At each age the memory of past metabolic experience contributes to determining current metabolic behaviour, to a greater or lesser degree, although the greatest impact appears to be related to experience during pre-natal life or in infancy.

One of the more important features of the observations made by Barker's group, which are often ignored, or misinterpreted, is that the changes described operate in a graded fashion, across the range of birth weights, which in the past have been considered to be normal. There has been the tendency to interpret the observations as being a feature of babies of lower birth weight, which has very easily been translated to a feature of babies of low birth weight, that is obviously pathological limitations in growth and development. The implication that the changes are graded across the normal range of birth weight, rather than a pathological feature which is expressed below some critical cut-off point has major implication which are often not appreciated, in terms of the basis of the changes and the implications which they carry for health during pregnancy and later in life for the offspring.

Despite the obvious dependence of fetal growth on the delivery of nutrients from the mother, it has been difficult to demonstrate simple relationships between maternal diet, energy or nutrient consumption, during pregnancy and the growth of the fetus. Although it has been possible to show relations between size at birth and the maternal intake of macronutrients, and selected micronutrients, the relative contribution to the variability in birth weight appears modest, explaining of the order of 3 to 5% of the variability in birth weight[22-24]. This is similar to the 5 to 7% of variation in birth weight explained by smoking[22]. When characterising the nutritional status of an individual, the dietary intake is only one part, and body composition and the functional ability or the metabolic state of adaptation also have to be taken into consideration[25]. Thus, relative to the explanatory power of dietary consumption, maternal fat mass during pregnancy showed a much stronger relationship with the blood pressure of the child at 11 years of age[26]. When measures of maternal metabolic function are used to assess the competence of the mother for carrying a pregnancy, the relationship with growth are much more evident. For example, the visceral mass of the mother shows a close relationship with the amount of protein which she synthesises on a daily basis, and this in turn is related to the growth of the fetus[27]. Thus, at least 20% of the variability in length of the newborn could be attributed to variations in maternal protein synthesis, a very strong explanatory variable. The importance of maternal body composition as a measure of her metabolic competence is further emphasised by findings of inter-generational relationships[28]. From studies carried out in Finland. Heart disease was most common in men who were born light, especially in those who were thin at birth. The risk was even greater in men who had mothers who were short, especially if the mothers were short and fat. The authors suggest that in societies, or individuals, in transition from poorer to improved social circumstance women move from being short and thin to being short and fat, before they become taller. They suggest that in this way the diseases of affluence mark the demographic transition, a biological marker of inter-generational competence and availability of food[29].

In all the epidemiological studies, there tends to be a loss in the associations between birth size and measures of metabolic competence until after 2-3 years of age, and again around adolescence until its completion. Both these time periods represent the transition between the different phases of growth: infant to child and child to adolescence. This raises the question of the need for an established drive to growth, or growth trajectory for exposing the relationships in population studies. It raises the possibility that during childhood a growth hormone drive is required to expose the potential limitation in the underlying metabolic capacity for specific functions, and it is for this reason that height itself is a good proxy for metabolic capacity.

6.   ANIMAL STUDIES

Even the most elegant and skilfully conducted epidemiological studies can only provide indirect evidence in support of the general hypothesis that early exposure programmes later metabolic function. The range of variables which have to be taken into consideration and the number of uncontrolled factors which play a part in determining the final outcome over long periods of time, means that if we are to move forward in providing reasonable proof, or in understanding the mechanistic basis of the associations, experimental studies must be carried out. Thus we and others have sought to reproduce the observations from human epidemiological studies in experimental animals. It is important to be clear about the objectives of this work, and its potential limitations. Firstly, in animal studies one is not necessarily seeking to reproduce a disease, but rather to try to modify the processes which are known to lead to disease under suitable circumstances. Secondly, as has been emphasised above, one of the more important feature of the observations which have been made in epidemiological studies is that the changes observed are seen across the normal range of variation and are not a special feature of extremes of size at birth or extremes of dietary intake in the mother. There are many studies in which animals have been provided with diets which have been severely restricted or deficient in one or other nutrient. The result has been offspring which have failed to grow and which have obvious abnormalities of function. The more important challenge is to determine whether it is possible to achieve significant variation in function, when the dietary intake of the animal is varied across a range which reflects the normal variability of dietary consumption. Thus, do the modest variations in macronutrient consumption, across the range usually seen amongst population groups, induce important differences in the growth, development and function of the offspring? The literature contains a number of examples in which extreme dietary manipulations have exerted marked effects upon physiologic and metabolic function. The studies of McCance and Widdowson[30] clearly established the general principle that diet during early life influences the rate of growth and development of form and function at later stages and identified the susceptibility of hypothalamic function during critical periods in early pregnancy. The idea of Winick and Noble that any particular tissue would be most sensitive to an insult, with irreversible effect, if the insult were to act during the period of most rapid cell division has dominated thinking in this area[31]. Whilst establishing basic principles each of these models has used extremes of dietary manipulations. Thus it can be shown that specific appetite for macronutrients in the offspring can be markedly influence by the macronutrient intake of the mother during pregnancy and lactation[32] Sexual dimorphism in growth, body composition, fat patterning and thyroid hormonal profiles were seen in the offspring from pregnancies where the total food intake was reduced to 50% during the first two thirds of pregnancy. The females offspring became relatively obese, whereas the males had evidence of preferential deposition of adipose tissue in intra-abdominal sites[33].

7.   MATERNAL MACRONUTRIENT CONSUMPTION AND PROGRAMMED METABOLIC FUNCTION

The remarkable aspect of the epidemiological work carried out by Barker and colleagues, is that the important observations have related to variations in function which lead to subsequent pathology within a range of maternal food intakes, birth weights and growth during infant which have in the past been considered to encompass a normal range function[4;21]. Therefore, we have been interested to develop an animal model within which to explore the possibility that relatively modest changes in maternal intake during pregnancy might exert an influence upon metabolic function in the offspring. The level of protein in the maternal diet has been shown to influence the development and function of the endocrine pancreas[34]. We have varied the protein intake during pregnancy in a range from adequate (about 20% protein) through marginally adequate to frankly inadequate (about 6% protein) and demonstrated a graded response to the programming of a wide range of metabolic functions. The dams are given different levels of protein in the diet before and/or during pregnancy. At birth they are placed onto normal laboratory chow and the offspring are weaned to chow diets. Therefore, the only exposure to nutritional constraint is pre-natal. With this model there is disproportionate growth of the fetus and placenta[35]. The altered body proportions in the pups are indicative of selective protection of brain growth at the expense of viscera and somatic tissues[35-36]. Postnatal growth is near normal except at the extremes of maternal dietary protein (6%)[37]. When offspring are allowed macronutrient self-selection up to 100 days, the animals exposed to 9% protein in utero are significantly heavier than those exposed to 18% protein[38]. The pattern of macronutrient selected is modified in the 9% protein group, with the males and females showing different responses. Females exposed to 9% protein have significantly increased adipose tissue in all regions, with increases of around 100% for intra-abdominal sites. Males have highly significant increases in omental and mesenteric sites[38].

Pre-natal exposure to low protein diets alters glucose tolerance[39;34]. There is a graded increase in blood pressure as the maternal dietary protein is decreased, which is identifiable from 4 weeks of age and persists for life[37]. There is altered anti-oxidant capability, inflammatory response and immune function[40]. Hepatic function is modulated with the appearance of direct effects upon the development of hepatic zonation[41], and there is impaired nephrogenesis[42]. Thus relatively changes in the maternal diet can exert wide-ranging effects, which are specific, not generalised, and represent fundamental changes in aspects of metabolic competence of which changes in growth and body composition are one manifestation.

There are other models, which have sought to relate changes in maternal diet during pregnancy to programmed changes in the offspring. Many of the dietary changes are extreme, but manipulationg the fatty acid composition of the diet also exerts significant programmed effects upon blood pressure[43], and immune function[44]. There is a great deal still to be learnt in this area.

8. PROGRAMMING OF THE HYPOTHALAMO-PITUITARY-ADRENAL AXIS

McCance and Widdowson had suggested that the critical influence exerted by nutrition during fetal life would be upon hypothalamic function[30]. Edwards and colleagues have suggested that blood pressure might be critically determined through the maternal glucocorticoid axis[45]. In dams given low protein diets, the activity of placental 11ßOH-steroid dehydrogenase was reduced by about one third, which would increase the likelihood of fetal over-exposure to maternal glucocorticoids[46]. The extent to which maternal glucocorticoids might directly contribute to programming fetal metabolism has been explored[47]. Maternal administration of metyrapone or maternal adrenalectomy during early pregnancy abolishes the effect of maternal low protein diets upon the blood pressure of offspring[47-48]. This provides direct evidence that part of the effect might be attributed to changes in the hypothalamo-pituitary-adrenal axis in the mother and/or the fetus. Further support comes from the observations that maternal low protein diets induce modulation of glucocorticoid sensitive enzymes in the fetal brain and liver[47-49]. There is differential regulation of glucocorticoid receptors in the brain, liver and aorta, and offspring of dams given 9% protein during pregnancy do not show a diurnal pattern of ACTH in blood, although diurnal changes in cortisol concentrations are maintained [47-49].

9. CONCLUSIONS

The nutritional determinant of the function of a mother and her fetus have to allow for at least four different levels of interaction: genetic endowment and intergenerational influences; early programming, shape, size and body composition at birth; growth and development interacting with lifetime experience; current plane of nutrition, lifestyle and diet. Her shape and size are a reflection of her genetic endowment, but may also represent the effect of inter-generational influences. In addition her body composition will relate to her chronic food intake and patterns of activity. The plane of nutrition will determine the nature of her metabolic adaptation. Her current food intake will determine the set of her homeostatic mechanisms at any particular point in time. Within these interaction it may be very difficult to differentiate genetic from inter-generational effects. For example, when the genetic model of rodent hypertension, the spontaneously hypertensive rat, is cross-fostered during lactation, the pups have a lifelong blood pressure which is in the normal range. The composition of the maternal milk appears to exert a major effect upon the development of "genetically predisposed" increases blood pressure[50]. Thus the early life origins of adult disease are set in train through an interaction amongst maternal body composition, pre-natal diet and post-natal diet. These directly determine the shape, size and body composition of the individual which interacts with the hormonal profiling and nutrient intake. There is clear evidence for hypothalamic programming playing a part in the process with evidence for a contribution from glucocorticoids, growth hormone, thyroid hormone, sex steroids and the autonomic nervous system.

Early growth determines later shape and size, which is probably a reflection of the adjustments required to protect brain growth and function over visceral function or somatic growth. Shape and size is related to metabolic function and entraining of weight can be related to a severe insult during the third trimester. Two processes interact with life style. During early pregnancy the growth trajectory is set, based upon the interaction of the genetic profile with the maternal hormonal milieu and the local availability of oxygen and nutrients. This sets or programmes the "fetal metabolic demand", probably at the level of the hypothalamus. During late gestation and infancy the achieved growth is a balance between the programmed fetal demand and the hormonal milieu (maternal and fetal) and the availability of energy and nutrients to the fetus. This interaction sets or programmes "fetal or infant metabolic competence". The metabolic competence determines the extent to which an individual might withstand an adverse lifestyle.

The next decade will see the complete unravelling of the human genome. The following period will require that we understand the factors which exert important influences upon the expression of genes. Programmed metabolic function is likely to be on of the more important variables about which we will need much more detailed knowledge and understanding.

REFERENCES

1. Jackson, A.A. (1996) Perinatal nutrition: the impact on postnatal growth and development. In: *Pediatrics and Perinatology*, edited by Gluckman, P.D. and Heymann, M.A.London:Arnold, p. 298-303.

2. Jackson, A.A. (1985) Nutritional adaptation in disease and recovery. In: *Nutritional adaptation in man*. edited by Blaxter, K. and Waterlow, J.C.London:John Libbey, p. 111-126.

3. Jackson, A.A. (1992) How can early diet influence later disease? *BNF Nutr Bull* **17**:23-30.

4. Barker, D.J.P. (1994) *Mothers, babies and disease in later life*. BMJ Publishiing Group.

5. Lucas, A. (1991) Programming by early nutrition in man. In: *The childhood environment and adult disease*, edited by Boch, G.R. and Whelan, J.Chichester:John Wiley & Sons, p. 38-55.

6. Jackson, A.A. and Wootton, S.A. (1990) The energy requirements of growth and catch-up growth. In: *Activity, Energy Expenditure and Energy Requirements of Infants and Children*. edited by Schurch, B. and Scrimshaw, N.S.Lausanne, Switzerland:IDECG, p. 185-214.

7. Uauy, R. and Alvear, J. (1992) Effects of protein-energy interactions on growth. In: *Protein-energy interactions*. edited by Scrimshaw, N.S. and Schurch, B.Lauşanne, Switzerland:International Dietary Energy Consultative Group, p. 151-190.

8. Karlberg, J., Jalil, F., Lam, B., Low, L., and Yeung, C.Y. (1994) Linear growth retardation in relation to the three phases of growth. *Eur J Clin Nutr* **48**(Supplement):S25-S44.

9. Jackson, A.A. (1983) Amino acids: essential and non-essential. *Lancet* ii:1034-1037.

10. Jackson, A.A. (1992) Protein metabolism in man. In: *The Contribution of Nutrition to Human and Animal Health*. edited by Widdowson, E.M. and Mathers, J.C. Cambridge:Cambridge University Press, p. 92-104.

11. Widdowson, E.M., Southgate, D.A.T., and Hey, E.M. (1979) Body composition of the fetus and infant. In: *Nutrition and Metabolism of the Fetus and Infant*. edited by Visser, H.A.K.The Hague:Martinus Nijhoff, p. 169-177.

12. Bennett, F.I. and Jackson, A.A. (1998) Glycine is not formed through the amino acid transferase reaction in human or rat placenta. *Placenta* **19**:329-331.

13. Barker, D.J.P. (1994) The fetal origins of adult disease. *Fetal and Maternal Medicine Review* **6**: 71-80.

14. Barker, D.J.P. and Osmond, C. (1986) Infant mortality, childhood nutrition, and ischaemic heart disease in England and Wales. *Lancet* i: 1077-1081.

15. Barker, D.J.P., Osmond, C., Simmonds, S.J., Wield, G.A. (1993) The relation of small head circumference and thinness at birth to death from cardiovascular disease in adult life. *BMJ* **306**: 422-426.

16. Osmond, C., Barker, D.J.P., Winter, P.D., Fall, C.H.D., Simmonds, S.J. (1993) Early growth and death from cardiovascular disease in women. *BMJ* **307**: 1519-1524.

17. Fall, C.H.D., Vijayakumar, M., Barker, D.J.P., Osmond, C., Duggleby, S. (1995) Weight in infancy and prevalence of coronary heart disease in adult life. *BMJ* **310**: 17-19.

18. Barker, D.J.P., Martyn, C.N., Osmond, C., Hales, C.N., Fall, C.H. (1993) Growth in utero and serum cholesterol concentrations in adult life. *BMJ* **307**: 1524-1527.

19. Fall, C.H.D., Osmond, C., Barker, D.J.P., et al. (1995) Fetal and infant growth and cardiovascular risk factors in women.. *BMJ* **310**: 428-432.

20. Martyn, C.N., Meade, T.W., Stirling, Y. and Barker, D.J.P. (1995) Plasma concentrations of fibrinogen and factor VII in adult life and their relation to intra-uterine growth. *Br J Haematol* **89**: 142-146.

21. Barker, D.J.P. (1998). *Mothers, babies and health in later life*. Edinburgh:Churchill Livingstone.

22. Haste, F.M., Brooke, O.G., Anderson, H.R., and Bland, J.M. (1991) The effect of nutritional intake on outcome of pregnancy in smokers and non-smokers. *Br J Nutr* **65**:347-354.
23. Godfrey, K., Robinson, S., Barker, D.J.P., Osmond, C. and Cox, V. (1996) Maternal nutrition in early and late pregnancy in relation to placental and fetal growth. *BMJ* **312**: 410-414.
24. Mathews, F., Yudkin, P., and Neil, A. (1999) Influence of maternal nutrition on outcome of pregnancy: prospective cohort study. *BMJ* **319**:339-343.
25. Blaxter, K. and Waterlow, J.C. (1985) *Nutritional adaptation in man.* London:John.A. Libbey.
26. Godfrey, K.M., Forrester, T., Barker, D.J.P., Jackson, A.A., Landman, J.P., Hall, J.S.E., and Cox, V. (1994) Maternal nutritional status in pregnancy and blood pressure in childhood. *Br J Obstet Gynaecol* **101**:398-403.
27. Duggleby, S.L. and Jackson, A.A. (2000) Whole body protein turnover during pregnancy, maternal body composiiton and fetal outcome. Proc Nutr Soc, in the press (abstr).
28. Godfrey, K., Barker, D.J.P., Robinson, S., and Osmond, C. (1997) Maternal birthweight and diet in pregnancy in relation to the infant's thinness at birth. *Br J Obstet Gynaecol* **104**:663-667.
29. Forsen, T., Eriksson, J.G., Tuomilehto, J., Teramo, K., Osmond, C., and Barker, D.J.P. (1997) Mother's weight in pregnancy and coronary heart disease in a cohort of Finnish men: follow up study. *BMJ* **315**:837-840.
30. McCance, R.A. and Widdowson, E.M. (1974) The determinants of growth and form. *Proc Roy Soc B* **185**:1-17.
31. Winick, M. and Noble, A. (1996) Cellular response in rats during malnutrition. J Nutr **89**:300-306.
32. Leprohon, C.E. and Anderson, G.H. (1980) Maternal diet affects feeding behaviour of self-selecting weanling rats. *Physiol Behav* **24**:553-559.
33. Anguita, R.M., Sigulem, D.M., and Sawaya, A.L. 1993. Intrauterine food restriction is associated with obesity in young rats. *J Nutr* **123**:1421-1428.
34. Dahri, S., Reusens, B., Remacle, C., and Hoet, J.J. (1995) Nutritional influences on pancreatic development and potential links with non-insulin-dependent diabetes. *Proc Nutr Soc* **54**:345-356.
35. Levy, L. and Jackson, A.A. (1993) Modest restriction of dietary protein during pregnancy in the rat: fetal and placental growth. *J Devel Physiol* **19**:113-118.
36. Langley-Evans, S.C., Gardner, D.S., and Jackson, A.A. (1996) Disproportionate fetal growth in late gestation is associated with raised systolic blood pressure in later life. *J Reprod Fertil* **106**:307-312.
37. Langley, S.C. and Jackson, A.A. (1994) Increased systolic blood pressure in adult rats caused by fetal exposure to maternal low protein diets. *Clin Sci* **86**:217-222.
38. McCarthy, H.D., Pickard, C.L., Speed, J., and Jackson, A.A. (1994) Sexual dimorphism of macronutrient selection and regional adipose tissue accumulation following *in utero* exposure to maternal low-protein diet. *Proc Nutr Soc* **53**:172A.
39. Pickard, C.L., McCarthy, H.D., Browne, R.F., and Jackson, A.A. (1996) Altered insulin response to a glucose load in rats following exposure to a low-protein diet *in utero.*. Proc Nutr Soc **55**:44A.
40. Langley, S.C., Seakins, M., Grimble, R.F., and Jackson, A.A. (1994) The acute phase response of adult rats is altered by in utero exposure to maternal low protein diets. *J Nutr* **124**:1588-1596.

41. Desai, M., Crowther, N.J., Ozanne, S.E., Lucas, A., and Hales, C.N. (1995) Adult glucose and lipid metabolism may be programmed during fetal life. Biochem Soc Transact **23**:331-335.

42. Langley-Evans, S.C., Welham, S.J.M., and Jackson, A.A. (1999) Fetal exposure to a meternal low protein diet impairs nephrogenesis and promotes hypertension in the rat. *Life Sciences* **64**:965-974.

43. Langley-Evans, S.C. (1996) Intrauterine programming of hypertension: nutrient interactions. *Comp Biochem Physiol A Physiol* **114A**:327-333.

44. Calder, P.C. and Yaqoob, P. (2000) The level of protein and type of fat in the diet of pregnant rats both affect lymphocyte function in the offspring. In the press.

45. Edwards, C.R.W., Benediktsson, R., Lindsay, R.S., and Seckl, J.R. (1993) Dysfunction of placental glucocorticoid barrier: link between fetal environment and adult hypertension. *Lancet* **341**:355-357.

46. Langley-Evans, S.C., Phillips, G.J., Benediktsson, R., Gardner, D.S., Edwards, C.R.W., Jackson, A.A., and Seckl, J.R. (1996) Protein intake in pregnancy, placental glucocorticoid metabolism and the programming of hypertension in the rat. *Placenta* **17**:169-172.

47. Langley-Evans, S.C. (1999) Impact of maternal nutrition on the renin-angiotensin system in the fetal rat. In: *Fetal Programming: Influences on Development and Disease in Later Life*, edited by O'Brien, P.M.S., Wheeler, T. and Barker, D.J.P. London:RCOG, p. 374-388.

48. Langley-Evans, S.C. and Jackson, A.A. (1966). Intrauterine programming of hypertension: nutrient-hormone interactions. *Nutriton Reviews* **54**: 163-169.

49. Gardner, D.S., Jackson, A.A., and Langley-Evans, S.C. (1998)The effect of prenatal diet and glucocorticoids on growth and systolic blood pressure in the rat. *Proc Nutr Soc* **57**:235-240.

50. McCarty, R. and Fields-Okotcha, C. (1994) Timing of preweanling maternal effects on development of hypertension in SHR rats. Physiol Behav **55**:839-844.

5

EARLY PROGRAMMING OF GLUCOSE METABOLISM, INSULIN ACTION AND LONGEVITY

C. N. Hales

Department of Clinical Biochemistry, University of Cambridge
Addenbrook's Hospital, Cambridge CB2 2GR England

1.   INTRODUCTION AND BACKGROUND

The studies which I review below were designed to test our hypothesis that restriction of growth during fetal and possibly early infant growth could lead to life-long programmed changes in glucose and insulin metabolism. A consequence of this, especially when combined with adult obesity we predicted would be glucose intolerance and type 2 diabetes[1]. This hypothesis in turn arose from epidemiological studies carried out in collaboration with Professor David Barker in Southampton examining the relationship of poor early growth (e.g. low birth weight or thinness at birth) with loss of glucose tolerance[2] or the presence in adult life of the insulin resistance syndrome[3]. It was found that low birth weight was related to an increased prevalence of impaired glucose tolerance and type 2 diabetes. Even more strongly low birth weight was related to a greatly increased odds ratio for developing the insulin resistance syndrome (also referred to as syndrome X or the metabolic syndrome). These findings have been reproduced in a wide variety of populations and ethnic groups world wide[4].

Short and Long Term Effects of Breast Feeding on Child Health
Edited by Berthold Koletzko *et al.*, Kluwer Academic/Plenum Publishers, 2000

Our "thrifty phenotype" hypothesis[1] was introduced and so named to be contrasted with the much earlier "thrifty genotype" hypothesis proposed by Neel[5]. Neel suggested that the lack of elimination of the (supposed at that time) genes which caused diabetes by natural selection indicated that in some circumstances these genes were beneficial and hence retained by natural selection. These conditions he proposed were those pertaining to much of human evolution namely a precarious and intermittent supply of macronutrients. Such genes had only recently had detrimental effects as a consequence of an overabundance of macronutrients and lack of exercise leading to obesity. At the time that Neel made his proposal the distinction between diabetes type 1 (early onset and relevant to reproduction and natural selection) and type 2 (late onset, predominately post reproductive and therefore protected from natural selection) was not clear. Despite this problem with how the thrifty genes might actually operate and a lack of insight as to which they might be this genetic theory of the aetiology of type 2 diabetes is probably the most generally accepted even at the present time.
Nevertheless it is clear that the effects of relatively poor fetal growth can effect susceptibility to type 2 diabetes independently of genetic factors. Beck-Nielson's group have studied identical twins discordant for type 2 diabetes. They found that the birth weights of the non-diabetic twin were significantly higher than those who had diabetes[6].

2.   ANIMAL MODELS

It has been known for many years that both in animals and humans poor protein nutrition could lead to a loss of glucose tolerance and reduction in insulin secretion and that these changes may be irreversible (reviewed in [1]). In a more recent example of this approach applied to the pregnant rat dam it was found that the β cell growth, replication, insulin secretion and glucose tolerance of offspring of such pregnancies - particularly if the protein deficient diet was also fed to the offspring for a while after weaning - were considerably impaired[7]. We therefore decided to adopt this model to explore the concepts and their potential underlying mechanisms proposed in the thrifty phenotype hypothesis. Most commonly we have fed pregnant and lactating rats an 8% protein isocaloric diet and compared their offspring with those of rats fed 20% protein diets. In the great majority of experiments all animals were weaned onto a normal diet and fed ad lib. In experiments where we combined the reduced protein diet with diet-induced adult obesity we continued the reduced protein diet to 70 days of age to reproduce exactly the conditions shown to have major effects on glucose tolerance[7]. We have also in a number of studies compared the effects of maternal restriction during pregnancy or lactation separately. We have reviewed the early findings of these studies[8] and therefore what follows is a brief summary of the main results.

3.   METABOLISM IN VIVO

The glucose tolerance of offspring from reduced protein pregnancies and lactation up to the age of 3 months was increased. This was associated with an increased insulin sensitivity since the fasting plasma insulin concentration like that of glucose was reduced. At one year of age there was no difference in glucose tolerance but by 15-18 months of age the offspring whose dams consumed a reduced protein diet had a significantly reduced glucose tolerance (but not frank diabetes). Overall therefore they showed a greater age dependant loss of glucose tolerance. In male animals this appeared to be associated with relative insulin deficiency whereas in females plasma insulin concentrations were reduced [review in 9]. The age dependency and different features between the male and female situation are consistent with what is observed in the human situation.

We have also observed changes in blood pressure but the pattern of changes differs depending on the exact dietary regime imposed and the composition of the weaning diet. The importance of the weaning diet on outcome has been emphasised by the research of other workers studying this aspect of the problem[10]. Most commonly we have observed a significant reduction in blood pressure. However in the experiments in which the reduced protein diet was prolonged to 70 days and then followed by diet-induced obesity hypertension was produced both by the reduced protein and by obesity. When the two were combined an additive effect resulted in severe hypertension[11].

Plasma lipid concentrations were most commonly reduced in the offspring of reduced protein pregnancies[12]. However obesity increased plasma triglyceride in both control and reduced protein offspring. As judged by the fasting plasma insulin concentration it also produced insulin resistance in both groups. The effects of obesity and reduced protein were not additive the latter if anything somewhat reducing the changes due to obesity per se.

Nevertheless it is still not clear how many of the features of the insulin resistance syndrome are simply secondary to coexistent (usually intra-abdominal) obesity and how many are expressions of a separate inherent series of other metabolic changes. Certainly offspring of reduced protein pregnancies with diet induced adult obesity exhibit many of the key features of the insulin resistance syndrome in humans. They are short, fat, glucose intolerant, insulin resistant, severely hypertensive and have hypertriglyceridaemia[11].

4.   METABOLISM IN VITRO

4.1   Liver

There were permanent changes in the key enzymes of glycolysis and gluconeogenesis. Glucokinase was reduced and phosphoenolpyruvate carboxykinase increased. Livers from reduced protein offspring when perfused with lactate put out more glucose. The effect of glucagon to stimulate glucose production was unexpectedly reduced but insulin's normal effect to inhibit this was initially reversed to an increase in glucose output. The reduced effect of glucagon may be due to a considerable reduction in its receptors. However insulin receptor numbers were increased.

In view of the reduction in glucagon action and receptors we wondered whether the animals might be resistant to ketosis after starvation. This is a well known feature of diabetes in countries such as India where poor nutrition is common. After 48 hours of starvation the offspring of reduced protein pregnancies had higher concentrations of non-esterified fatty acids but lower concentrations of β hydroxybutyrate than controls. This finding is consistent with their being ketosis resistant.

The changes in hepatic metabolism which we have observed are also consistent with a proposal of the thrifty phenotype hypothesis, namely that they are adapted to better withstand starvation. Increased gluconeogenesis and non-esterified fatty acid concentration but with a lower production of ketone bodies would be beneficial to the maintenance of fuel supply without an enhanced risk of acidosis. It is unclear exactly what are the mechanisms leading to these hepatic changes. It is clear that they are profound and are accompanied by structural changes which include an increase in size and decrease in number of the liver lobules[13].

4.2   Muscle

Glucose uptake by isolated muscle strips from reduced protein offspring at 3 months of age was increased but could be returned to normal by a 1 hour pre-incubation in the absence of insulin. Under the latter conditions the effect of an intermediate submaximal concentration of insulin was enhanced suggesting an increased sensitivity to insulin. The latter may be at least in part due to a considerable increase in the number of insulin receptors. These observations may again at least in part explain the increased glucose tolerance and insulin sensitivity of these animals in vivo.

4.3   Adipose tissue

The basal glucose uptake of isolated adipocytes of 3 month old reduced protein offspring was increased. Since in preparation these cells have already been pre-incubated in the absence of insulin this finding differs from that in muscle. A further difference is that stimulation by insulin increased the maximum glucose uptake above that of controls whereas in muscle an equal maximum was reached for both groups of animals. In contrast to this enhancement of glucose metabolism there was a reduction of the effect of insulin to inhibit catecholamine-stimulated lipolysis. There was also an enhanced stimulation of lipolysis by a catecholamine in the fat cells of reduced protein offspring. The factors mediating these changes are not entirely clear. As with liver and muscle an increased number of insulin receptors was seen. Of the components of the insulin signalling system examined to date the greatest change observed was in the cell's content of the p110 β catalytic subunit of phosphatidyl inositol-3-kinase. This was drastically reduced in the cells of the reduced protein offspring. We have speculated that the latter subunits may be involved in insulin's antilipolytic action and the α subunit in its effects to increase glucose uptake. Thus by a change in the relative amounts of the subunits expressed the balance of metabolic control in adipose tissue could be shifted to enhanced uptake and storage of glucose as fat coupled with an increased release of fatty acids as an alternative fuel[14]. Again one could argue that when carbohydrate was intermittently available it would be metabolically advantageous to take it up rapidly and convert it to a long-term energy store.

Indeed Neel in proposing the thrifty genotype hypothesis speculated that one of the features might be a very rapid and high insulin response to intermittent nutrition. In this way again long-term storage of nutrient could be achieved. It is therefore very interesting that in our model of the thrifty phenotype essentially the same outcome is achieved but by a general increase in the expression of the insulin receptor rather than a large increase in insulin output.

5.   LONGEVITY

In our more recent studies we have become very interested in the effect of changes in fetal and post natal growth on life span. This interest was raised by our observation that in male rats life span could be increased or decreased depending upon whether growth was retarded post natally or during fetal life respectively. In female rats the pattern of changes was the same but much smaller and hence did not reach statistical significance[9].

We have repeated these observations in a further round of experiments in which we sought to widen the growth differences still further by manipulation of litter size. Male rats born from normally fed dams were cross-fostered to lactating females on the reduced protein diet but (unlike the previous experiment in which all litters were culled to a uniform number of 8) litters were not culled resulting in an average size of 13 thus maximising competition for already limited nutrition. Conversely male offspring of reduced protein pregnancies were cross fostered to normally fed lactating dams but the litters culled to 4 thus further enhancing the switch to abundant nutrition. Under these conditions similar changes of survival were observed but with much smaller numbers of animals.

We hypothesised that the changes in longevity which we observed could be due to changes in the rate of telomere shortening in tissues crucial for long term survival. Telomeres are nucleoprotein structures at the ends of each chromosome. They serve a number of functions. It has been suggested that one of these is to control the number of cell divisions which a cell can undergo. In the absence of the enzyme telomerase which appears to be the main, but perhaps not sole, method of maintaining telomere length, telomeres shorten with each cell division. When telomeres reach a critical shortness it is suggested that cell cycling is arrested, cell senescence occurs and this may be followed by cell death. The evidence that this process accounts for the senescence of mortal cells in tissue culture is now very impressive [reviewed in[15]. The evidence that telomere shortening may be linked to cell senescence and longevity in vivo is much less clear.

We therefore carried out a study of our male "cross over" rat experiments with the object of determining whether i) rat telomeres shorten significantly with age ii) they shorten such that significant numbers reach a critical shortness (1-4 kb) by the age at which they start to die iii) our animals which die young have significantly shorter telomeres than those with an increased life span. We found that the telomeres of kidney and liver but not the brain (the three tissues studied) shortened significantly and sufficiently to be involved in cell survival in these organs. The telomeres of the kidney but not the liver were significantly longer in the animals with an increased compared with the animals with a decreased life span. This is particularly interesting since male rats predominately die of renal failure. We have speculated that differences in telomere length determine the rate of renal cell senescence, hence renal failure and death of the animal[16]. Further experiments are in progress to monitor closely the relationship of renal function to telomere length.

6.   CONCLUSION

It is clear from these experiments in animal models that early programming of glucose metabolism, insulin action and longevity does occur in the rat. The changes which occur are quite complex and widespread. They may include structural changes in differentiated tissues but probably occur at the stage of differentiation. The changes in metabolism are the consequence of changes in expression of hormone receptors, components of hormone signalling pathways and the expression of key regulatory enzymes. It seems probable that these in turn reflect changes in gene expression which are established early in life and then continue into adult life. The consequences of the progress in understanding in this area is that much more attention to and insight into the optimisation of early growth is required in order to improve long term human health. Areas of particular importance are the growth and health of females, good nutrition pre and post conception and the harmonisation of post natal nutrition and growth with the growth potential established during fetal life. Our studies in rats would suggest that it is unwise to force post natal catch up growth in situations where fetal growth has been retarded leading to a reduced post natal growth potential.

ACKNOWLEDGMENTS

Our research reported above was supported by grants from the British Diabetic Association, Medical Research Council, Parthenon Trust and the Wellcome Trust.

REFERENCES

1. Hales CN and Barker DJP, 1992, Type 2 (non-insulin-dependent) diabetes mellitus: the thrifty phenotype hypothesis. *Diabetologia* 35: 595-601.
2. Hales CN, Barker DJP, Clark PMS, Cox LJ, Fall C, Osmond C & Winter PD, 1991, Fetal and infant growth and impaired glucose tolerance at age 64 years. *Brit. Med. J.* 303: 1019-1022.
3. Barker DJP, Hales CN, Fall CHD, Osmond C, Phipps K & Clark PMS, 1993, Type 2 (non-insulin-dependent) diabetes mellitus, hypertension and hyper-lipideamia (syndrome X): relation to reduced fetal growth. *Diabetologia* 36: 62-67
4. Phillips DIW & Hales CN, 1996, The intrauterine environment and susceptibility to non-insulin dependent diabetes and the insulin resistance syndrome. *The Diabetes Annual* 10: 1-13
5. Neel JV (1962) Diabetes mellitus: "a thrifty" genotype rendered detrimental by "progress". *Am J Hum Genet* 14: 353-362.
6. Poulsen P, Vaag A, Kyvik KO, Moller-Jansen, Beck-Nielsen H, 1997, Low birth weight is associated with non-insulin-dependent diabetes mellitus in discordant monozygotic and dizygotic twin pairs. *Diabetologia* 40: 439-446
7. Snoek A, Remacle C, Reusens B & Hoet JJ, 1990, Effect of a low protein diet during pregnancy on the fetal rat endocrine pancreas. *Biol Neonate* 57: 107-118.
8. Desai M & Hales C N, 1997, Role of fetal and infant growth in programming metabolism in later life. *Biol. Rev* 72: 329-348.
9. Hales CN, Desai M, Ozanne SE & Crowther NJ, 1996, Fishing in the steam of diabetes: From measuring insulin to the control of fetal organogenesis. *Biochem Soc Trans* 24: 341-350.
10. Langley-Evans S & Jackson A, 1996, Intrauterine programming of hypertension: Nutrient-hormone interactions. *Nutrition Reviews* 54 No 6: 163-169.
11. Petry CJ, Ozanne SE, Wang CL & Hales CN, 1997, Early protein restriction and obesity independently induced hypertension in year old rats. *Clin Science* 93: 147-152.
12. Lucas A, Baker BA, Desai M & Hales CN 1996 Nutrition in pregnant or lactating rats programs lipid metabolism in the offspring. *Brit J Nutrition* 76: 605-612.
13. Burns SP, Desai, Cohen RD, Hales CN, Iles RA, Germain JP, Going TCH & Bailey RA, 1997 Glucogeogenesis, glucose handling, and structural changes in livers of the adult offspring of rats partially deprived of protein during pregnancy and lactaiton. *J Clin Invest* 100: 1768-1774.
14. Ozanne SE & Hales CN (1999) The Long term consequences of intrauterine protein malnutrition for glucose metabolism. Proc Nutr Soc. (In press).
15. de Lange T, 1998, Telomeres and senescence: Ending the debate. *Science* 279: 334-335.
16. Jennings BJ, Ozanne SE, Dorling MW & Hales CN,1999, Early growth determines longevity in male rats and may be related to telomere shortening in the kidney. *FEBS Letters* 448(1): 4-8.

6

THE MAMMARY GLAND—INFANT INTESTINE IMMUNOLOGIC DYAD

[1]L Å Hanson, [1,2]L Ceafalau, [2]I Mattsby-Baltzer, [1]M Lagerberg, [1]A Hjalmarsson, [3]R Ashraf, [3]S Zaman and [3]F Jalil
[1]Department of Clinical Immunology,[2]Department of Clinical Bacteriology, Göteborg University, Guldhedsgatan 10, SE-413 46 Göteborg, Sweden. [3]Department of Social and Preventive Paediatrics, King Edward Medical College, Lahore, Pakistan.

Key words: Breastfeeding, passive protection, active protection, secretory IgA antibodies, lactoferrin, leptin, antisecretory factor

Abstract: The human infant has a very small immune system and needs the support of the mother with the transplacentally arrived IgG antibodies to protect tissues with inflammatogenic and energy-consuming defense. The mucous membranes, where most infections occur, need support via the specialized secretory IgA antibodies and the many other mucosal defense mechanisms provided via the mother's milk. This defense is not inflammatogenic and energy-consuming.

We learn about additional defense factors in the milk, like the anti-secretory factor, which seems to protect against diarrhoea. The milk contains numerous growth factors and cytokines, like leptin, which may promote the development of the intestine as well as the immune system.

Results are appearing giving interesting evidence for enhanced protection against infection also after the termination of breastfeeding. This may occur via the priming of the infant's immune system after uptake of anti-idiotypic antibodies and lymphocytes from the milk.

A breastfeeding motivation study in a large Pakistani village resulted in a 50% decrease of diarrhoea and infant mortality. Deep interviews with the mothers and the traditional birth attendants suggested that even better results may be obtained.

Short and Long Term Effects of Breast Feeding on Child Health
Edited by Berthold Koletzko *et al.*, Kluwer Academic/Plenum Publishers, 2000

65

1.   THE SMALL IMMUNE SYSTEM OF THE NEWBORN

A newborn mouse has only 1% of the immune system of an adult animal[1]. In man the information is less complete, but Brandtzaeg has shown how strikingly especially the IgA-producing B cells increase in number in the intestinal mucosa during the first several weeks – months of life[2]. The newborn can be compared with a germ-free, but not antigen-free, animal where one can see a 10-fold increase in the number of lymphocytes in the gut mucosa after colonization even with one single bacterial strain[3, 4]. These observations give a relatively good picture of the size of the whole immune system since about 2/3 of that is found in the intestinal mucosa[5].

Not only has the newborn an immune system of limited size, but it is also somewhat functionally deficient at birth. Switching through the immuno-globulin isotype genes is inefficient and early antibody responses are mainly composed of IgM antibodies[1]. Immunologic memory is reported to be sparse and several cytokines are only produced in small amounts like IFN-γ (interferon-γ) and IL-4 (interleukin-4). Phagocytes also have a decreased function. Even if newborns are sensitive to infections they are still apt at protective immune responses quite early. They are not like an immunodeficient individual who cannot respond. For instance newborns can mount a memory T_H1 response to BCG-vaccine of a magnitude similar to that in adults[6]. On the other hand the newborn can only produce 10% of adult levels of IFN-γ, known to be important in defense against Mycobacteria.

2.   INTESTINAL COLONIZATION OF THE NEWBORN AND THE IMMUNE SYSTEM

The strongest stimulus expanding the immune system seems to be the colonization of the intestinal mucosa with bacteria after birth[7]. It may also be one reason why the intestine grows with some 20-25 cm in the first few days, but here growth factors and cytokines in the mother's milk may well be important also.

In an adult the anaerobic bacterial flora provides "colonization resistance" which makes it difficult for new bacterial strains to settle in the gut. At that time the anaerobs make up >98% of the flora. However, in early life aerobs dominate till they have consumed the oxygen in the gut to an extent that anaerobes can settle and grow. Before 4 months of age the ratio of anaerobes to aerobes is still only 1.5[8]. Only slowly do the anaerobes increase. This may mean that potentially pathogenic aerobes may reach relatively high numbers in early life since there is less competition from the anaerobes.

Furthermore, there is today a much changed order of bacterial colonization and other species in the gut of the newborn than previously recorded[7]. This is reviewed by A. Wold in the present volume. She also brings up the effects of breastfeeding on the intestinal flora.

3.   THE ENTEROMAMMARIC LINK – MILK   IgA ANTIBODIES AND THEIR ROLE

The mother's milk consistently contains SIgA antibodies against numerous *Escherichia coli* 0 and K antigens[9, 10], as well as other intestinal microbes[11]. The explanation is now well understood. Microbes in the gut are sampled by the M cells covering the Peyer's patches bringing them into contact with the antigen-presenting and lymphoid cells of the patches[5]. After antigen exposure lymphoid cells committed to production of IgA-dimers + J (joining) chain will leave the patches to migrate, or "home", to various mucosae such as in the gut, where the IgA dimers produced will bind to the poly Ig receptor on the basal portion of the gut epithelium via the J chain. The complex formed will pass through the epithelial cells appearing on its surface as SIgA antibodies protective against mucosal infections. But the lymphoid cells from the Peyer's patches will also home to exocrine glands like the lactating mammary glands where they will produce the IgA dimer-J chain which are transported into the milk via the poly Ig receptor and appears in considerable amounts as the complete, stable SIgA[5].

As a consequence of this underscore{enteromammaric link} the breastfed infant will be able to cover its intestinal epithelium with SIgA antibodies to the microflora which the mother has been exposed to both most recently, and also a long time ago responding again in the mammary gland via her memory lymphocytes migrating there during lactation[5]. This way the infant will be well covered against the microbes of its milieux; which are those which are most likely to colonize the infant's mucosae. It is likely that this way the infant's encounter with the early colonizers is dampened. Thus intestinal bacteria in breastfed infants are covered by SIgA antibodies which may possibly limit their numbers in the gut and diminish their adherence to mucosal receptors.

These milk SIgA antibodies have been shown to provide significant protection against intestinal infections caused by *Vibrio cholerae*, enterotoxigenic *Escherichia coli, Campylobacter, Shigella* and *Giardia lamblia*[12-16].

By now, it is well accepted that breastfeeding protects against otitis media, respiratory tract infections, gastroenteritis, urinary tract infections, neonatal septicemia and necrotizing enterocolitis[17]. The SIgA antibodies may play a role in all of these infections, but this has not been formally proven.

4.   OTHER DEFENSE FACTORS IN MILK ACTING IN THE INFANT'S GUT

It is unknown whether or not the limited amounts of IgG and IgM antibodies present in the maternal milk play a measureable role in the mucosal defense of the infant.

In early colostrum the major milk protein is SIgA, in mature milk it is lactoferrin (LF) at the level of 2-5 g/l[5]. LF is a single chain glycoprotein. Its peptide chain contains 692 aminoacids and folds into two globular lobes; each of these contains an iron-binding site[18]. LF has many functions besides binding iron. It is bacteriostatic and bactericidal for many species. It also inhibits certain viruses, kills yeasts and even certain tumour cells in vitro[18, 19]. Enzymic degradation gives rise to peptides, especially the lactoferricin (LF-cin), which are efficiently bactericidal[20].

LF and LF-cin are also anti-inflammatory, e.g. by inhibiting production of anti-inflammatory cytokines like IL-1, IL-6, IL-8, TNF-α[18, 21, 22]. Furthermore, it can bind to B-cells and inhibit antibody synthesis, affect T cell proliferation, interfere with the complement system, interfere with the cytotoxic effects of NK cells and block histamin release from mast cells[22-24].

There are data to suggest that LF and LF peptides come out in the urine of preterm breastfed infants[25, 26]. Milk SIgA antibodies coat the enteric bacteria which are usually the cause of urinary tract infections by entering the urinary tract from below. The anti-adherence effects of these antibodies may help preventing such a course. Breastfed infants also have a higher level of oligosaccharide receptor analogues in the urine than non-breastfed[27-29]. Furthermore, breastfeeding may result in a selection of less virulent bacteria in the gut [30-32]. All these factors may help explaining how breastfeeding can protect against urinary tract infections[33, 34].

We have studied the possible protective role of orally given human LF and LF peptides against urinary tract infections caused by *E. coli* in the mouse[35]. The LF structures were given 30 minutes after the introduction of the bacteria into the urinary tract. The LF reduced the number of bacteria in the bladder and the kidneys compared to the control 24 hours after the start of the infection (p<0.0001 and p=0.006). One of the peptides also reduced the number of bacteria in the kidneys. The LF could reduce the levels of the inflammatogenic IL-6 both in the urine and the blood (p<0.05 and p<0.02). Thus it seems that milk LF may reach the urinary tract presumably after binding to the LF receptors in the intestinal brush-border[23]. Such a transport may also involve some of the peptides resulting from enzymic degradation of the relatively resistant LF in the gut.

Using experimental colitis in mice as another *in vivo* model we could also show protective effects of LF[36]. Thus there were significant effects delaying the appearance of blood in the stool (p<0.001) and macroscopic bleedings from the rectum (p=0.008). The length of the colon was not reduced in the LF treated group as in the untreated controls (p<0.05) and there were fewer changes in the histologic picture (p=0.012). Synthetic peptides derived from LF seemed also able to reduce the inflammatory changes including the number of MHC II positive cells. High levels of LF could be shown in serum and also in urine of the LF-treated animals. Thus it may be that LF provided via breastfeeding may have an anti-inflammatory activity in the gut.

Most of the anti-viral effects of milk seem to be connected with LF, although there are also SIgA antibodies to viruses like parainfluenzae, influenzae A, rhinovirus, rotavirus, poliovirus, cytomegalovirus and respiratory syncytial virus. Why breastfeeding, which protects so well against many other enteric infections, does not provide more than a delaying or partial defense against rotavirus infections is not quite clear[37-39].

The lactadherin which is a 46kDa mucinrelated glycoprotein can bind rotavirus and seemed to be protective in a study of rotavirus infections in Mexican children[40]. This has been debated[41].

There are several other protective components in human milk than antibodies and LF, but their protective capacity need further studies. This is true for the 90K, Mac2 binding protein in milk, which has been claimed to protect against viral infections in the respiratory tract[42]. Its possible effect on enteric viruses does not seem to have been studied.

The presence of leptin in the milk[43] may be of significance for the infant's host defense since leptin has the structure and several functions of a cytokine[44, 45]. It stimulates haematopoeitic and lymphoid cells, especially T_H1 cells which produce IFN-γ, it enhances phagocytosis and may upregulate inflammatory cytokines[45]. However, the role of milk leptin for the offspring has not yet been investigated, when it comes to its possible role for the immune system.

Certain bacterial enterotoxins induce a regulatory peptide, anti-secretory factor (AF), which turns off diarrhoea[46]. A structurally closely related group of peptides called feed-induced lectins (FIL) reduces the prevalence of post-weaning diarrhoea in piglets[47]. A proper mix of sugars and aminoacids, or processed cereals can induce FIL. With such a diet we were recently finally able to control devastatingly voluminous and frequent diarrhoeas in a patient with hypogammaglobulinemia on immunoglobulin prophylaxis, but without AF in his intestinal mucosa.

Furthermore, using Western blot we have been able to demonstrate the presence of AF/FIL in milk from Pakistani and Guatemalan mothers, but not from Swedish mothers [48]. Presumably the Swedish mothers had not been exposed to microbial enterotoxins as the other mothers presumably had. It is possible that the presence of AF/FIL in maternal milk can be yet another factor which protects against diarrhoeal disease in the offspring. We do not know whether it is possible to induce AF/FIL in the milk via the mother's diet.

There are numerous cytokines and growth factors present in human milk[49-51]. Especially IFN-γ, TGF-β (Transforming Growth Factor-β) and G-CSF (Granulocyte-Colony Stimulating Factor) are present in high amounts in milk. These components may well be functional in the infant. This is suggested for TGF-β1 by the fact that fosterfeeding rescued gene-disrupted newborn mice to early survival and normal development[52].

5.   LONG TERM EFFECTS OF BREASTFEEDING

By now several studies have provided evidence that breastfeeding provides enhanced protection against infection also for years after the termination of breastfeeding[49]. This has been suggested for otitis media[53], respiratory tract infections[54], *Haemophilus influenzae* type b infections[55, 56], diarrhoea[57] and wheezing bronchitis in non-atopic children[58, 59]. This enhanced protection may last from 3-10 years and the protection seems to be increased for each week of breastfeeding.

There is also evidence that vaccinations may be enhanced during and after breastfeeding against e.g. BCG[60], tetanus and diphteria toxoids and poliovirus vaccines[61]. However, this effect is not seen against all vaccines which has been discussed[49].

Studies of the mechanisms behind this indicate that anti-idiotypic antibodies and lymphocytes from the mother's milk are taken up in the infant's gut and can obviously prime its immune system. Anti-idiotypes given to neonatal mice via the milk clearly primes, enhancing subsequent immune responses[62, 63].

Anti-idiotypic antibodies are present in human milk and might have a similar effect[64].

Several studies indicate that milk lymphocytes are taken up and found in the gut mucosa, mesenteric lymph nodes and even in small numbers in spleen and lungs[65-69]. Quite remarkable is that the offspring becomes tolerant to the maternal MHC thus becoming able to accept these milk cells which then might be able to transfer immunological information. One striking consequence is that this tolerance to maternal MHC results in significantly better results of renal transplantation using the mother as the donor and the child (even as an adult) as a recipient. The results are much better than if the donor is the father or a mother who has not breastfed[70-72]. In agreement with this breastfed children have a significantly lower precursor frequency of cytotoxic T lymphocytes reactive against maternal HLA than non breastfed[73].

6.　　BREASTFEEDING IN REALITY

This was the title of the key note presentation of the first author at our Conference in Oaxaca 1986. At that time we reviewed the data from our studies of the mode of feeding in Pakistan illustrating all the problems with delayed onset of breastfeeding, consistent addition of other foods and fluids before and during breastfeeding (prelacteals) with a heavy exposure to various microbes in early life as a consequence[74]. On the basis of our findings we instituted in one village with a population of 6500 a breastfeeding motivation campaign as part of a health care program. After 3 years we have evaluated some of the outcomes. The results were striking with a 50% reduction both in the prevalence of diarrhoea and in infant mortality (Ashraf, Zaman, Jalil et al, unpublished results). Previously all children were given prelacteals like cleared butter, a herb concoction, sugar or salt water etc. and only 50% of the children had had any breastmilk at 48 hours after delivery[74]. After the motivation campaign prelacteals were more often avoided and 90% the children started to breastfeed within the first 24 hours. The median delay after birth was 6 hours.

The decline in the prevalence of diarrhoeal illnesses was presumably not only due to the introduction of colostrum, but also to continued exclusive breastfeeding and avoidance of the bottle (which were messages during the motivation campaign and later). The avoidance of the prelacteals may have reduced neonatal septicaemia and other related infections in early postnatal age. The longterm effect of optimal brestfeeding practices seem to impact the attained length at the age of two years where we can see that this new cohort of children have "gained" at least 3-4 cms in length and that the "gain" starts as early as 3-6 months of life.

However, deep interviews with the mothers and the traditional birth attendants (TBA:s) who had been informed about the advantages of breastfeeding still showed that some misconceptions remained. It was conceived by some that the breast was empty till the 2nd or 3rd day and that the baby should only be put to the breast at that time. It was also mentioned that the colostrum had been in the breast for a long time, was not clean, good, or digestible and should not be given as suggested by elders. Giving prelacteals is a tradition, about 2000 years old[75], and it was considered needed since the breast was empty after delivery. Still this tradition is obviously being applied much less now.

The many benefits of breastfeeding were well known to the TBA:s as, well as the mothers.

These early results which are still incomplete show a striking improvement in early health, but also demonstrates that the information to the TBA:s and mothers need to be expanded to make obvious the importance of an immediate start of breastfeeding after delivery to stimulate milk production and a strict avoidance of prelacteals, which we previously have shown to add to the early intestinal colonization with bacteria of the infants[76]. This is a definitely dangerous factor, most likely partly explaining the high risk of 2% of e.g. neonatal septicemia with a mortality of some 60%[77]. Even partial breastfeeding was found to protect against neonatal septicemia with an odd's ratio of 18 in this setting[78].

These observations illustrate the obvious importance of early onset of breastfeeding in poor communities, but also show what improvements can be attained. Especially rewarding was the fact that the mothers in general had received the information so positively in the motivation study. The resulting empowerment of these women was evident.

REFERENCES

1. Adkins B. T-cell function in newborn mice and humans. Immunol Today 1999:20:330-5.
2. Brandtzaeg P, Nilssen DE, Rognum TO, and Thrane PS. Ontogeny of the mucosal immune system and IgA deficiency. Gastroenterol Clin North Am 1991:20:397-439.
3. Crabbé PA, Bazin H, Eyssen H, and Heremans JF. The normal microbial flora as a major stimulus for proliferation of plasma cells synthesizing IgA in the gut. Int Arch Allergy 1968:34:362-75.
4. Crabbé PA, Nash DR, Bazin H, Eysseb H, and Heremans JF. Immunohistochemical observations on lymphoid tissues from conventional and germ-free mice. Lag Invest 1970:22:448-57.
5. Goldblum RM, Hanson LÅ and Brandtzaeg P. The mucosal defense system. In: Stiehm E R, ed. Immunologic Disorders in Infants and Children. Philadelphia: W B Saunders, 1996:159-99.
6. Marchant A, Goetghebuer T, Ota MO, Wolfe I, Ceesay SJ, De Groote D, Corrah T, Bennett S, Wheeler J, Huygen K, Aaby P, McAdam KP, and Newport MJ. Newborns develop a Th1-type immune response to Mycobacterium bovis bacillus Calmette-Guerin vaccination. J Immunol 1999:163:2249-55.
7. Adlerberth I, Wold AE and Hanson LÅ. The ontogeny of the intestinal flora. In: Sanderson I R, et al, eds. Development of the gastrointestinal tract. Ontario: B C Decker, 1999.

8. Ellis-Pegler RB, Crabtree C and Lambert HP. The fecal flora of children in the United Kingdom. J Hyg (Camb) 1975:75:135-42.
9. Carlsson B, Kaijser B, Ahlstedt S, Gothefors L, and Hanson LÅ. Antibodies against *Escherichia coli* capsular (K) antigens in human milk and serum: their relation to the *E. coli* gut flora of the mother and neonate. Acta Paediatr Scand 1982:71:313-8.
10. Carlsson B, Ahlstedt S, Hanson LÅ, Lidin-Janson G, Lindblad B, and S S. *Escherichia coli* O antibody content in milk from healthy Swedish mothers and mothers from a very low socio-economic group of a developing country. Acta Paediatr Scand 1976:65:417-23.
11. Hanson LÅ, Carlsson B, Jalil F, Hahn-Zoric M, Karlberg J, Mellander L, Shaukat RK, Lindblad B, Thiringer K, and Zaman S. Antiviral and antibacterial factors in human milk. In: Hanson LÅ, ed. Biology of Human Milk. New York: Raven Press, 1988:141-57.
12. Glass RI, Svennerholm AM, Stoll BJ, Khan MR, Hossain KM, Huq MI, and Holmgren J. Protection against cholera in breast-fed children by antibodies in breast-milk. N Engl J Med 1983:308:1389-92.
13. Cruz JR, Gil L, Cano F, Caceres P, and Pareja G. Breast-milk anti-*Escherichia coli* heat-labile toxin IgA antibodies protect against toxin-induced infantile diarrhoea. Acta Paediatr Scand 1988:77:658-62.
14. Ruiz-Palacios GM, Calva J and Pickering LK. Protection of breast-fed infants against *Campylobacter* diarrhoea by antibodies in human milk. J Pediatr 1990:116:707-13.
15. Hayani KC, Guerrero ML, Morrow AL, Gomez HF, Winsor DK, Ruiz-Palacios GM, and Cleary TG. Concentration of milk secretory immunoglobulin A against *Shigella* virulence plasmid-associated antigens as a predictor of symptom status in *Shigella*-infected breast-fed infants. J Pediatr 1992:121:852-6.
16. Walterspiel JN, Morrow AL, Guerrero ML, Ruiz-Palacios GM, and Pickering LK. Secretory anti-*Giardia lamblia* antibodies in human milk: Protective effect against diarrhea. Pediatrics 1994:93:28-31.
17. Hanson LÅ and Telemo E. Immunobiology and epidemiology of breastfeeding in relation to prevention of infections from a global perspective. In: Ogra PL, et al, eds. Mucosal Immunology. San Diego: Academic Press, 1999:1501-10.
18. Lönnerdal B and Iyer S. Lactoferrin: Molecular structure and biologocal function. Annu Rev Nutr 1995:15:93-110.
19. Brock J. Lactoferrin: a multifunctional immunoregulatory protein? Imm Today 1995:16:417-9.
20. Tomita M, Takase M, Wakabayashi H, and Bellamy W. Antimicrobial peptides of lactoferrin. In: T W Hutchens et al, ed. Lactoferrin, Structure and Function. New York: Plenum Press, 1994.
21. Mattsby-Baltzer I, Roseanu A, Motas C, Elverfors J, Engberg I, and Hanson LÅ. Lactoferrin or a fragment thereof inhibits the endotoxin-induced interleukin-6 response in human monocytic cells. Pediatr Res 1996:40:257-62.
22. Ferenc Levay P and Viljoen M. Lactoferrin: A general review. Haematologica 1995:80:252-67.
23. Iyer S and Lönnerdal B. Review. Lactoferrin, lactoferrin receptors and iron metabolism. European Journal of Clinical Nutrition 1993:47:232-41.
24. Zimecki M, Mazurier J, Spik G, and Kapp JA. Human lactoferrin induces phenotypic and functional changes in murine splenic B cells. Immunmology 1995:86:122-7.
25. Hutchens TW, Henry JH, Yip T-T, Hachey DL, Schanler RJ, Motil KJ, and Garza C. Origin of intact lactoferrin and its DNA-binding fragments found in the urine of human milk-fed preterm infants. Evaluation by stable isotopic enrichment. Pediatr Res 1991:29:243-50.

26. Goldblum RM, Schanler RJ, Garza C, and Goldman AS. Human milk feeding enhances the urinary excretion of immunologic factors in low birth weight infants. Pediatr Res 1989:25:184-8.

27. Wold A and Hanson LÅ. Defence factors in human milk. Curr Opin Gastroenterol 1994:10:652-8.

28. Rudloff S, Pohlentz G, Diekmann L, Egge H, and Kunz C. Urinary excretion of lactose and oligosaccharides in preterm infants fed human milk or infant formula. Acta Paediatr 1996:85:598-603.

29. Coppa GV, Gabrielli O, Giorgi P, Catassi C, Montanari MP, Varaldo PE, and Nichols BL. Preliminary study of breastfeeding and bacterial adhesion to uroepithelial cells. Lancet 1990:335:569-71.

30. Slaviková M, Lodinová-Zadniková R, Adlerberth I, Hanson LÅ, Svanborg C, and Wold A. Increased mannose-specific adherence and colonizing ability of *Escherichia coli* O83 in breast-fed infants. Adv Exp Med Biol 1995:371A:421-4.

31. Gothefors L, Olling S and Winberg J. Breastfeeding and biological properties of faecal *Escherichia coli* strains. Acta Paediatr Scand 1975:64:807-12.

32. Tullus K. Fecal colonization with P-fimbriated *Escherichia coli* between 0 and 18 months of age. Epidemiol Infect 1988:100:185-91.

33. Pisacane A, Graziano L, Mazzarella G, Scarpellino B, and Zona G. Breast-feeding and urinary tract infection. J Pediatr 1992:120:87-9.

34. Mårild S, Jodal U and Hanson LÅ. Breastfeeding and urinary-tract infection. Lancet 1990:336:942.

35. Ceafalau LA, Engberg I, Dolphin G, Baltzer L, Hanson LÅ, and Mattsby-Baltzer I. Lactoferrin and peptides derived from a surface exposed helical region prevent experimental *Escherichia coli* urinary tract infection in mice. 1999. (In manuscript).

36. Ceafalau LA, Dolphin G, Baltzer L, Hanson LÅ, and Mattsby-Baltzer I. Anti-inflammatory activities of human lactoferrin and synthetic peptides thereof in experimental dextran-sulphate induced colitis in mice. 1999. (In manuscript).

37. Espinoza F, Paniagua M, Hallander H, Svensson L, and Strannegård Ö. Rotavirus infections in young Nicaraguan children. Pediatr Infect Dis J 1997:16:564-71.

38. Jayashree S, Bhan M, Kumar R, Bhandari N, and Sazawal S. Protection against neonatal rotavirus infection by breast milk antibodies and trypsin inhibitors. J Med Virol 1988:26:333-8.

39. Clemens J, Rao M, Ahmed F, Ward R, Huda S, Chakraborty J, Yunus M, Khan M, Ali M, and Kay Bea. Breast-feeding and the risk of life-threatening rotavirus diarrhea: Prevention or postponement? Pediatrics 1993:92:680-5.

40. Newburg DS, Peterson JA, Ruiz-Palacios GM, Matson DO, Morrow AL, Shults J, Guerrero ML, Chaturvedi P, Newburg SO, Scallan CD, Taylor MR, Ceriani RL, and Pickering LK. Role of human-milk lactadherin in protection against symptomatic rotavirus infection. Lancet 1998:351:1160-4.

41. Black ME and Armstrong D. Human-milk lactadherin in protection against rotavirus. Lancet 1998:351:1815-6.

42. Fornarini B, Iacobelli S, Tinari N, Natoli C, De Martino M, and Sabatino G. Human milk 90K (Mac-2 BP): possible protective effects against acute respiratory infections. Clin Exp Immunol 1999:115:91-4.

43. Casabiell X, Pineiro V, Tome MA, Peino R, Dieguez C, and Casanueva FF. Presence of leptin in colostrum and/or breast milk from lactating mothers: a potential role in the regulation of neonatal food intake. J Clin Endocrin Metab 1997:82:4270-3.

44. Mantzoros CS. The role of leptin in human obesity and disease: a review of current evidence. Ann Intern Med 1999:130:671-80.

45. Loffreda S, Yang SQ, Lin HZ, Karp CL, Brengman ML, Wang DJ, Klein AS, Bulkley GB, Bao C, Noble PW, Lane MD, and Diehl AM. Leptin regulates proinflammatory immune responses. FASEB J 1998:12:57-65.

46. Lönnroth I and Lange S. Inhibition of cyclic AMP-mediated intestinal hypersecretion by pituitary extracts from rats pretreated with cholera toxin. Med Biol 1984:62:290-4.

47. Göransson L, Lange S and Lönnroth I. Post weaning diarrhoea: focus on diet. Pig News Inform 1995:16:89-91.

48. Hanson LÅ, Lönnroth I, Lange S, Bjersing J, and Dahlgren U. Nutritional resistance to viral propagation. 1999. In: Nutrients and Viral Infections, from Molecular Biology to Public Health. Nutr Rev (In press).

49. Hanson LÅ. Breastfeeding provides passive and likely long-lasting active immunity. Ann Allergy Asthma Immunol 1998:81:523-33.

50. Hawkes JS, Bryan D-L, James MJ, and Gibson RA. Cytokines (IL-1β, IL-6, TNF-α, TGF-β1, and TGF-β2) and prostaglandin E2 in human milk during the first three months postpartum. Pediatr Res 1999:46:194-9.

51. Bryan D-L, Hawkes JS and Gibson RA. Interleukin-12 in human milk. Pediatr Res 1999:45:858-9.

52. Letterio JJ. Maternal rescue of transforming growth factor-β1 null mice. Science 1994:264:1936-8.

53. Saarinen UM. Prolonged breast feeding as prophylaxis for recurrent otitis media. Acta Pediatr Scand 1982:71:567-71.

54. Wilson AC, Forsyth JS, Greene SA, Irvine L, Hau C, and Howie PW. Relation of infant diet to childhood health: seven year follow up of cohort of children in Dundee infant feeding study. BMJ 1998:316:21-5.

55. Silfverdal SA, Bodin L, Hugosson S, Garpenholt O, Werner B, Esbjorner E, Lindquist B, and Olcen P. Protective effect of breastfeeding on invasive Haemophilus influenzae infection: a case-control study in Swedish preschool children. Int J Epidemiol 1997:26:443-50.

56. Silfverdal SA, Bodin L and Olcen P. Protective effect of breastfeeding: an ecologic study of Haemophilus influenzae meningitis and breastfeeding in a Swedish population. Int J Epidemiol 1999:28:152-6.

57. Howie PW, Forsyth JS, Ogston SA, Clark A, and V FC. Protective effect of breast feeding against infection. BMJ 1990:300:11-6.

58. Burr ML, Limb ES, Maguire MJ, Amarah L, Eldridge BA, Layzell JC, and Merrett TG. Infant feeding, wheezing, and allergy: a prospective study. Arch Dis Child 1993:68:724-8.

59. Porro E, Indinnimeo L, Antognoni G, Midulla F, and Criscione S. Early wheezing and breast feeding. J Asthma 1993:30:23-8.

60. Pabst HF, Grace M, Godel J, Cho H, and spady DW. Effect on breastfeeding on antibody response to BCG vaccination. Lancet 1989:I:295-7.

61. Hahn-Zoric M, Fulconis F, Minoli I, Moro G, Carlsson B, Böttiger M, Räihä N, and Hanson LÅ. Antibody responses to parenteral and oral vaccines are impaired by conventional and low protein formulas as compared to breast-feeding. Acta Paediatr Scand 1990:79:1137-42.

62. Stein KE and Söderström T. Neonatal administration of idiotype or anti-idiotype primes for protection against *Escherichia coli* K13 infection in mice. J Exp Med 1984:160:1001-11.

63. Okamoto Y, Tsutsumi H, Kumar NS, and Ogra PS. Effect of breast feeding on the development of anti-idiotype antibody response to F glycoprotein of respiratory syncytial virus in infant mice after post-partum maternal immunisation. J Immunol 1989:142:2507-12.

64. Hahn-Zoric M, Carlsson B, Jeansson S, Ekre O, Osterhaus AD, Roberton DM, and Hanson LÅ. Anti-idiotypic to poliovirus in commercial immunoglobulin, human serum and human milk. Pediatr Res 1993:33:475-80.

65. Weiler IJ, Hickler W and Sprenger R. Demonstration that milk cells invade the suckling neonatal mouse. Am J Reproduct Immunol 1983:4:95-8.

66. Sheldrake RF and Husband AJ. Intestinal uptake of intact maternal lymphocytes by neonatal rats and lambs. Res Vet Science 1985:39:10-5.

67. Kumar SN, Stewart GL, Steven WM, and Seelig LL. Maternal to neonatal transmission of T-cell mediated immunity to Trichinella spiralis during lactation. Immunology 1989:68:87-92.

68. Tuboly S, Bernáth S, Glávits R, Kovács A, and Megyeri Z. Intestinal absorption of colostral lymphocytes in newborn lambs and their role in the development of immune status. Acta Vet Hungar 1995:43:105-15.

69. Gustafsson E, Arvola M, Svensson L, Mattsson A, and Mattson R. Postnatally transmitted maternal B cells can cause long-term maintenance of serum IgG in B cell-deficient mice nursed by phenotypically normal dams. 1997. In manuscript.

70. Kois WE, Campbell DA, Jr., Lorber MI, Sweeton JC, and Dafoe DC. Influence of breast feeding on subsequent reactivity to a related renal allograft. J Surg Res 1984:37:89-93.

71. Deroche A, Nepomnaschy I, Torello S, Goldman A, and Piazzon I. Regulation of parental alloreactivity by reciprocal F1 hybrids. The role of lactation. J Reprod Immunol 1993:23:235-45.

72. Campbell DA, Jr., Lorber MI, Sweeton JC, Turcotte JG, Niederhuber JE, and Beer AE. Breast feeding and maternal-donor renal allografts. Possibly the original donor-specific transfusion. Transplantation 1984:37:340-4.

73. Zhang L, van Bree S, van Rood JJ, and Claas FHJ. Influence of breast feeding on the cytotoxic T cell allorepertoire in man. Transplantation 1991:52:914-6.

74. Hanson LÅ, Adlerberth I, Carlsson B, Jalil F, Karlberg J, Lindblad BS, Mellander L, Khan SR, Hasan R, Sheiku AK, and Söderström T. Breast feeding in reality. In: Hamosh M, et al, eds. Human Lactation 2. Maternal-Environmental Factors: Raven Press, 1986:1-12.

75. Fildes VA. Breast, Bottles and Babies: A History of Infant Feeding. 1986: Edinburgh University Press.

76. Adlerberth I, Carlsson B, de Man P, Jalil F, Khan SR, Larsson P, Mellander L, Svanborg C, Wold AE, and Hanson LÅ. Intestinal colonization with *Enterobacteriaceae* in Pakistani and Swedish hospital-delivered infants. Acta Paediatr Scand 1991:80:602-10.

77. Jalil F, Lindblad BS, Hanson LÅ, Khan SR, Yaqoob M, and Karlberg J. Early child health in Lahore, Pakistan: IX. Perinatal events. Acta Paediatr Suppl 1993:390:95-107.

78. Ashraf R, Jalil F, Zaman S, Karlberg J, Khan SR, Lindblad BS, and Hanson LÅ. Breast feeding and protection against neonatal sepsis in a high risk population. Arch Dis Child 1991:66:488-90.

7

BREAST FEEDING AND THE INTESTINAL MICROFLORA OF THE INFANT— IMPLICATIONS FOR PROTECTION AGAINST INFECTIOUS DISEASES

A. E. Wold and I. Adlerberth

Department of Clinical Immunology, Göteborg University, Guldhedsgatan 10, SE-413 46 Göteborg, Sweden

Key words: Milk, human IgA, secretory, large intestine, bacterial adherence

Abstract: Human breast milk contains an array of factors with anti-infectious potential, such as immunoglobulins (especially secretory IgA), oligosaccharides and glycoproteins with anti-adhesive capacity, and cytokines. Breast-feeding is associated with protection from the following infections or infection-related conditions: gastroenteritis, upper and lower respiratory tract infection, acute otitis media, urinary tract infection, neonatal septicaemia and necrotizing enterocolitis. Some of the protective effects may derive from an altered mucosal colonization pattern in the breast-fed infant. In other instances breast-fed infants develop less symptoms to the same microbe which causes disease in the bottle-fed infant. An example of an altered colonization pattern is that breast-fed infants have less P-fimbriated, but more type 1-fimbriated *E. coli*. This may protect against urinary tract infection in the breast-fed infant since P fimbriae are the major virulence factor for urinary tract infection. An example of changed consequences of the same microbial colonization is that secretory IgA in the breast-milk protects very efficiently from translocation of intestinal bacteria across the gut mucosa by coating intestinal bacteria and blocking their interaction with the epithelium. This mechanism may protect the infant from septicaemia of gut origin and, possibly, necrotizing enterocolitis. Breast-milk is also highly anti-inflammatogenic and contains hormone like factors which counteract diarrhea. Thus, breast-fed infants may be colonized by recognized diarrheal pathogens and still remain healthy. Due to a less virulent intestinal microflora and decreased translocation breast-fed infants will obtain less stimuli for the gut immune system, resulting, in e.g., lower salivary IgA antibody titres.

1.   INTRODUCTION

Breast-feeding is associated with protection from a range of infections or infection-related conditions (Table 1). For infants in developing countries, breast-feeding is in many cases life saving[2], but also in developed countries excess morbitity due to lack of breast-feeding may be substantial[3]. Some of the protective effects may derive from an altered mucosal colonization pattern in the breast-fed infant. In other instances breast-fed infants develop less symptoms to the same microbe which causes disease in the bottle-fed infant. This might relate either to a changed behaviour of the colonizing microbe, e.g. alteration of toxin or adhesin production, or to altered host responsiveness. For example, anti-diarrheal hormones or anti-inflammatogenic compounds in the milk might render the infant less sensitive to microbes and their toxins. Some mechanisms of importance for the protection of the breast-fed infants against infection will be reviewed here.

2.   COMPONENTS OF HUMAN MILK WITH POTENTIAL TO AFFECT MICROBES OR HOST RESPONSES TO THEM

An adult human being produces approximately 2-3 g of secretory IgA per day. The fully breast-fed infant is supplemented with 0.5-1 g per day. Thus, the breast-fed infant's mucosal membranes are equally effectively covered by secretory IgA as are those of an adult, despite a very low production of secretory IgA by the newborn infant. Secretory IgA in the milk derives from dimeric IgA produced by plasma cells in the mammary gland which acquires secretory component during passage through the mammary gland duct epithelial cells. Secretory IgA is highly resistant to proteolytic degradation in the gastrointestinal tract[4, 5]. IgA antibodies do not activate complement or other inflammatogenic effector functions, but are thought to exert their action by agglutinating bacteria and blocking their too close interaction with mucosal epithelial cells. IgM and IgG antibodies together make up only a few per cent of milk immunoglobulin. Breast milk antibodies are directed against a multitude of antigens: microbial surface structures, toxins and food proteins.

A component of human milk with potential capacity to influence microbial colonization and pathogenicity is the large amounts of receptor-active structures both in the form of soluble oligosaccharides and as protein- or lipid-bound glycosyl chains. Human breast milk contains 4-6 g/l of complex oligosaccharides, which are virtually absent from cow's milk[6]. The free oligosaccharides consist of a variety of linear and branched structures based on milk lactose, comprising a total of more than a hundred different oligosaccharide structures. Fucosylated oligosaccharides can function as receptors for the hemagglutinin of *Vibrio cholerae* of the classical biotype[7]. Other free oligosaccharides in milk inhibit the adherence of pneumococci to retropharyngeal epithelial cells[8].

In addition, glycoproteins in the milk have N- and O-linked oligosaccharide chains that may possess receptor activity towards intestinal microbes. The mannose-containing N-linked oligosaccharide chains of secretory IgA are receptors for type 1-fimbriated *E. coli*[9]. The O-linked oligosaccharide chains of the IgA1 subclass are receptors for *Actinomyces naeslundii* that are part of dental plaques[10], and the very complex oligosaccharide chains of secretory component[11] interact with *Helicobacter pylori*[12] as well as type 1 fimbriated *E. coli*[9]. Other milk glycoproteins carry oligosaccharide receptors for *Haemophilus influenzae*[8] or S-fimbriated *E. coli*[13], which are associated with urinary tract infection and neonatal sepsis/meningitis[14].

Human milk also contains quite high levels of cytokines , mainly of the types derived from macrophages[15-21]. Cytokines may actually survive the passage through the gastrointestinal canal with retained physiologic activity[22], which opens the possibility that they may influence intestinal physiology and the development of the infant's immune system. In addition, a variety of hormones and growth factors are found in the milk, which may affect the function and structure of the developing gut.

3. PRINCIPLES OF NEONATAL COLONIZATION AND ESTABLISHMENT OF A COMPLEX INTESTINAL MICROFLORA

The gastrointestinal tract which is sterile at birth becomes colonized by a successively larger number of bacterial species during the first years of life. The pattern of such colonization has recently been reviewed[23]. Within a few days, enterobacteria such as *E. coli*, *Klebsiella* or *Enterobacter*, enterococci or staphylococci can be cultured from the rectum of most infants. During the first week(s) such bacterial species, collectively called facultative bacteria because they can grow both in the absence and presence of ambient oxygen, dominate the intestinal microflora. Anaerobic bacteria, such as bifidobacteria, *Bacteroides*, clostridia and other genera reach high bacterial numbers somewhat later. This occurs when the facultative bacteria have consumed the oxygen in the intestine and rendered this habitat suitable for the anaerobes, most of which are very oxygen sensitive and die rapidly in contact with air.

As more and more anaerobic species establish in the intestine, they will in turn impede the capacity of the facultatives to proliferate. This suppression of faculative population numbers is a complex and incompletely understood process which relates to the limited availability of metabolizable substrate in combination with a complete lack of oxygen and the presence of a range of growth-inhibiting substances produced by anaerobic bacteria such as H_2S, organic acids etc.[24]. Freter showed that some 95 different anaerobic species were needed in order to replicate the suppressive effect of a full intestinal microflora[24]. The adult individual who harbours several hundred anaerobic species has population levels of *E. coli* and other facultatives which are a hundred to a thousandfold lower than those seen in the newborn infant due to this suppressive effect. Since it takes several years until all anaerobic species have established in the intestine[25], young infants tend to have higher levels of facultative bacteria, including *E. coli*, compared with adults[26].

Self-evidently, an infant can only be colonized by a bacterial species if she/he is exposed to that particular species. Contrary to what most people believe, most infants born in "modern" societies are not colonized from their mother's intestinal, vaginal or perineal microflora, but rather from the environment. At least this is true for *E. coli* and other enterobacteria, which is the only group of bacteria that has been systematically studied in this respect. Only one third or less of infants born in developed countries derive their intestinal *E. coli* from their mother's fecal flora[27]. The most common source of such bacteria is instead a cross-colonization between infants cared for by the same staff at the maternity ward[28, 29]. Since such spread of bacteria is much dependent on hygienic routines and environmental conditions, infants born in developing countries are earlier colonized with enterobacteria than infants born in developed countries[30] and also display a more rapid turn-over of enterobacterial strains in their microflora during infancy[31].

4. INFLUENCE OF FEEDING MODE ON INTESTINAL MICROFLORA COMPOSITION

Infant feeding practice may affect the intestinal colonization pattern in two ways: by influencing which microbes that are available, and by influencing the intestinal milieu to become hostile to some bacteria but favourable for others.

During breast-feeding the infant will suckle not only milk, but also bacteria on or around the nipple. Thus, the infant swallows typical skin flora bacteria, such as *Staph. epidermidis* and *Staph. aureus*. Such bacteria are also found in banked mother's milk[32]. Conversely, the bottle fed infant may ingest

bacteria contaminating the feeds, such as enterobacteria, especially in developing countries with poor hygienic conditions[31].

We have recently summarized the results of 25 studies that compare the
intestinal flora of breast-fed and bottle-fed infants[23]. The results from six of
these studies are shown in Table 2. The most consistently observed differences are that bottle-fed infants have more enterococci and more clostridia
than breast-fed infants. Instead, breast-fed infants tend to have more staphylococci, especially at an early age.

In some studies, breast-fed infants have lower counts of enterobacteria
than bottle-fed infants, but more consistently they have less enterobacteria
other than *E. coli*, e.g. *Klebsiella*, *Enterobacter* and *Citrobacter*, as compared with bottle-fed infants. Breast-fed infants also have fewer *E. coli*
strains at a certain time point and over a period of time as compared with
bottle-fed infants[33-35]. Among *E. coli* strains, those expressing type 1 fimbriae with mannose-specific adhesins seem to be selectively favoured in the
suckling infant[36, 37], while *E. coli* with adhesins conferring mannose-resistant
hemagglutination and P-fimbriated *E. coli* are disfavoured by breast-feeding[35, 38]. There are also studies showing that breast-fed infants less often
than bottle-fed ones tend to be colonized with *E. coli* strains that are resistant
to the bactericidal effect of human serum[39], or carry the K1 capsule[33], the
latter being a virulence factor for neonatal sepsis/meningitis[40]. Collectively,
these factors contribute to a less virulent composition of the enterobacterial
flora of the breast-fed infant.

Already a century ago, Tissier reported that breast-fed infants had a
microflora dominated by bifidobacteria, while this was not the case with artificially fed infants[41]. Such a pronounced difference has not been noted in
most recent studies, for unknown reasons[23].

5. INFLUENCE OF BREAST-FEEDING ON TRANSLOCATION AND INFLAMMATION

In germ-free animals that are monocolonized with, e.g., *E. coli*, live bacteria pass across the intestinal barrier to reach the mesenteric lymph nodes,
blood stream and other organs, a process termed translocation[42]. Translocation depends strongly on the population numbers in the intestine of bacteria
with capacity to translocate, such as *E. coli*, enterococci, lactobacilli and
staphylococci. Above a population level of 10^9 per gram feces of a certain
species, translocation of such bacteria is readily detectable in experimental
animals[43, 44]. The high levels of facultative bacteria in the intestinal flora of
the neonate may predispose for translocation. Thus, transient bacteremia was

detected in a number of healthy newborn infants during their first week of life[45]. This may be the mechanism underlying neonatal septicaemia[46].

Another reason for the susceptibility of the newborn to bacterial translocation is under-developed host defenses. Protection from translocation is afforded by T cells[47, 48] and by secretory IgA (see below). As both these defence systems mature in response to the intestinal microflora[49, 50], the newborn infants has a paucity of both intestinal T cells and IgA producing plasma cells.

Breast-feeding seems to protect very efficiently against translocation[51-54]. The most important mechanism is probably that milk secretory IgA coats the intestinal bacteria whose translocation is thereby prevented[55]. Thus, supplementation of formula by secretory IgA from rabbit milk abrogates translocation[56, 57], while neither IgG nor lactoferrin has any effect[57]. Other mechanisms may, however, contribute, since the breast milk contains such an endless array of components with the capacity to influence gut function. For example, epidermal growth factor, which is present in human milk, was shown to significantly decrease bacterial translocation when administered to newborn rabbits together with formula[58]. Peroral treatment with IL-6, a cytokine present in the breast-milk protects mice from translocation[59].

Probably as a consequence of both a less varied intestinal microflora and less translocation, breast fed infants have fewer T cell blasts in their circulation and their lymphocytes are less responsive to antigen stimulation[60]. Several studies show a more rapid and prominent increase of salivary or serum IgA in bottle-fed infants[61-64], although there are also studies which report the opposite[65]. A more rapid rise in serum IgM antibodies against *E. coli* has been reported in bottle-fed as compared to breast-fed infants[66].

6.   MECHANISMS OF PROTECTION AFFORDED BY BREAST-FEEDING ON INFECTIONS AND RELATED DISEASES

6.1   Septicaemia

Breast feeding has a dramatic protective effect against infant septicaemia. As septicaemia might strike 2% of newborn infants in a developing country and kill 1%, this disease is second only to diarrhea as a global killer[67]. Infant septicaemia may result from translocation of intestinal bacteria across the intestinal barrier. Thus, the same bacterial strain has been recovered from blood and feces in cases of septicaemia due to *E. coli*[68] as well as other enterobacteria[69]. The extremely efficient protection from septicaemia afforded by breast-feeding is likely to depend primarily on prevention of translocation by means of milk secretory IgA.

6.2   Gastroenteritis

Breast-feeding offers significant protection from gastroenteritis (Table 1). A range of substances could mediate such an effect. Secretory IgA antibodies against many diarrheal pathogens and their toxins are present in the milk. To delineate which types of anti-microbial antibodies of the secretory IgA isotype that afford protection against gastroenteritis, the mouse backpack tumour model was developed[70]. Plasma cell tumours making dimeric IgA with anti-microbial specificity are constructed and injected into non-immune mice where they establish and produce their immunoglobulins. Since dimeric IgA is transported into secretions, these mice will obtain a "natural" secretory IgA response on their mucosae, the specificity of which is determined by the tumour. The protection afforded by secretory IgA with various specificities can thus be determined[70].

6.2.1   Rotavirus infection

Rotavirus infects mature intestinal epithelial cells and is the major cause of diarrhea in infants and young children world-wide. It does not seem as breast-feeding offers significant protection against rotavirus infection in the young infant[71-73]. However, infections may more often be asymptomatic in the breast-fed infant[74], and breast-feeding may delay the time-point for infection[75].

Rotavirus induced diarrhea in mice can be prevented by giving the mice plasma cell tumours secreting dimeric IgA which is transported to the intestinal lumen via the intestinal epithelial cells[76]. IgA anti-rotavirus antibodies seem to function by neutralizing virus within the cells during this process[77]. Since maternal secretory IgA antibodies from the milk are delivered in the intestinal lumen and are not transported through the epithelium, virus neutralization within the epithelial cell is not likely to occur.

Other milk components than secretory IgA may bind and neutralize rotavirus, e.g. mucin molecules[78, 79].

6.2.2   Bacterial diarrheal pathogens

In backpack tumour models, secretory IgA antibodies against *Vibrio cholerae* bacteria protect tumour bearing mice against cholera-induced diarrhea[70]. Antibodies against bacterial LPS are very effective, whereas antibodies against the toxin are relatively inefficient[80]. Probably, the anti-bacterial antibodies prevent attachment to small intestinal epithelium[81], which is the prerequisite for efficient delivery of the toxin[82], and hence, for diarrhea to occur.

In a similar way, backpack tumours secreting antibodies against a carbohydrate epitope on the *Salmonella* surface protect mice against peroral challenge with this organism[83]. Anti-salmonella immunity is also transferred via the breast-milk of immune mothers and protects the suckling pups[84].

The effectiveness of antibacterial antibodies against colonization of the small intestine with diarrheal pathogens contrasts sharphly with the complete ineffectiveness of anti-bacterial antibodies to clear organisms from the colonic micoflora. Thus, at this site most bacteria are coated with IgA and persist unaffected[85]. This relates to the fact that the vigorous peristalis of the small intestine requires that bacteria adhere avidly to the mucosal surface in order to remain[24, 86]. In contrast, for persistence in the colonic microflora with its vasts populations of resident bacteria, adherence to the mucosa is not mandatory, although certain adhesins, most notably P fimbriae in *E. coli*, promote long-term colonization[87].

Fully breast-fed infants may be colonized with several diarrheal pathogens and still remain healthy[88, 89]. Anti-secretory factor refers to a group of proteins whose synthesis is induced after an episode of diarrhea, and which protect against new diarrheal challenge[90]. Anti-secretory factor is found in the pituitary gland, where the protein has also been identified in humans[91], but also in the milk of rats and pigs. Anti-secretory factor in sow's milk confers protection on the piglets from diarrhea, caused by toxin-producing *Escherichia coli*[92]. Anti-secretory factor appears to be present in milk of mothers from areas where diarrheal diseases are endemic (unpublished data).

6.3   Urinary tract infection

Urinary tract infection may occur after colonization of the periurethral area by intestinal bacteria, mainly *E. coli*, which subsequently spread to the urinary tract. P fimbriae are the major virulence associated trait for urinary tract infection - such adhesins bind to urinary tract epithelial cells which both facilitates colonization and triggers an inflammatory response[93]. P fimbriae are also a colonization factor in the human large intestine - *E. coli* expressing P fimbriae have better capacity to persist in the microflora than strains lacking such adhesins[94-96]. Susceptibility to urinary tract infection correlates with carriage of P-fimbriated strains in the intestinal microflora[97].

Breast-feeding is moderately protective against urinary tract infection (Table 1) and the effects lasts for some time after breast-feeding has ceased[98, 99]. There is therefore reason to believe that a modulation of the intestinal microflora may be responsible for this effect. Indeed, as mentioned above, breast-fed infants less frequently than bottle-fed infants carry P fimbriated *E. coli* in their microflora[35].

6.4 Acute otitis media

Breast-fed infants are protected from acute otitis media, an effect which seems to be independent of other known risk factors such as sibling or day care contact and parental smoking[100]. The mechanism for protection is unclear - there are antibodies in the milk against pneumococcal polysaccharides, but such antibodies do not seem to prevent the infant to be colonized by pneumococci or contract otitis[101]. In contrast, antibodies against non-typeable *Haemophilus influenzae*, the second major cause of otitis, in the breast-milk were associated with a lower colonization rate in the infant, but the correlation was very weak, -0.27[102], and thus of questionable biological significance.

Breast milk contains both a factor that inhibits binding of pneumococci and another factor which prevents adherence of *Haemophilus* to nasopharyngeal epithelium[8]. It would thus seem logical if breast-fed infants would be less often colonized by these organisms, but this has not been observed[103].

6.5 Necrotizing enterocolitis

Necrotizing enterocolitis is the most common gastrointestinal emergency in premature infants. It affects between 1 and 8% of all neonatal intensive care admissions in the United States[104, 105] and mortality remains between 20 and 40% with frequent sequelae in the survivors[106]. Symptoms include abdominal distention and rectal bleeding and in severe cases the intestinal wall is perforated. The pathogenesis of necrotizing enterocolitis is unknown, but is thought to derive from a detrimental interaction between intestinal bacteria and the premature gut, expecially under conditions of poor blood perfusion. The clustering of cases have suggested that certain bacteria could be causative agents, but the microbes isolated from the affected infants are normal flora bacteria typical of the age group, e.g., *E. coli*, *Klebsiella* and clostridia[104].

Necrotizing enterocolitis almost exclusively occurs in bottle-fed infants. The beneficial effect of maternal milk could be due to interference with direct contact between bacteria and mucosa, in combination with the anti-inflammatory properties of human milk. For example, human colostrum has been shown to protect cell monolayers from injury by activated polymorphonuclear leukocytes[107, 108]. IgA antibodies are not only non-inflammatogenic, but also counteract inflammation by down-regulating oxidative burst and secretion of proinflammatory cytokines from phagocytic cells[109, 110]. Growth factors in the milk may contribute to development of the neonatal gut leading to increased resistance to damage by microbes or their products[111].

Table 1. Infections and infection-related diseases in which breast-feeding has been proven to exert protection.

Disease country	Risk ratio	References
Overall mortality		
Guinea Bissau	3.5	112
Gastroenteritis		
Developing countries	2-10	Reviewed in 113
Industrialized countries	2-8	Reviewed in 114
Dehydration due to diarrhea	6	115
Death in diarrhea	14	2
Sepsis		
Pakistan	18	116
Sweden	n.d.	117
Pneumonia (deaths)		
Brazil	4	2
Otitis media		
Finland	>3[a]	118
U.S.A.	2	119
U.S.A.	2	100
Upper respiratory infections		103
Urinary tract infection		
Italy	3-5[b]	120
Sweden	n.d.	99
Necrotizing enterocolitis		
Great Britain	20[c]	121

n.d. = not determined.
a.   Relative risk 3 times for falling ill before 1 year of age, comparing children breast-fed 6 months or more versus bottle-fed infants. Before 6 months of age 0% of the fully breast-fed infants fell ill, versus 10% in the bottle-fed group.
b.   Relative risk 5 times if considering feeding mode at referral, 3 times if considering ever breast-fed versus never breast-fed.
c.   In infants born after at least 30 weeks gestation.

Table 2. Examples of observed differences in intestinal colonization pattern between breast- and bottle-fed infants.

Species	Relation breast/bottle-fed infants	Studies with significant differences	Difference but not significant	Negative studies
Staphylococci	1000	122-124[a]		
Enterococci	0.01	123-125		
Clostridia	0.01	123[b], 124[c]		
Enterobacteriaceae	0.1	126[d]		127
Bifidobacteria	10		123, 125	
Bacteroides	0.1		125	123

a. Significant by 4w (not by 2 or 6w).
b. Significant day 14, 28 (not d4).
c. Significant by 2w, 4w, not by 6w.
d. Significant by 2w, not by 4w. Significant only for the frequency colonized, not for the number of CFU in the different groups.

REFERENCES

1. Defense factors in human milk. Wold AE, Hanson LÅ Curr.Opin. Gastroenterol.1994,10:652.
2. Evidence for protection by breast-feeding against infant deaths from infectious diseases in Brazil. Victora CG, Smith PG, Vaughan JP, et al. Lancet 1987,ii:319.
3. Health care costs of formula-feeding in the first year of life. Ball TM, Wright AL Pediatrics 1999,103 (4 Pt 2):870.
4. Proteolytic degradation of exocrine and serum immunoglobulins. Brown WR, Newcomb RW, Ishizaka IK J. Clin. Invest. 1970,49:1374.
5. Studies on the structural and conformational basis for the relative resistance of serum and secretory immunoglobulin A to proteolysis. Underdown BJ, Dorrington KJ J. Immunol. 1974,112:949.
6. Biological functions of oligosaccharides in human milk. Kunz C, Rudloff S Acta Paediatr. 1993,82:902.
7. Receptor-like glycocompounds in human milk that inhibit classical and El Tor *Vibrio cholerae* cell adherence (hemagglutination). Holmgren J, Svennerholm AM, Lindblad M Infect. Immun. 1983,39:147.
8. Inhibition of attachment of *Streptococcus pneumoniae* and *Haemophilus influenzae* by human milk and receptor oligosaccharides. Andersson B, Porras O, Hanson LÅ, Lagergård T, Svanborg Edén C J. Infect. Dis. 1986,153:232.
9. Secretory immunoglobulin A carries oligosaccharide receptors for *Escherichia coli* type 1 fimbrial lectin. Wold AE, Mestecky J, Tomana M, et al. Infect. Immun. 1990,58:3073.

10. Secretory immunoglobulin A heavy chains presents Gal□/GalNAc□ binding structures for *Actinomyces naeslundii* genospecies 1. Bratt P, Borén T, Strömberg N J. Dent. Res. 1999,78:1238.

11. Structure of the carbohydrate moieties of secretory component purified from human milk. Mizoguchi A, Mizouchi T, Kobata A J. Biol. Chem. 1982,257:9612.

12. Attachment of *Helicobacter pylori* to gastric epithelium mediated by blood group antigens. Borén T, Falk P, Roth KA, Larsson G, Normark S Science 1994,262:1892.

13. Inhibition of adhesion of S-fimbriated *E. coli* to buccal epithelial cells by human skim milk is predominantly mediated by mucins and depends on the period of lactation. Schroten H, Plogmann R, Hanish FG, Hacker J, Nobis-Bosch R, Wahn V Acta Paediatr. 1993,82:6.

14. Serotypes, hemolysin production and receptor recognition of *Escherichia coli* strains associated with neonatal sepsis and meningitis. Korhonen TK, Valtonen MV, Parkkinen J, et al. Infect. Immun. 1985,48:486.

15. Isolation of interleukin-1 from human milk. Söder O Int. Arch. Allergy Appl. Immunol. 1987,83:19.

16. Tumor necrosis factor-alpha in human milk. Rudloff HE, Schmalstieg FC, Mushtaha AA, Palkowetz KH, Liu SK, Goldman AS Pediatr. Res. 1992,31:29.

17. Interleukin-6 in human milk. Rudloff HE, Schmalstieg Jr FC, Palkowetz KH, Paszkiewicz EJ, Goldman AS J. Reprod. Immunol. 1993,23:13.

18. Presence of interferon-gamma and interleukin-6 in colostrum of normal women. Bocci V, von Bremen K, Corradeschi F, Franchi F, Luzzi E, Paulesu L Lymphokine Cytokine Res. 1993,12:21.

19. Interleukin-10 in human milk. Garofalo R, Chheda S, Mei F, et al. Paediatr. Res. 1995,37 (4 Pt 1):444.

20. Human milk contains granulocyte colony stimulating factor. Gilmore WS, McKelvey-Martin VJ, Rutherford S, et al. Eur. J. Clin. Nutr. 1994,48:222.

21. Interleukin-12 in human milk. Bryan DL, Hawkes JS, Gibson RA Pediatr. Res. 1999,45:858.

22. Oral cytokine administration. Rollwagen FM, Baqar S Immunol. Today 1996,17:548.

23. Adlerberth I, Hanson LÅ, Wold AE. The ontogeny of the intestinal flora. In *Development of the gastrointestinal tract*, Edited by Sanderson IR, Walker WA. Hamilton, Ontario: B.C. Decker; 1999:

24. Freter R. Mechanisms that control the microflora of the large intestine. In *Human intestinal microflora in health and disease*, Edited by Hentges DJ. New York: Academic Press; 1983: 33.

25. Midtvedt A-C. The establishment and development of some metabolic activities associated with the intestinal microflora in healthy children. Thesis. Stockholm, 1994.

26. The fecal flora of children in the United Kingdom. Ellis-Pegler RB, Crabtree C, Lambert HP J. Hyg. (Camb.) 1975,75:135.

27. Influence of maternal gut flora and colostral and cord serum antibodies on presence of *Escherichia coli* in faeces of the newborn infant. Gothefors L, Carlsson B, Ahlstedt S, Hanson LÅ, Winberg J Acta Paediatr. Scand. 1976,65:225.

28. The acquisition of *Escherichia coli* by newborn babies. Bettelheim KA, Lennox-King SMJ Infection 1976,4:174.

29. Importance of the environment and the faecal flora of infants, nursing staff and parents as sources of Gram-negative bacteria colonizing newborns in three neonatal wards. Fryklund B, Tullus K, Berglund B, Burman LG Infection 1992,20:253.

30. Intestinal colonization with *Enterobacteriaceae* in Pakistani and Swedish hospital-delivered infants. Adlerberth I, Carlsson B, de Man P, et al. Acta Paediatr. Scand. 1991,80:602.

31. High turn-over rate of *Escherichia coli* strains in the intestinal flora of infants in Pakistan. Adlerberth I, Jalil F, Carlsson B, et al. Epidemiol. Infect. 1998,121:587.

32. Reduction in bacterial contamination in banked human milk. Asquith MT, Harrod JR J. Pediatr. 1979,95:993.

33. *Escherichia coli* serogroups in breast-fed and bottle-fed infants. Orskov F, Biering Sorensen K Acta Path. Microbiol. Scand. Sect. B 1975,83:25.

34. Effect of iron on serotypes and hemagglutination patterns of *Escherichia coli* in bottle-fed infants. Mevissen-Verhage EAE, Marcelis JH, Guiné PAM, Verhoe J Eur. J. Clin. Microbiol. 1985,4:570.

35. Fecal colonization with P-fimbriated *E. coli* between 0 and 18 months of age. Tullus K Epidemiol. Infect. 1988,100:185.

36. The antibody response in breast-fed and non-breast-fed infants after artificial colonization of the intestine with *Escherichia coli* O83. Lodinová-Zádníková R, Slavíková M, Tlaskalová-Hogenová H, et al. Pediatr. Res. 1991,29:396.

37. Increased mannose-specific adherence and colonizing ability of *E. coli* O83 in breast-fed infants. Slaviková M, Lodinová-Zadniková R, Adlerberth I, Hanson LÅ, Svanborg C, Wold AE Adv. Exp. Med. Biol. 1995,371A:421.

38. Mannose-resistant hemagglutination (MRHA) and haemolysin production of strains of *Escherichia coli* isolated from children with diarrhoea: effect of breastfeeding. Giugliano LG, Meyer CJ, Arantes LC, Ribeiro ST, Giugliano R J. Trop. Pediatr. 1993,39:183.

39. Breast feeding and biological properties of faecal *E. coli* strains. Gothefors L, Olling S, Winberg J Acta Paediatr. Scand. 1975,64:807.

40. *Escherichia coli* K1 capsular polysaccharide associated with neonatal meningitis. Robbins JB, McCracken GHJ, Gotschlich EC, Orskov F, Orskov I, Hanson LÅ N. Engl. J. Med. 1974,290:1216.

41. Tissier H. Recherches sur la flore intestinale des nourrissons (état normal et pathologique). Paris, 1900.

42. Berg RD. Translocation of indigenous bacteria from the intestinal tract. In *Intestinal microflora in health and disease*, Edited by Hentges DJ. New York: Acad. Press; 1983: 333.

43. Role of *Escherichia coli* P fimbriae in intestinal colonization in gnotobiotic rats. Herías MV, Midtedt T, Hanson LÅ, Wold AE Infect. Immun. 1995,63:4781.

44. *Escherichia coli* K5 capsule expression enhances colonization of the large intestine in the gnotobiotic rat. Herías MV, Midtvedt T, Hanson LÅ, Wold AE Infect. Immun. 1997,65:531.

45. Asymptomatic bacteriemia in the newborn infant. Albers WH, Tyler CW, Boxerbaum B J. Pediatr. 1966,69:193.

46. Bacterial translocation in the neonate. Van Camp JM, Tomaselli V, Coran AG Curr. Opin. Pediatr. 1994,6:327.

47. Bacterial translocation from the gastrointestinal tract of athymic (nu/nu) mice. Owens WE, Berg RD Infect. Immun. 1980,27:461.

48. Bacterial translocation from the gastrointestinal tracts of thymectomized mice. Owens WE, Berg RD Curr. Microbiol. 1982,7:169.

49. The normal microbial flora as a major stimulus for proliferation of plasma cells synthesizing IgA in the gut. Crabbé PA, Bazin H, Eyssen H, Heremans JF Int. Arch. Allergy 1968,34:362.

50. Immunohistochemical observations on lymphoid tissues from conventional and germ-free mice. Crabbé PA, Nash DR, Bazin H, Eysseb H, Heremans JF Lab. Invest. 1970,22:448.

51. Effect of early nutritional deprivation and diet on translocation of bacteria from the gastro-intestinal tract in the newborn rat. Steinwender G, Schimpl G, Sixl B, et al. Pediatr. Res. 1995,39:415.

52. Breast milk protects the neonate from bacterial translocation. Go LL, Albanese CT, Watkins SC, Simmons RL, Rowe MI J. Pediatr. Surg. 1994,29:1059.

53. Quantitative and morphologic analysis of bacterial translocation in neonates. Go LL, Ford HR, Watkins SC, et al. Arch. Surg. 1994,129:1184.

54. *Escherichia coli* S fimbriae in intestinal colonization and translocation. Herías MV, Robertson A-K, Midtvedt T, Wold AE In manuscript 1999,

55. Effect of secretory IgA on transepithelial passage of bacteria across the intact ileum in vitro. Albanese CT, Smith SD, Watkins S, Kurkchubasche A, Simmons RL, Rowe MI J. Am. Coll. Surg. 1994,179:679.

56. The protective role of enteral IgA supplementation in neonatal gut origin sepsis. Maxson RT, Jackson RJ, Smith SD J. Pediatr. Surg. 1995,30:231.

57. Immunoglobulin A supplementation abrogates bacterial translocation and preserves the architecture of the intestinal epithelium. Dickinson EC, Gorga JC, Garrett M, et al. Surgery 1998,124:284.

58. The effect of epidermal growth factor on bacterial translocation in newborn rabbits. Okuyama H, Urao M, Lee D, Drongowski RA, Coran AG J. Pediatr. Surg. 1998,33:225.

59. Systemic sepsis following hemorrhagic shock: alleviation with oral interleukin-6. Rollwagen FM, Li YY, Pacheco ND, Baqar S Mil. Med. 1997,162:366.

60. Differential modulation of the immune response by breast- or formula-feeding of infants. Pabst HF, Spady DW, Pilarski LM, Carson MM, Beeler JA, Krezolek MP Acta Pediatr 1997,86:1291.

61. Serum immunoglobulins in preterm infants: comparison of human milk and formula feeding. Savilahti E, Jarvenpaa AL, Raiha MC Pediatrics 1983,72:312.

62. Serum and saliva Ig-levels in infants of non-atopic mothers fed breast milk or cow's milk-based formulas. Ostergaard PA Acta Paediatr. Scand. 1985,74:555.

63. Breastfeeding conditions a differential developmental pattern of mucosal immunity. Gleeson M, Cripps AW, Clancy RL, Hensley MJ, Dobson AJ, Firman DW Clin. Exp. Immunol. 1986,66:216.

64. Development of secretory immunity in breast fed and bottle fed infants. Stephens S Arch. Dis. Child. 1986,61:263.

65. Immunoglobulin A subclasses in infants' saliva and milk from their mothers. Fitzsimmons SP, Evans MK, Pearce CL, Sheridan MJ, Wientzen R, Cole MF J. Pediatr. 1994,124:566.

66. In-vivo immune responses of breast- and bottle-fed infants to tetanus toxoid antigen and to normal gut flora. Stephens S, Kennedy CR, Lakhani PK, Brenner MK Acta Paediatr. 1984,73:426.

67. Early child health in Lahore, Pakistan: X. Mortality. Khan SR, Jalil F, Zaman S, Lindblad BS, Karlberg J Acta Paediatr. Suppl. 1993,390:109.

68. Epidemiology of *Escherichia coli* K1 in healthy and diseased newborns. Sarff LD, McCracken Jr GH, Schiffer MS, et al. Lancet 1975,i:1099.

69. Molecular analysis provides evidence for the endogenous origin of bacteremia and meningitis due to *Enterobacter cloaceae* in an infant. Lambert-Zechovsky N, Bingen E, Denamur E, et al. Clin. Infect. Dis. 1992,15:30.

70. New models for analysis of mucosal immunity: intestinal secretion of specific monoclonal immunoglobulin A from hybridoma tumors protects against *Vibrio cholera* infection. Winner III L, Mack J, Weltzin R, Mekalanos JJ, Kraehenbuhl JP, Neutra MR Infect. Immun. 1991,59:977.

71. Influence of breast milk on nosocomial rotavirus infections in infants. Berger R, Hadziselimovic F, Just M, Reigel F Infection 1984,12:171.

72. Effect of breast-feeding on morbidity in rotavirus gastroenteritis. Weinberg RJ, Tipton G, Klish WJ, Brown MR Pediatrics 1984,74:250.

73. Rotavirus serology and breast-feeding in young children in rural Guinea-Bissau. Gunnlaugsson G, Smedman L, da Silva MC, Grandien M, Zetterstrom R Acta Paediatr. Scand. 1989,78:62.

74. Rotavirus infections in young Nicaraguan children. Espinoza F, Paniagua M, Hallander H, Svensson L, Strannegard O Pediatr. Infect. Dis. J. 1997,16:564.

75. Breast-feeding and the risk of life-threatening rotavirus diarrhea: prevention or postponement? Clemens J, Rao M, Ahmed F, et al. Pediatrics 1993,92:680.

76. Antirotavirus immunoglobulin A neutralizes virus in vitro after transcytosis through epithelial cells and protects infant mice from diarrhea. Ruggeri FM, Johansen K, Basile G, Kraehenbuhl JP, Svensson L J. Virol. 1998,72:2708.

77. Protective effect of rotavirus VP6-specific IgA monoclonal antibodies that lack neutralizing activity. Burns JW, Siadat-Pjouh M, Krishnaney AA, Greenberg HB Science 1996,272:104.

78. Human milk mucin inhibits rotavirus replication and prevents experimental gastroenteritis. Yolken RH, Peterson JA, Vonderfecht SL, Fouts ET, Midthun K, Newburg DS J. Clin. Invest. 1992,90:1984.

79. Role of human-milk lactadherin in protection against symptomatic rotavirus infection. Newburg DS, Peterson JA, Ruiz-Palacios GM, et al. Lancet 1998,351:1160.

80. Analysis of the roles of antilipopolysaccharide and anti-cholera toxin immunoglobulin A (IgA) antibodies in protection against *Vibrio cholerae* and cholera toxin by use of monoclonal IgA antibodies in vivo. Apter FM, Michetti P, Winner III LS, Mack JA, Mekalanos JJ, Neutra MR Infect. Immun. 1993,61:5279.

81. Studies on the mechanism of action of intestinal antibody in experimental cholera. Freter R Texas Rep. Biol. Med. 1969,27 (Suppl. 1):299.

82. Growth advantage and enhanced toxicity of *Escherichia coli* adherent to tissue culture cells due to restricted diffusion of products secreted by the cells. Zafriri D, Oron Y, Eisenstein B, Ofek I J. Clin. Invest. 1987,79:1210.

83. Monoclonal secretory immunoglobulin A protects mice against oral challenge with the invasive pathogen *Salmonella typhimurium*. Michetti P, Mahan MJ, Slauch JM, Mekalanos JJ, Neutra MR Infect. Immun. 1992,60:1786.

84. Passive secretory immunity against Salmonella typhimurium demonstrated with foster mouse pups. Shope SR, Schiemann DA J. Med. Microbiol. 1991,35:53.

85. In vivo IgA coating of anaerobic bacteria in human feces. van der Waaij LA, Limburg PC, Mesander G, van der Waaij D Gut 1996,38:348.

86. Observations on the pathogenic properties of the K88, HLY and ENT plasmids of *Escherichia coli* with particular reference to porcine diarrhoea. Smith HW, Linggood MA J. Med. Microbiol. 1971,4:467.

87. Wold AE. Role of bacterial adherence in the establishment of the normal intestinal microflora. In *Probiotics, other nutritional factors, and intestinal microflora*, Edited by Hanson LÅ, Yolken RH. Philadelphia: Vevey/Lipincott-Raven Publishers; 1999: 47. Nestlé Nutrition Workshop Series; vol 42).

88. The uniqueness of human milk. Host resistance to infection. Mata LJ, Wyatt RG Am. J. Clin. Nutr. 1971,24:976.

89. Mata JL. The children of Santa María Cauqué. A prospective field study of health and growth.Cambridge, Massachussets: MIT Press, 1978:395. ; vol XVII).

90. The antisecretory factors: inducible proteins which modulate secretion in the small intestine. Lönnroth I, Lange S, Skadhauge E Comput. Biochem. Physiol. 1988,90A:611.

91. A hormone-like protein from the pituitary gland inhibits intestinal hypersecretion induced by cholera toxin. Lönnroth I, Lange S Regulatory Peptides Suppl. 1985,4:216.

92. Evidence of protection against diarrhoea in suckling piglets by a hormone-like protein in the sow's milk. Lönnroth I, Martinsson K, Lange S J. Vet. Med. 1988,35:628.

93. Bacterial virulence versus host resistance in the urinary tracts of mice. Svanborg Edén C, Hagberg L, Hull R, Hull S, Magnusson K-E, Öhman L Infect. Immun. 1987,55:1224.

94. Resident colonic *Escherichia coli* strains frequently display uropathogenic characteristics. Wold AE, Caugant DA, Lidin-Janson G, de Man P, Svanborg C J. Inf. Dis. 1992,165:46.

95. The importance of P and type 1 fimbriae for the persistence of *Escherichia coli* in the human gut. Tullus K, Kühn I, Ørskov I, Ørskov F, Möllby R Epidemiol. Infect. 1992,108:415.

96. P fimbriae and other adhesins enhance intestinal persistence of *Escherichia coli* in early infancy. Adlerberth I, Svanborg C, Carlsson B, et al. Epidemiol. Infect. 1998,121:599.

97. Intestinal carriage of P-fimbriated *Escherichia coli* and the susceptibility to urinary tract infection in young children. Plos K, Connell H, Jodal U, et al. J. Infect. Dis. 1995,171:

98. Breastfeeding and urinary tract infection. Piscane A, Graziano L, Zona G Lancet 1990,336:50.

99. Breast-feeding and urinary-tract infection. Mårild S, Jodal U, Hanson LÅ Lancet 1990,336:942.

100. Exclusive breastfeeding protects against bacterial colonization and day care exposure to otitis media. Duffy LC, Faden H, Wasiliewski R, Wolf J, Krystofik D Pediatrics 1997,100:E7.

101. Antibodies to pneumococcal polysaccharides in human milk: lack of relationship to colonization and acute otitis media. Rosen IA, Hakansson A, Aniansson G, et al. Pediatr. Infect. Dis. J. 1996,15:498.

102. Human milk secretory IgA antibodies to nontypeable Haemophilus influenzae: possible protective effects against nasopharyngeal colonization. Harabuchi Y, H. F, Yamanaka N, Duffy L, Wolf J, Krystofik D J. Pediatr. 1994,124:193.

103. A prospective cohort study on breast-feeding and otitis media in Swedish infants. Aniansson G, Alm B, Andersson B, et al. Pediatr. Infect. Dis. J. 1994,13:183.

104. Epidemiology of necrotizing enterocolitis. Kosloske AM Acta Paediatr. Scand. Suppl. 1994,396:2.

105. Necrotizing enterocolitis. Albanese CT, Rowe MI Semin. Pediatr. Surg. 1995,4:200.

106. Necrotizing enterocolitis in infancy. Kleinhaus S, Weinberg G, Gregor MB Surg. Clin. North Am. 1992,72:261.

107. Antioxidant properties of human colostrum. Buescher ES, McIlheran SM Pediatr. Res. 1988,24:14.

108. Further characterization of human colostral antioxidants. Buescher ES, McIlheran SM, Frenck RW Pediatr. Res. 1989,25:266.

109. Inhibition of receptor-dependent and receptor-independent generation of the respiratory burst in human neutrophils and monocytes by human serum IgA. Wolf HM, Vogel E, Fischer MB, Rengs H, Schwartz HP, Eibl MM Pediatr. Res. 1994,36:235.

110. Anti-inflammatory properties of human serum IgA: induction of IL-1 receptor antagonist and Fc alpha R (CD89)-mediated down-regulation of tumour necrosis factor-alpha (TNF-alpha) and IL-6 in human monocytes. Wolf HM, Hauber I, Gulle H, et al. Clin. Exp. Immunol. 1996,105:537.

111. Neonatal necrotizing colitis, a disease of the immature intestinal mucosal barrier. Israel EJ Acta Paediatr. Suppl. 1994,396:27.

112. Prolonged breast feeding, diarrhoeal disease, and survival of children in Guinea-Bissau. Molbak K, Gottschau A, Aaby P, Hojlyng N, Ingholt L, da Silva AP BMJ 1994,308:1403.

113. Mortality and infectious disease associated with infant-feeding practices in developing countries. Jason JM, Nieburg P, Marks JS Pediatrics 1984,74:702.

114. Review of the epidemiologic evidence for and association between infant feeding and infant health. Kovar MG, Sedula MK, Marks JS, Frase DW Pediatrics 1984,74:615.

115. Case-control study of risk of dehydrating diarrhoea in infants in vulnerable period after full weaning. Fuchs SC, Victora CG, Maritnez J BMJ 1996,313:391.

116. Breast feeding and protection against neonatal sepsis in a high risk population. Ashraf RN, Jalil F, Zaman S, et al. Arch. Dis. Child. 1991,66:488.

117. Does breast milk protect against septicemia in the newborn? Winberg J, Wessner G Lancet 1971,i:1091.

118. Prolonged breast feeding as prophylaxis for recurrent otitis media. Saarinen UM Acta Paediatr. Scand. 1982,71:567.

119. Exclusive breast-feeding for at least 4 months protects against otitis media. Duncan B, Ey J, Holberg CJ, Wright AL, Martinez FD, Taussig LM Pediatrics 1993,91:867.

120. Breast-feeding and urinary tract infection. Piscane A, Graziano L, Mazzarella G, Scarpellino B, Zona G J. Pediatr. 1992,120:87.

121. Breast milk and neonatal necrotising enterocolitis. Lucas A, Cole TJ Lancet 1990,336:1519.

122. The composition of the faecal microflora in breastfed and bottle fed infants from birth to eight weeks. Lundequist B, Nord CE, Winberg J Acta Paediatr. Scand. 1985,74:45.

123. Diet and faecal flora in the newborn: breast milk and infant formula. Balmer SE, Wharton BA Arch. Dis. Child. 1989,64:1672.

124. Effect of feeding on infants' faecal flora. Simhon A, Douglas JR, Drasar BS, Soothill JF Arch. Dis. Child. 1982,57:54.

125. The microbial ecology of the large bowel of breast-fed and formula-fed infants during the first year of life. Stark PL, Lee A J. Med. Microbiol. 1982,15:189.

126. Diet and faecal flora in the newborn: nucleotides. Balmer SE, Hanvey LS, Wharton BA Arch. Dis. Child. 1994,70:F137.

127. Effect of various milk feeds on numbers of *Escherichia coli* and *Bifidobacterium* in the stools of new-born infants. Hewitt JH, Rigby J J. Hyg., Camb. 1976,77:129.

8

OPSONOPHAGOCYTOSIS VERSUS LECTINOPHAGOCYTOSIS IN HUMAN MILK MACROPHAGES

Horst Schroten, Frank Kuczera, Henrik Köhler and Rüdiger Adam

University Children's Hospital, Heinrich Heine Universität Düsseldorf, Düsseldorf Germany

Key words: Human milk, milk macrophages, opsonophagocytosis, lectinophagocytosis, neonate immunity

Abstract: Some important immunoprotective effects of human breast milk have been attributed to the presence of macrophages. We investigated the generation of superoxide anion (O_2^-) by monocytes and human milk macrophages after stimulation with opsonized and unopsonized zymosan in the absence and presence of mannose as an inhibitor to investigate lectinophagocytic and opsonophagocytic properties. Peripheral blood monocytes generated more O_2^- than human milk macrophages ($417,4 \pm 79,1$ nmol O_2^-/ mg protein vs. $216,1 \pm 15,1$ nmol O_2^-/ mg protein, $p<0,05$) after stimulation with opsonized zymosan. When unopsonized zymosan was used as a serum-independent stimulus monocytes generated slightly less O_2^- in comparison to human milk macrophages ($150,8 \pm 34,5$ nmol / mg protein vs. $176,1 \pm 18$ nmol O_2^- / mg protein, $p<0,05$). These findings demonstrate that the proportion of opsonin-independent phagocytosis in human milk macrophages is higher than in monocytes (82% vs. 36%). When mannose was used as an inhibitor a significantly higher reduction of O_2^- generation occurred in human milk macrophages compared to monocytes stimulated with opsonized zymosan, whereas no difference was found when unopsonized zymosan was used. These results indicate that human milk macrophages are stimulated to a greater extent by opsonin-independent mechanisms than blood borne monocytes. As the colostrum and the intestinal environment of the neonate offers only a little amount of opsonins like complement and immunoglobulin G, such a differentiation to lectinophagocytic properties could bear a great advantage for protective fuctions of human milk macrophages.

1.   INTRODUCTION

Preferation of breast milk feeding is in all infants is based on various advantages. Besides its well known nutritional benefits antimicrobial properties are of great importance. The presence of soluble factors such as secretory immunoglobulins (especially sIgA), lactoferrin, lysozym and a variety of additional humoral defense factors such as complement, oligosaccharides and other non-cellular components contribute to the beneficial effects. In addition large numbers of viable cells are present in human breast milk with a high proportion of macrophages likely being responsible for some antiinfectious properties.

These mother milk macrophages are of 18 to 40 µm in diameter with a high amount of phagocytosed lipids. Morphological and cytochemical properties are similar to differentiated macrophages. They bear Fc-receptors for different subclasses of IgG and C3b-receptors (Balkwill and Hogg 1979, Schroten *et al* 1987), synthesize various humoral defensive factors such as complement factors (C2, C3, C4), cytokines (Interleukin 1), lactoferrin, lysozyme and more (Ogra and Greene 1982, Cole *et al* 1982, Speer and Kreikenbaum 1993). Human milk macrophages are antigen presenting cells with a capacity of phagocytosis comparable to circulating macrophages (Mori and Hayward 1982, Leyvan-Cobián and Clemente 1984, Speer *et al* 1986) while antibody dependend cytotoxicity was reported to be reduced (Mandyla *et al* 1982). They have been shown to phagocytose and kill certain bacteria, virus and yeast (Speer *et al* 1986 & 1993). In comparison to peripheral blood monocytes milk macrophages show a lower capacity of adherence and chemotaxis (Clemente *et al* 1986, Speer and Kreikenbaum 1993) whereas production of reactive oxygen intermediates was reported to be equal in these cells (Cummings *et al* 1982, Tsuda *et al* 1984 , Speer *et al* 1986).

Studies on the pH-resistance showed relative resistance of human milk macrophages to alkali conditions similar to those in the small intestine (Blau *et al* 1983) and to conditions with a pH < 3 (Speer *et al* 1986) so it seems very likely that they can develop their immunoprotective functions within the gastrointestinal tract of the breastfed baby.

Due to a lower availability of opsonizing factors in the milk (Vassao and Carneiro-Sampaio 1989) and the gastrointestinal tract of the infant human milk macrophages are supposed to be activated by other mechanisms than blood monocytes.

Different patterns of recognition and ingestion of invading pathogens can be clearly distinguished in phagocytic cells. Interaction of macrophage membrane receptors with complentary coating substances on the surface of the pathogenetic particle is well described as *opsonophagocytosis*. These coatings (opsonins), derived from various sites of the hosts immune system, consist of bridging serum factors such as immunoglobulins, iC3b-fragment of the C3-complement factor, C-reactive protein, surface protein A and D and the mannose binding protein.

Interaction of carbohydrate binding proteins, lectin receptors, with complementary carbohydrate chains are another main mechanism of enhancing uptake of pathogens. This phagocytic process, known as serum independent- or *lectinophagocytosis*, is mediated for example through the mannose receptor or a lectin-site on the CD11b/CD18 (MAC-1) integrin, the beta-glucan-receptor.

Aim of this study was the investigation of opsono- and lectinophagocytic properties of human milk macrophages by measuring the superoxide anion (O_2^-) production in comparison to human blood monocytes after stimulation with opsonized and unopsonized zymosan particles in the absence and presence of D-mannose as a relevant inhibitor.

2. MATERIAL AND METHODS

2.1 Collection, preparation, and culture of cells

Human milk was collected from 38 healthy lactating women 1-6 days post partum by hand expression at the Department of Gynecology and Obstetrics, Heinrich Heine Universität Düsseldorf, Germany after having obtained informed consent. The samples were stored at room temperature in sterile containers until they were cultured within 4h.

Degreasement of milk was performed by 1:1 dilution with PBS and centrifugation at 4°C and 600 g for 10 min. For purification the sediment was resuspended in 25 ml PBS, layered on 25 ml Ficoll-Hypaque (Pharmacia, Uppsala, Schweden) and then centrifuged at 20°C and 1000 g for 20 min. The mononuclear interface cell layer was washed in PBS and RPMI (Gibco) (supplemented with penicillin, gentamicin, Hepes, fetal calf serum FCS and glutamin) and resuspended in RPMI (with supplements). Purity (> 90%) of monocytes macorphages was assessed by naphtylacetate-esterase staining. Cells were enumerated by cell counter (Coulter, Krefeld Germany) and adjusted at a concentration of 2.5×10^5 cells / ml. Monocytic viability of $\geq$ 95 % was assured by the trypan blue exclusion test. Two ml of the cell-suspension were prepared in plastic culture dishes and cells were allowed to adhere for 2h at 37°C and 5 % CO, then washed vigorously with PBS to remove nonadherent cells.

Monocytes were isolated from heparinized human blood from healthy volunteers as described above by Ficoll-Hypaque gradient and then treated like the milk macrophages.

In both tissue dishes with monocytes and macrophages the protein content was determined according to the method described by Lowry (Lowry *et al* 1951). Only samples with a protein content between 40 and 100 µg were used because of an unacceptable variability in superoxide anion production in samples containing less than 35 µg (Johnston *et al* 1978). Until the essay was performed the cells were stored in PBS on ice (max. 15 min.).

2.2   Superoxide anion production

Superoxide anion production was measured by reduction of superoxide dismutase (SOD) sensitive cytochrome C. Stimulation of the cells was achieved by adding 100µl opsonized or unopsonized zymosan with 200 µl cytochrome C solution.   Addition of 2 ml N-ethylmaleimid stopped the induced oxidative metabolism after 30 min. Reduction of cytochrom C was quantified spectrophotometrically (550 nm). The assay was repeated with SOD to correct for oxygen independent reduction of cytochrome C. Results were expressed in nmol O_2^- / mg protein.

2.3   Stimulating agents

Opsonized and unopsonized zymosan (Sigma Chemicals, St. Louis, USA) was used as a stimulus. For opsonization serum from healthy donors was taken. The zymosan particles (2×10^5/µl) were autoclaved for 30 min, washed twice with PBS and resuspended in PBS. The samples were adjusted to 2×10^5 particles /µl and stored at -70° C until being used in the assay.

2.4   Inhibitor

Mannose (Sigma Chemicals) was used as a potential inhibitor. It was incubated with the isolated cells for 15 min at 37°C prior to the stimulation assay. Mannose was used in 0.1-, 0.25- and 0.5-molar solution. All assays were performed in duplicate.

2.5   Expression of mannose-receptor

To visualize possible expression of the mannose receptor, phagocytes were stained with a murine antibody generated against the human mannose receptor (Pharmingen, San Diego, USA). Human bloodborne monocytes and milk macrophages were prepared as described above until incubated for ten minutes, washed with PBS, centrifuged with 300 g at 20°C for 10 min.. Detection of staining was performed with a fluorescence microscope (Zeiss Optics, Göttingen, Germany).

2.6   Statistics

Statistical analysis was performed by using the Student t-test. An alpha-error of p<0,05 was regarded as significant.

3.   RESULTS

3.1   Stimulation without inhibitors

Without any additional stimuli superoxide anion production was 40 ± 3 nmol O_2^-/mg Protein/30 min (nmol O_2^-/mg P/30') in milk macrophages and 47 ± 4.7 nmol O_2^-/mg P/30' in blood monocytes.

After stimulation with <u>opsonized</u> zymosan peripheral monocytes generated 417 ± 79 O_2^-/mg P/30' while 216 ± 15 nmol nmol O_2^-/mg P/30' could be measured in the assay with milk macrophages in the absence of potential inhibitors. When <u>unopsonized</u> zymosan was used, blood monocytes produced 150 ± 35 nmol O_2^-/mg P/30' and milk macrophages generated 176 ± 18 nmol O_2^-/mg P/30'. Thus peripheral blood monocyes released a higher absolute amount of superoxide anions than human milk macrophages when stimulated with opsonized zymosan while O_2^--production after activation with unopsonized zymosan demonstrated approximately equal release of the measured oxygen metabolites. When looking at the relations between opsonin-dependent and opsonin-independent stimulation human milk macrophages revealed a much higher proportion of superoxide anion generation (100% to 82 %) than bloodborne monocytes (100% to 36%) when stimulated with unopsonized zymosan as a serum-independent particle.

Stimulation after preincubation with Mannose

After addition of D-mannose in concentrations of 0.1, 0.25 and 0.5 m prior to stimulation with <u>opsonized zymosan</u> blood monocytes reacted with a significant reduction of O_2^--generation to 302 ± 62, 247 ± 58 and 162 ± 53 nmol O_2^-/mg P/30' (p<0.05). Milk macrophages showed lowering of superoxide anion production to 139 ± 18, 84 ± 14 and 39 ± 1 nmol O_2^-/mg P/30' after preincubation with the above mentioned concentrations of D-mannose (p<0.0005). This reduction was significantly concentration-dependent (p<0.0005). Comparison of the different cell types revealed a significantly greater relative decrease in O_2^- generation in milk macrophages compared to blood monocytes after stimulation with opsonized zymosan and mannose treatment. When inhibiting with a 0.5 molar mannose solution, reduction of 61% could be demonstrated in the assay with blood monocytes and a reduction of 82% in the milk macrophages. Milk macrophages can thus be inhibited to a greater extent by mannose than blood monocytes under conditions of serum-opsonization (figure 1).

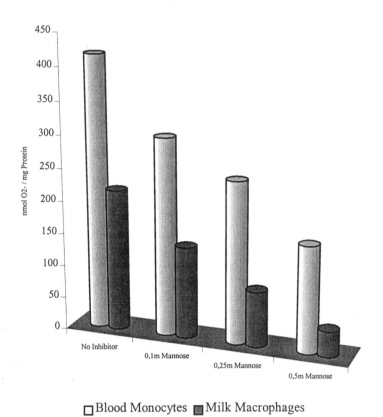

Figure 1: Stimulation with opsonized zymosan and inhibition with mannose.

Preincubation of D-Mannose after stimulating with <u>unopsonized zymosan</u> revealed a decrease in oxygen radical output to 89 ± 15, 63 ± 11 and 30 ± 5 nmol O_2^-/mg P/30' in blood monocytes, 80 % with 0.5m mannose, (p<0.05) and a reduction to 99 ± 13, 58 ± 7 and 32 ± 5 nmol O_2^-/mg P/30' in milk macrophages, 82 % with 0.5 m mannose (p<0.0005). No significant difference could be found between the two cell population when unopsonized zymosan was used - blood monocytes and milk macrophages could be equally inhibited with mannose in the absence of opsonizing particles.

4. DISCUSSION

4.1 Stimulation without inhibitors

Superoxide anion production in human milk macrophages has been reported to be equal to blood monocytes after stimulation with phorbol myristate acetate (PMA) (Cummings *et al* 1985) and when challenged with PMA or opsonized zymosan (Tsuda *et al* 1984, Speer *et al* 1986). In all publications though the generation of superoxide anions were related to the amount of cells in the sample (nmol $O_2^-/5x10^5-10^6$ cells). Since milk macrophages are much bigger in diameter than monocytes and thus have a greater surface, a greater number of relevant receptors per cell should principally be assumed. This fact could account for a bias with the measurement of a too elevated O_2^--production in milk macrophages. According to a publication by Johnston and co-workers an unacceptable variability in the determination of superoxide anion production occurs in samples with a protein content below 35 µg protein so that the O_2^--generation should be related to the absolute amount of protein instead of the quantitiy of cells (Johnston *et al* 1978).

In our study we compared opsonized and unopsonized particles and were able to demonstrate that monocytes exhibited a greater O_2^--release than milk macrophages when stimulated with <u>opsonized zymosan</u> in correlation with the absolute amount of protein in the sample (nmol O_2^-/mg protein/30 min.). After stimulation with <u>unopsonized zymosan</u> an equal superoxide anion-production was measured.

Comparison of the relation between *opsonophagocytosis* and opsonin-independent phagocytosis within the different cell subpopulations leads to the observation that human breast milk macrophages exhibit a higher proportion of *lectinophagocytosis* than blood borne monocytes (82 vs. 36%).

Different patterns of receptors on the surface of the phagocytes regarding their number and quality (e.g. Fc-receptor and CR-3 on one hand, mannose-receptor and ß-glucan-receptor on the other) could be a possible indication for this specialization. Reduced amount of opsonins such as complement and immunoglobulins in the colostrum (Vassao and Carneiro-Sampaio 1989) and the gastrointestinal tract of the neonate could have lead to a relatively better serum-independent stimulation of milk macrophages being of favour for the early defense line in breast fed children.

Systematic suppression of maternal immune responses could also play a role in differentiation of milk macrophages towards better stimulation by nonopsonic factors. Opsonic activities of the mother in the second and third trimester of pregnancy and in neonatal sera have been reported to be reduced (Everaerts *et al* 1985, Sebring *et al* 1989) and studies on the distribution of the Fc-receptor showed reduced density of this recognition moiety on human milk macrophages in comparison to blood monocytes (Rivas *et al* 1994).

4.2   Stimulation after preincubation with mannose

Zymosan as a derivative of the cell wall of *Saccharomyces cerevisiae* is composed of α-D-mannan and ß-D-glucan, two carbohydrate polymers with glucan being the most abundant component (Di Carlo and Fiore 1958, Bacon *et al* 1969).

Binding and phagocytosis of unopsonized zymosan was reported to be dependend on the expression of the mannose receptor on human (Speert and Silverstein 1985) and murine macrophages (Warr 1980, Sung *et al* 1983). Other studies showed the dependency of superoxide anion release in murine and rabbit macrophages on the mannose receptor (Berton 1983, Klegeris *et al* 1996].

Besides difficulties in the direct transfer of research results derived from different species some aspects of our study indicate that the mannose receptor might not play a major role but that another type of membrane receptor is responsible for zymosan signalling and consecutive respiratory burst activites in human blood monocytes and milk macrophages.

Monocytes do not express the mannose receptor until they are cultured for several days (Moekoena and Gordon 1985, Ezekowitz *et al* 1990, Stahl and Ezekowitz 1998). We confirmed this by demonstrating negative staining of blood monocytes with FITC-labelled anti-human mannose receptor monoclonal antibodies within the cultivation periods of monocytes used in our experiments. In our assay both types of cells produced approximately equal amounts of O_2^- when challenged with zymosan particles without any opsonizing serum factors. Furthermore addition of D-mannose in different concentrations resulted in inhibition of superoxide anion release to the same extent in both types of cells. Since the mannose receptor is absent on the surface of blood monocytes and they still show the same reactions to stimulation and inhibition as milk macrophages who do bear mannose receptors on their membrane (as shown by staining with moAbs), an involvment of this type of receptor seems to be unlikely in the production of superoxide anions, even though the process of internalization *per se* might be induced by different means. These findings are supported by a recent report of Astarie-Dequeker *et al.* who showed that phagocytosis of unopsonized zymosan through the mannose receptor did not result in triggering of O_2^--production (Astarie-Dequeker *et al* 1999). These investigators could demonstrate that the uptake of zymosan particles by human monocyte derived macrophages was dependend on the mannose receptor as well as on another membrane component, the ß-glucan receptor, which is located on the complement receptor type three (CR3). Even though internalization of unopsonized zymosan was also mediated by the mannose receptor, an observation which has been confirmed by other authors (Lombard *et al* 1994), the O_2^--generation itself was triggered only by phagocytosis via the ß-glucan receptor.

This lectin-like ß-glucan receptor has been located on the $\alpha_m\beta_2$ integrin CR3 (CD11b/CD18, Mac-1) It has been shown to be functionally independed from the complement receptor type 1 (CR1) and the receptor for IgG (FcR) (Czop and Austen 1985). Another ß-glucan receptor not localized on the CR3 has been postulated on human monocytes and a myelomonocytic cell line (Czop and Kay 1991), but its existence is discussed controversially (Thornton *et al* 1996).

Some laboratories found the binding of zymosan particles to the ß-glucan receptor to be inhibited by a variety of glucan-containing polysaccharides in human and murine mononuclear phagocytes whereas mannose-monomers, mannose-homoglycans or methylmannoside failed to block this lectine site (Czop and Austen 1985, Janusz *et al* 1989, Thornton *et al* 1996, Xia *et al* 1999). In murine peritoneal macrophages pretreatment with ß-glucans reduced release of reactive oxigen metabolites after stimulation with unopsonized zymosan (Adachi *et al* 1993).

Recently Thornton *et al.* used a soluble zymosan polysaccharide (SZP) to evaluate the sugar specifity of the ß-glucan receptor. Their investigations revealed the lectin site of CR 3 to have a broader specifity for certain polysaccharides than originally appreciated. SZP, which blocked the binding site to the same extent as various ß-glucan preparations, was unexpectedly found to consist primarily of mannose. In addition a specifity for N-acetyl-D-glucosamin (NADG) and glucose could be demonstrated (Thornton *et al* 1996).

Our results with stimulation by unopsonized zymosan and inhibition with D-mannose to the same extent in both types of cells could be the consequence of an equal distribution of the ß-glucan receptor on blood monocytes and milk macrophages. Considering the sugar specifity of this lectin-site the demonstrated concentration dependend functional impairment of zymosan-induced superoxide anion production could be explained in the inhibition of the ß-glucan receptor by D-mannose. Even though mannose did not alter SZP binding to the ß-glucan receptor (Thornton *et al* 1996) it could possibly interfere with the binding of unopsonized zymosan. A reason for the discrepant results of mannose-exerted inhibition of the ß-glucan receptor could also be found in the fact that ß-glucan triggered production of reactive hydrogen metabolites is regulated differently from signalling pathways for phagocytosis of ß-glucans (Okazaki *et al* 1996). Also the different concentrations of inhibitors used in the assays could contribute to differing results.

In the opsonization of zymosan the participation of both alternative and classical complement pathways as well as immunoglobulins has been demonstrated in a study on respiratory burst in human granulocytes (Cheson and Morris 1981). Zymosan specific IgG antibodies have been identified to enhance alternative pathway activities in human serum (Schenkein and Ruddy 1981). According to Valletta *et al.* superoxide anion production in rodent macrophages was dependend upon immunoglobulins as well (Valletta and Berton 1987).

Complement factors such as C3b or iC3b are also necessary in the opsonization of zymosan (Xia *et al* 1999). A concerted interaction between CR3 and the ß-glucan lectin site with the complement receptor being the primary binding site and the ß-glucan-receptor being the function triggering moiety has been postulated for example in the synthesis of platelet-activating-factor (PAF) in human monocytes (Elstad *et al* 1994). In human neutrophils binding of complement-opsonized yeast is related to complement receptor 1 (CR1) and the binding site for iC3b on CR3 whereas ingestion and respiratory burst depepend on coupling with the ß-glucan binding site (Cain *et al* 1987). Respiratory burst in rodent macrophages was reported to be inhibited by complement receptor blockade (Klegeris and McGeer 1994).

Monocytes have been shown to secrete the essential factors for activation and propagation of the alternative complement pathway (factors C3, B, D, H and I) (Hetland and Eskeland 1986) so they are capable of local zymosan opsonization via autocrine liberation of complement factors (Ezekowitz *et al* 1984 & 1985).

In our studies challenge of blood monocytes and milk macrophages with opsonized zymosan resulted in a high stimulation of blood monocytes with a release of superoxide anions being twofold higher than after stimulation with unopsonized zymosan. Milk macrophages' liberation of oxygen metabolites was about equal with and without opsonization. Since similar numbers of CR3-receptors have been postulated in the two cell subpopulations, a different type of opsonin-receptor would possibly account for the effect of this uneven stimulation and inhibition in connection with opsonized zymosan. Equal inhibition of the CR3-dependend opsonophagozytosis by mannose on one hand and a higher amount of FcR-dependend *opsonophagocytosis* not being mannose inhibitable on the other then result in the better stimulation of blood monocytes and lower inhibition by mannose under opsonin challenge in blood monocytes in comparison to milk macrophages. A decreased equipment of milk macrophages with Fc-receptor has been described by Rivas and co-workers supporting the idea of an uneven distribution of this recognition site (Rivas et al 1994).

Summa summarum the undertaken study has shown that the macrophage population in human milk is capable of reacting with the release of superoxide anions to both opsonized and unopsonized particles. The higher amount of lectinophagocytic responses possibly reflects the spezialization of these phagocytes to the specific neonatal environment.

REFERENCES

Adachi, Y., Ohno, N., Yadomae, T., 1993, Inhibitory effect of beta-glucans on zymosan-mediated hydrogen peroxide production by murine peritoneal macrophages in vitro. Biol Pharm Bull 16: 462-467.

Astarie-Dequeker, C., N'Diaye, E., Le Cabec, V., Rittig, M. G., Prandi, J., Maridonneau-Parini, I., 1999, The mannose receptor mediates uptake of pathogenic and nonpathogenic mycobacteria and bypasses bactericidal responses in human macrophages. Infect Immun 67, 469-477.

Bacon, J. S. D., Farmer, V. C., Jones, D., Taylor, I. F., 1969, The glucan components of the cell wall of baker's yeast (*Saccharomyces cerevisiae*) considered in relation to ist ultrastructure. Biochem J 114: 557.

Balkwill, F. R. and Hogg, N.,1979, Characterization of human breast milk macrophages cytostaitc for human cell lines. J Immunol 123: 1451-1456.

Berton, G., Gordon, S., 1983, Modulation of macrophage mannosyl-specific receptors by cultivation on immobilized zymosan. Effects on superoxide-anion release and phagocytosis. Immunology 49: 705-715.

Blau, H., Passwell, H., Levanon, M., Davidson, J., Kohen, F., Ramot, B., 1983, Studies on human milk macrophages: effect of activation on phagocytosis and secretion of prostaglandin E2 and lysozyme. Pediatr Res 17: 241-245.

Cain, J. A., Newman, S. L., Ross, G. D., 1987, Role of complement receptor type three and serum opsonins in the neutrophil response to yeast. Complement 4: 75-86.

Cheson, B. D., Morris, S. E., 1981, The role of complement and IgG on zymosan opsonization. Int Arch Allergy Appl Immunol 66: 48-54.

Clemente, J., Clerici, N., Espinosa, M. A., Leyva-Cobiàn, F., 1986, Defective chemotactic response of human alveolar and colostral macrophages. Immunol Lett 12: 271-276.

Cole, F.S., Schneeberger, E. E., Lichtenberg, N. A. and Colten, H. R., 1982, Complement biosynthesis in human breast milk macrophages and blood monocytes. Immunology 46: 429-441.

Cummings N. P., Neifert, M. R., Pabst M. J., Johnston R. B., 1985, Oxidative metabolic response and micorbicidal activity of human milk macrophages: effect of lio

Czop, J. K., Austen, K. F., 1985, A beta-glucan inhibitable receptor on human monocytes: its identity with the phagocytic receptor for particulate activators of the alternative complement pathway. J Immunol 134: 2588-2593.

Czop, J. K., Kay, J., 1991, Isolation and characterization of ß-glucan receptors on human mononuclear phagocytes. J Exp Med 173: 1511-1520.

Di Carlo, F. J., Fiore, J. V., 1958, On the composition of zymosan. Science 127: 756.

Elstad, M. R., Parker, C. J., Cowley, F. S., Wilcox, L. A., McIntyre, T. M., Prescot, S. M., Zimmerman, G. A., 1994, CD11b/CD18 integrin and a beta-glucan receptor act in concert to induce the synthesis of platelet-activating factor by monocytes. J Immunol 152: 220-230.

Everaerts, M. C., Van den Berghe, G., Saint-Remy, J. M., Corbeel, L., 1985, Effect of age-dependent enzymatic degradation of zymosan into oligosaccharides during incubation with serum on its opsonization by complement. Pediatr Res 19: 1293-1297.

Ezekowitz, R. A., Sim, R. B., Hill, M., Gordon, S., 1984, Local opsonization by secreted macrophage complement components. Role of receptors for complement in uptake of zymosan. J Exp Med 159: 244-260.

Ezekowitz, R. A., Sim, R. B., MacPherson, G. G., Gordon , S., 1985, Interaction of human monocytes, macrophages and polymorphonuclear leukocytes with zymosan in vitro. Role of type 3 complement receptors and macrophage-derived complement. J Clin Invest 76: 2368-2376.

Ezekowitz, R. A. B., Sastry, K., Bailly, P., Warner, A., 1990, Molecular characterization of the human macrophages mannose receptor: demonstration of multiple carbohydrate recognition-like domains and phagocytosis of yeasts in Col-1 cells. J Exp Med 172, 1785-1794.

Hetland, G., Eskeland, T., 1986, Formation of the functional alternative pathway of complement by human monocytes in vitro as demonstrated by phagocytosis of agarose beads. Scand J Immunol 23: 301-308.

Janusz, M. J., Austen, K. F., Czop, J. K., 1989, Isolation of a yeast heptaglucoside that inhibits monocyte phagocytosis of zymosan particles. J Immunol 142: 959-965.

Johnston, R. B., Godzik, C. A., Cohn, Z. A., 1978, Increased superoxide anion production by immunologically activated and chemically elicited macrophages. J Exp Med 148, 115-127.

Klegeris, A., McGeer, P. L., 1994, Inhibition of respiratory burst in macrophages by complement receptor blockade. Eur J Pharmacol 260: 271-277.

Klegeris, A., Budd, T. C., Greenfield, S. A., 1996, Acetylcholinesteraose-induced respiratory burst in macrophages: evidence for the involvement of the macrophage mannose-fucose receptor. Biochim Biophys Acta 1289: 159-168.

Leyva-Cobián, F., Clemente, J., 1984, Phenotypic characterization and functional activity of human milk macrophages. Immunol Lett 8: 249-256.

Lombard, Y., Giamis, J., Makaya-Kumba, M., Fonteneau, P., Poindron, P., 1994, A new method for studying the binding and ingestion of zymosan particles by macrophages. J Immunol Methods 174: 155-165.

Lowry, O. H., Rosebrough, N. J., Farr, A. L., Randall, R. J.1951: Protein measurement with the folin phenol reagent. J Biol Chem 193:265.

Mandyla, H., Xanthou, M., Maravelias, C., Baum, D., Matsaniotis, N., 1982, Antibody dependent cytotoxicity of human colostrum phagocytes. Pediatr Res 16: 995-999.

Mokoena, T., Gordon, S., 1985, Human macrophage activation. J Clin Invest 75: 624-631.

Mori, M., Hayward, A. R., 1982: Phenotype and function of human milk monocytes as antigen presenting cells. Clin Immunol Immunopathol 23: 94-99.

Ogra, P. K. and Greene, H. L., 1982, Human milk and breast feeding: an update on the state of the art. Pediatr Res 16: 266-271.

Okazaki, M., Chiba, N., Adachi, Y., Ohno, N., Yadomae, T., 1996, Signal transduction pathway on beta-glucans-triggered hydrogen peroxide production by murine peritoneal macrophages in vitro. Biol Pharm Bull 19: 18-23.

Rivas, R. A., el-Mohandes, A., A., Katona, I. M., 1994, Mononuclear phagocytic cells in human milk: HLA-DR and Fc gamma R ligand expression. Biol Neonate 66: 195-204.

Schenkein, H. A., Ruddy, S., 1981, The role of immunoglobulins in alternative complement pathway activation by zymosan. I Human IgG with specifity for zymosan enhances alternative pathway activation by zymosan. J Immunol 126: 7-10.

Schroten, H., Uhlenbruck, G., Hanisch, F. G. and Mil, A., 1987, Varying rates of phagocytosis of human blood monocytes and breast milk macrophages: effect of intralipid and milk fat globules. Monatsschr Kinderheilk 135: 36-40.

Sebring, P. E., Bender, J. G., Van Epps, D. E., 1989, Decreased opsonic activity for Staphylococcus aureus in neonatal and late gestation maternal sera. Inflammation 13: 571-582.

Speer, C. P., Gahr, M., Pabst, M.J., 1986, Phagocytosis-associated oxidative metabolism in human milk macrophages. Acta Paediatr. Scand. 74: 444-451.

Speer, C. P., Hein-Kreikenbaum, H., 1993, Immunologic importance of breast milk. Monatsschr Kinderheilkd 141, 10-20.

Speert, D. P., Silverstein, S. C., 1985, Phagocytosis of unopsonized zymosan by human monocyte-derived macrophages: maturation and inhibition by mannan. J Leukoc Biol 38: 655-658, 1985.

Stahl, P. D., Ezekowitz, R. A. B., 1998, The mannose receptor is a pattern recogition receptor involved in host defense. Curr Opinion Immunol 10: 50-55.

Sung, S. J., Nelson, R. S., Silverstein, S., C., 1983, Yeast mannans inhibit binding and phagocytosis of zymosan by mouse peritoneal macrophages. J Cell Biol 96: 160-166.

Thornton, B. P., Vetvicka, V., Pitman, M., Goldman, R. C., Ross, G. D., 1996, Analysis of the sugar specifity and molecular location of the ß-glucan-binding lectin site of complement receptor type 3 (CD11b/CD18). J Immunol 156: 1235-1246.

Tsuda, H., Dickey, W. D., Goldman, A. S., 1984, Separation of human colostral macrophages and neutrophils on gelatin and collagen serum substrata. Cell Struct Funct 8: 367-371.

Valletta, E. A., Berton, G., 1987, Desensitization of macrophage oxygen metabolism on immobilized ligands: different effect of immunoglobulin G and complement. J Immunol 15: 4366-4373.

Vassao, R. C., Carneiro-Sampaio, M. M., 1989, Phagocytic activity of human colostrum macrophages. Braz J Med Biol Res 22: 457-464.

Warr, G. A., 1980, A macrophage receptor for (mannose/glucosamine)-glycoproteins of potential importance in phagocytic activity. Biochem Biophys Res Commun 93: 737-745.

Xia, Y., Vetvicka V., Yan, J., Hanikyrova, M., Mayadas, T., Ross, G. D., 1999, The ß-glucan-binding lectin site of mouse CR3 (CD11b/CD18) and its functions in generating a primed state of the receptor that mediates cytotoxic activation in response to iC3b-opsonized target cells. J Immunol 162: 2281-2290.

9

IS ALLERGY A PREVENTABLE DISEASE?

Bengt Björkstén
Karolinska Institute, Centre for Allergy Research, Stockholm

1.   INTRODUCTION

There is now an almost universal consensus that the prevalence of allergic diseases has increased considerably in western industrialised countries, particularly since the Second World War[1]. The reasons for the increase are largely unknown. Until recently, most of the interest has focused on identifying risk factors, i.e. environmental factors that would increase the likelihood for sensitisation. Thus, excessive exposure to indoor allergens, particularly house dust mites, tobacco smoke and poor indoor ventilation, have all been suggested as major risk factors. As a consequence, primary prevention has focussed on reducing exposure to these putative risk factors. None of the suggested risk factors can more than marginally explain the large regional differences on allergy prevalence, however, and the results of intervention studies have largely been disappointing.

As sensitisation to ubiquitous environmental allergens usually occur in early childhood and the increase in allergy prevalence has been particularly pronounced in children, much of the interest has been focussed on this age group. Over the past few years, novel discoveries related to the maturation of the immune system has resulted in an interest in identifying factors that protect against the development of manifest allergic disease, rather than studying risk factors. Such studies were prompted by the discovery that normal pregnancy in mammals, including man, is accompanied by an immune deviation towards Th2 type immunity[2]. As a consequence, the immune system of the new-born baby is also skewed towards Th2-type immunity[3]. Thus, an "allergy-type" immunity is normal early in life. The development of a balanced Th1/Th2 immunity is achieved in early childhood by the influence of the environment.

The tendency to develop allergic disease is strongly influenced by genetic factors, environmental influences, age and the conditions under which exposure takes place. The environment has undergone major changes in recent years. "Environment" and "life style" are much more than emissions from traffic and exposure to mites, however. The concept of "life style" should therefore be expanded considerably, since an altered life style also includes dietary changes, the microbial environment, extensive travelling to new environments, stress and much more. Furthermore, the mother is a little discussed, but significant "environmental factor" in early infancy.

Primary allergic sensitisation to environmental allergens most commonly occurs early in life, often even before birth[3-4]. Animal studies suggest that the neonatal mucosal tolerance induction mechanisms are malfunctional[5]. Moreover, cross-sectional[6-7] and prospective[8] studies strongly indicate that exposure to allergens early in life may have an impact on the incidence of allergy many years later. Thus, an understanding of the development of immune responses to allergens is a prerequisite for the understanding of why the prevalence of allergy is increasing in developed countries and for the implementation of primary prevention. In this review, the potential for primary prevention of allergy is discussed in the light of epidemiological observations and recent studies on the development of immune responses to allergens. Also, the role of the mother as an "environmental factor" will be discussed.

2.   EPIDEMIOLOGICAL ASPECTS

The increasing prevalence and severity of atopic diseases seen in industrialised countries are in marked contrast with the low prevalence of allergy among children in the formerly socialist countries of Europe with a life style similar to that prevailing in Western Europe 30-40 years ago[9-11]. These and other regional differences were recently confirmed in two large epidemiological surveys. In the European Community Respiratory Health Survey (ECRHS) the prevalence of asthma related symptoms were studied in young adults aged 20-44 years, mainly in Europe. Carefully validated questionnaires were used in populations who were selcected in an identical manner in all the study centres[12]. The findings were confirmed by lung function tests and analysis of IgE antibodies to allergens in representative subpopulations[13]. The International Study of Asthma and Allergy (ISAAC) comprised almost 800,000 children aged 6/7 and 13/14 years in over 150 centres in over 50 countries over the world[14-17]. Both the ECRHS and the ISAAC confirmed that that there are large variations in the prevalence of allergy and that these variations can not be explained by similar variations in any known life style and other environmental factors.

3. PRE- AND POSTNATAL DEVELOPMENT OF IMMUNE RESPONSES TO ALLERGENS

Immune responses to allergens are characterised by a cross-regulation between competing IFNγ-secreting T helper 1 (Th1)-like cell populations and IL-4-producing Th2-like cell populations. As already mentioned, pregnancy is associated with a strong skewing towards Th2 type immunity and if this does not occur in time, there is an increased risk for abortion[2]. As a consequence neonatal immunity is Th2-skewed and allergen specific T-cell responses are common already at birth[3]. Probably, these responses are normal and do not indicate future allergy.

During the first years of life, the neonatal immune responses towards inhalant allergens deviate towards a balanced Th1 and Th2 like immunity, resulting in low levels of IgG antibodies and low level T cell responses to inhalant allergens in non-allergic children and adults[4]. These T cell responses are predominantly Th1-like. This process seems largely to be completed at around 5 years of age[18]. In contrast, immune responses to foods are generally suppressed.

Temporary low-level IgE responses to food and inhalant allergens are common during the first years of life[19]. They are then down regulated in non atopic individuals, while they continue to increase in children who develop allergic manifestations. In a prospective study, the development of serum IgE and IgG subclass antibodies to β-lactoglobulin, ovalbumin, birch and cat was analysed from birth up to 8 years of age[20]. The levels of IgG-subclass antibodies to β-lactoglobulin peaked at 6 months and to ovalbumin at 18 months and then decreased, while the IgG-subclass antibody levels to the inhalant allergens generally increased with age. The kinetics of IgG antibodies to allergens was largely similar in Sweden with a high, and

Estonia, with a low prevalence of allergic disease, except for low levels of maternally derived IgG_4 antibodies to the inhalant allergens in cord blood in the latter babies[21]. The findings indicate that Th2 dependent antibody responses are normally down regulated in non atopic individuals.

In contrast, recent studies show that the atopic phenotype is associated with a prolonged period of Th2 type immune responses to allergens early in life[3,18]. Thus, the maturation process seems to proceed at a slower pace in infants with an atopic family history and/or who develop allergic disease, as compared to non atopic babies. The findings confirm on the T cell level the previous observations showing that humoral immune responses to food and inhalant allergens are common during the first years of life[19]. The difference between individuals with and without a genetically determined atopic propensity may thus be how readily the neonatal Th2-skewed immunity deviates towards a Th1 type response. Therefore, it seems reasonable to look for postnatal environmental factors affecting the incidence of allergy, rather than to advocate allergen avoidance during pregnancy.

4. MICROBIAL INFLUENCES

Rook and Stanford recently suggested two major syndromes that could be the result of inadequate microbial stimulation early in life; inadequate priming of T helper cells, leading to an incorrect cytokine balance and a failure to fine-tune the T cell repertoire in relation to epitopes that are cross-reactive between self and microorganisms[22]. The authors coined the expressions "input deprivation syndrome" and "uneducated T-cell regulation syndrome".

Infections can have long-lasting non-specific systemic effects on the nature of the immune response to unrelated antigens. It has been suggested that recurrent infections during early childhood may protect against allergy, as suggested by several studies reporting an inverse relationship between the incidence of atopy and family size, particularly the number of older siblings[23-25]. It has also been suggested that vaccination against pertussis may be increasing the incidence of Th2-mediated disease, although in a recent prospective study this was shown not to be the case[26]. From an immunological point of view, however, respiratory infections would not be expected to exert such continuous strong pressure on the maturing immune system as to induce immune deviation.

The microflora of the large gut may have important roles in both human health and disease. This perspective is by no means a new concept, as Metchnikoff already a century ago indicated the clinical importance of the host colonic microflora[27]. Rapid advancements have have been made, particularly over the past 10 years and the bacterial microflora of the human gut is now accepted as an integral component of the host defence system.

The total mucosal surface area of the adult human gastrointestinal tract is up to $300m^2$, making it the largest body area interacting with the environment. It is colonised with over 10^{14} micro-organisms, weighing over 1 kg and corresponding to more than 10 times the total number of cells in the body.

The gastrointestinal tract of the new-born baby is sterile. Soon after birth, however, it is colonised by numerous types of micro-organisms. Colonisation is complete after approximately one week but the numbers and species of bacteria fluctuate markedly during the first three months of life. When the microflora has been established it is surprisingly stable over time and environmental changes, e.g. a treatment period with antibiotics only temporary changes the composition of the microflora.

Microbial stimulation, both from normal commensals and pathogens in the gastrointestinal and respiratory tract, is important for normal postnatal maturation of immune functions. We recently observed that the gut flora of Estonian and Swedish infants differ in several respects[28]. The gut flora of Estonian infants is similar to the flora of European children some 20-30 years ago and more often comprises *Lactobacilli* and *Eubacteria*, and the numbers are higher than in Swedish infants. The potential significance of these findings were supported by an observation that colonisation with lactobacilli appears to be more intense in non allergic as compared to allergic children[29].

5. THE INFLUENCE OF MATERNAL IMMUNITY

The immune system of the newborn infant is influenced by maternal immunity, both transplacentally and via the breast milk. Thus, there is a close immunological interaction between the mother and her baby during gestation and during the period of breast-feeding, where the mother may provide protective factors and immune modifying components, as well as antigenic stimulation.

As already discussed, the fetomaternal interface is surrounded by high levels of the Th2 cytokines IL-4 and IL-10 [2], probably in order to divert the maternal immune response away from damaging Th1-mediated immune responses[30]. The tendency of atopics to express Th2-like immunity may thus be of reproductive advantage, and we have recently observed a higher number of children among atopic mothers as compared to non-atopic mothers[31]. The higher cord blood IgE levels seen in newborns of atopic mothers as compared to newborns with a paternal or no atopic history may depend on a possibly stronger placental Th2 shift in atopic mothers. The Th2 polarisation during pregnancy may influence the offspring for variable periods postnatally, as evidenced by the selective expansion of Th2 memory cells in antigen challenged newborn mice[32]. This could conceivably explain the well known higher penetration of maternal than paternal heredity of allergic disease.

Maternal IgG antibodies are transplacentally transferred via an active transport, providing a passive protection for infections in the baby. High levels of cord blood IgG antibodies to β-lactoglobulin have been reported to protect against the development of cow's milk allergy, although this was not confirmed in another study[33]. Low levels of IgG antibodies to cat and birch in cord blood are associated with an increased prevalence of sensitvity to cat, as well as asthma at 8 years of age[34]. If high levels of maternal allergen-specific IgG antibodies indeed are protective, this may be an alternative explanation to the observations in several epidemiological studies showing an increased risk for allergy to seasonal allergens in children born before the relevant pollen[6-7]. Birth at this time of the year would provide low levels of cord serum IgG antibodies. Furthermore, high levels of IgG anti-IgE antibodies in cord blood are associated with less allergy during the first 18 months of life, particularly in babies with a strong family history of allergy[35].

The precise relation between breast-feeding and infant allergy is poorly understood. Any allergy-preventing effect of human milk, if true, seems to be limited to babies with a genetically determined increased risk for atopic disease[36]. The capacity to influence infant immunity may also vary between mothers. Breast milk cell supernatants from atopic mothers stimulate higher levels of cord blood IgE secretion *in vitro* than cell supernatants from non-atopic mothers[37]. We have recently been able to demonstrate that breast-milk from non-atopic mothers contain higher levels of ovalbumin-specific secretory IgA antibodies than breast-milk from atopic mothers, as measured by a sensitive enzyme amplified ELISA (Casas *et al*, unpublished).

During early infancy there is a close immunological interaction between the mother and her offspring, through the breast milk but relatively little is known about the exchange of immunological information. Besides numerous components that help in the protection against infection, human milk contains components that enhance the maturation of the immune system of the new-born infant. Observations include an early stimulation of IgA antibody synthesis in breast-fed infants[38] and transfer of cell-mediated immunity and cytokines[39]. Thus, human milk would not only provide passive protection against infections, but also actively stimulate infant immunity. There are considerable individual variations in the composition of human milk, however. This may explain the controversy with regard to the possible allergy-preventive effects of breast feeding. If individual variations in the milk modulate the development of immunity in the neonate, then maternal immunity may represent an environmental factor, which would influence the risk for allergic manifestations in her child, possibly even several years later.

Human milk also contains foreign antigens, e. g. food antigens eaten by the mother and these may sensitise the baby[40]. A maternal hypoallergenic diet during the lactation period is associated with less atopic eczema in the children, but does not reduce the prevalence of other atopic manifestations during the first four years of life[41].

Low levels of total IgA and cow's milk specific IgA[42-43] in breast milk have been reported to be associated with cow's milk allergy in the infants. This was not confirmed, however, in a carefully controlled prospective study[44].

There are several reports in the literature suggesting that allergic disease is associated with an abnormal metabolism of long chain fatty acids. A disturbed composition of polyunsaturated fatty acids (PUFA) has been reported in milk from mothers of atopic infants. For example, the levels of the essential fatty acid linoleic acid (LA), as well as its metabolites were lower in early mature milk from atopic, as compared to non-atopic mothers and the ratio between n-6 and n-3 fatty acids was higher[45]. Differences in the fatty acid composition of human milk seems to have a relevance for the breast fed infants. Thus, lower levels of the n-3 fatty acids, EPA DPA and DHA have been observed in mothers of infants who developed allergic disease during the first year of life as compared to mothers of babies who did not develop any allergic manifestations[46]. These differences were independent of maternal allergy. Similarly low levels of certain polyamines have been observed in milk from atopic mothers[39]. As these compounds are required for optimal DNA synthesis, variations in the levels could affect immune responses to foreign antigens in breast fed infants.

6.   PRIMARY PREVENTION OF ALLERGY

Prospective intervention studies of allergy prevention have so far at best only shown modest effects. There are as many studies showing slightly reduced incidence of allergy among breast fed infants as compared to formula fed babies as there are studies showing no effect, or even more allergy in the former infants[36,39]. Efforts to prevent allergy in infancy and early childhood through substituting regular cow's milk based infant formulae with extensively hydrolysed products have only shown a slight reduction in the incidence of cow's milk allergy, while there was no effect on respiratory allergies[47].

Studies have also been devoted to the prevention of childhood allergy through manipulation of the maternal diet during pregnancy and the lactation period. The conclusion of these studies is that allergen avoidance during pregnancy[44] does not seem to have any effects on allergy incidence in the offspring, nor did a maternal diet rich in cow's milk increase the likelihood of tolerance induction[48]. In contrast, maternal avoidance of allergenic foods during the first three months of lactation was associated with a reduced incidence of atopic eczema in their babies during the first year of life[40,49].

It is well established that exposure to tobacco smoke in infancy and early childhood is associated with an increased risk for respiratory infections and wheezing, as well as for sensitisation to inhalant allergens[50]. Other measures, like efforts to reduce the levels of indoor allergens like house dust mites and pets have largely been disappointing[51]. Recent studies even suggest that the contrary may be true, i.e. that exposure to allergens during infancy may reduce the prevalence of allergic asthma in school children[52].

7.   CONCLUSIONS

Environmental factors, e. g. Western life style associated factors and maternal immunity, including the cytokine milieu at the placenta, transfer of IgG antibodies via the placenta and IgA antibodies and cytokines via the breast-milk, may all influence the development of immune responses to allergens. The first encounters with allergens occur during the first year of life, or even before birth. T- and B-cell reactivity to food allergens peak early in life and are then down regulated, whereas the responses to inhalant allergens increase with age. Atopic children may have a bias to allergen-stimulated production of type 2 cytokines, as reflected by higher levels of IgE and IgG_4 responses to allergens.

Currently recommended measures for primary prevention of allergy are at best only modestly effective. The avoidance of exposure to tobacco smoke is at present the only recommendation that is reasonably well documented by evidence based medicine. Primary prevention of allergy may in the future include measures to enhance the induction of immune deviation and clinical tolerance. Such studies are currently performed and the outcome will be known in a few years.

REFERENCES

1. Björkstén, B., 1997, The environment and sensitisation to allergens in early childhood. *Ped. Allergy Immunol.* **8 (suppl 10)**: 32-39.
2. Wegmann, T., Lin, H., Guilbert, L., and Mosmann, T.,1993, Bidirectional cytokine interactions in the maternal-fetal relationship: is successful pregnancy a Th2 phenomenon? *Immunol. Today* **14**: 353-356.
3. Björkstén, B., 1999, The intrauterine and postnatal environment. *J Allergy Clin Immunol*: **In press.**
4. Holt, P.G., Yabuhara, A., Prescott, S., Venaille, T., Macaubas, C., Holt, B.J., Björkstén, B., and Sly, P.D., 1997, Allergen recognition in the origin of asthma. *Ciba Foundation Symposium* **206**: 35-49.
5. Nelson, D., McMenamin, C., Wilkes, L., and Holt, P.G., 1991, Postnatal development of respiratory mucosal immune function in the rat: Regulation of IgE responses to inhaled allergen. *Pediatr. Allergy Immunol.* **4**: 170-177.
6. Aalberse, R., Nieuwenhuys, E., Hey, M., and Stapel, S., 1992, Horoscope effect not only for seasonal but also for nonseasonal allergens. *Clin. Exp. Allergy* **22**: 1003-1006.
7. Björkstén, B., Suoniemi, I., and Koski, V., 1980, Neonatal birch-pollen contact and subsequent allergy to pollen. *Clin. Allergy* **10**: 585-591.
8. Sporik, R., Holgate, S.T., and Cogswell, J.J., 1991, Natural history of asthma in childhood-a birth cohort study. *Arch. Dis. Childh.* **66**: 1050-3.
9. Bråbäck, L., Breborowicz, A., Dreborg, S., Knutsson, A., Pieklik, H., and Björkstén, B., 1994, Atopic sensitization and respiratory symptoms among Polish and Swedish schoolchildren. *Clin. Exper. Allergy* **24**: 826-835.
10. Bråbäck, L., Breborowicz, A., Julge, K., Knutsson, A., Riikjärv, M., Vasar, M., and Björkstén, B., 1995, Risk factors for respiratory symptoms and atopic sensitization in the Baltic area. *Arch. Dis. Child.* **72**: 487-493.
11. von Mutius, E., Fritzsch, C., Weiland, S. K., Röll, G., and Magnussen, H., 1992, Prevalence of asthma and allergic disorders among schoolchildren in united Germany: a descriptive comparison. *Br. Med. J* . **305**: 1395-9.
12. Burney, P., Luczinska, C., Chinn, S., and Jarvis, D., 1994, The European Community Respiratory Health Survey. *Eur. Respir. J.* **7**: 954-960.

13. Burney, P., Malmberg, E., Chinn, S., Jarvis, D., Luczynska, C., and Lai, E., 1997, The distribution of total and specific serum IgE in the European Community Respiratory Health Survey. *J. Allergy Clin. Immunol.* **99**: 314-22.
14. Asher, M., Andersson, H., Crane, J., Stewart, A., Anabwani, G., Beasley, R., Björkstén, B., Burr, M., Keil, U., Lai, C., Mallol, J., Martinez, F., Mitchell, E., Pearce, N., Montefort, S., Robertson, C., Strachan, D., von Mutius, E., Sibbald, B., Weiland, S., Williams, H., Ait-Khaled, N., and Shah, J., 1998, Worlwide variations in the prevalence of asthma symptoms: International study of asthma and allergies in childhood (ISAAC). *Eur. Resp. J.* **12**: 315-335.
15. Beasley, R.K.U., von Mutius, E., Pearce, N., Anabwani, G., Andersson, H.R., Asher, M.I., Björkstén, B., Burr, M.L., Crane, J., Lai, C., Mallol, J., Martinez, F.D., Mitchell, E.M., Montefort, S., Robertson, C., Shah, J.R., Sibbald, B., Stewart, A.W., Strachan, D., Weiland, S.K., and Williams, H.C., 1998, Worlwide variation in the prevalence of asthma and allergies: The International Study of Asthma and Allergies in Childhood (ISAAC). *Lancet* **351**: 1225-1232.
16. Strachan D, Weiland, S.K., Anabwani, G., Andersson, H.R., Asher, M.I., Beasley, R., Björkstén, B, Burr, M.L., Crane, J., Keil, U., Lai, C., Mallol, J., Martinez, F.D., Mitchell, E.M., von Mutius, E., Montefort, S., Pearce, N., Robertson, C., Stewart, A.W., Williams, H.C., Ait-Khaled, N., and Shah, J.R., 1997, Worlwide variations in the prevalence of allergic rhinoconjunctivitis in children: International study of asthma and allergies in childhood (ISAAC). *Pediatr. Allergy Immunol* .**8**: 161-176
17. Williams, H., Stewart, A., Ait-Khaled, N., Anabwani, G., Andersson, R., Asher, I., Beasley, R., Björkstén, B., Burr, M., Clayton, T., Crane, J., Ellwood, P., Keil ,U., Lai, C., Mallol, J., Martinez, F., Mitchell, E., Montefort, S., Pearce, N., Sibbald, B., Strachan, D., von Mutius, E., and Weiland, S.K., 1999, Worlwide variations in the prevalence of atopic eczema in children from the International study of asthma and allergies in childhood (ISAAC). *J Allergy Clin Immunol* **103**:125-38.
18. Prescott, S.D., Macaubas, C., Smallacombe, T., Holt, B.J., Sly, P.D., and Holt, P.G., 1999, Development of allergen-specific T-cell memory in atopic and normal children. *Lancet* **353**: 196-200.
19. Hattevig, G., Kjellman, B., and Björkstén, B., 1993, Appearance of IgE antibodies to ingested and inhaled allergens during first 12 years of life in atopic and non-atopic children. *Pediatr. Allergy Immunol* . **4**:182-189.
20. Jenmalm, M., and Björkstén, B., 1999b, Exposure to cow's milk during the first three months of life results in failure to downregulate IgG subclass antibodies to B-lactoglobulin up to eight years. *J. Allerg. Clin. Immunol.*: **In press**.
21. Julge, K., 1998, Humoral immune responses to allergens in early childhood. Thesis No 558, Linköping University, Sweden.
22. Rook, G., and Stanford, J., 1998, Give us this day our daily germs. *Immunol. Today* **19**: 113-116.
23. Strachan, D., 1989, Hay fever, hygiene and household size. *Br. Med. J.* **289**: 1259-60.
24. Strachan, D., Taylor, E., and Carpenter, R., 1996, Family structure, neonatal infection and hay fever in adolescense. *Arch. Dis. Childhood* **74**: 422-426.
25. von Mutius, E., Martinez, F.D., Fritzsch, C., Nicolai, T., Reitmeir, P., and Thiemann, H.H., 1994, Skin test reactivity and number of siblings. *Brit. Med. J.* **308**: 692-5.
26. Nilsson, L., Kjellman, N.-I., and Björkstén, B., 1998, A randomized controlled trial of the effect of pertussis vaccines on atopic disease. *Arch. Pediatr. Adolesc. Med.* **152**: 734-738.
27. Metchnikoff, E., 1907, The prolongation of life. William Heinemann, London.
28. Sepp, E., Julge, K., Vasar, M., Naaber, P., Björkstén, B., and Mikelsaar, M., 1997, Intestinal microflora of Estonian and Swedish infants. *Acta Paediatr.* **86**: 956-961.

29. Björkstén, B., Naaber, P., Sepp, E., and Mikelsaar, M., 1999, The intestinal microflora in allergic Estonian and Swedish 2-year old children.*Clin. Exp. Allergy* **29**:342-346.
30. Marzi, M., Vigano, A., and Trabattoni, D., 1996, Characterization of type 1 and type 2 cytokine production profile in physiologic and pathologic human pregnancy. *Clin. Exp. Immunol.* **106**: 127-133.
31. Nilsson, L., Kjellman, N.-I., and Björkstén, B., 1997, Parity among atopic and non-atopic mothers. *Pediatr. Allergy Immunol*.**8**: 134-137.
32. Barrios, C., Brawand, P., Berney, M., Brandt, C., Lambert, P., and Siegrist, C., 1996, Neonatal and early life immune responses to various forms of vaccine antigens qualitatively differ from adult responses: predominance of a Th2-biased pattern which persists after adult boosting. *Eur J. Immunol.* **26**, 1489-1496.
33. Fälth-Magnusson, K., Öman, H., and Kjellman, N.-I. M., 1987, Maternal abstention from cow milk and egg in allergy risk pregnancies. Effect on antibody production in the mother and the newborn. *Allergy* **42**: 64-73.
34. Jenmalm, M., and Björkstén, B., 1999a, Cord blood levels of IgG subclass antibodies to food and inhalant allergens in relation to maternal atopy and the development of atopic disease during the first eight years of life. *Clin. Exp. Allergy:* **In press**.
35. Vassella, C., Odelram, H., Kjellman, N.-I.M., Borres, M., Vanto, T., and Björkstén, B., 1994, High anti-IgE levels at birth are associated with a reduced allergy incidence in early childhood. *Clin. Exper. Allergy* **24**: 771-777.
36. Björkstén, B., 1983, Does breast feeding prevent the development of allergy? *Immunol. Today* **4**: 215- 217.
37. Allardyce, R., 1984, Breast milk cell supernatants from atopic donors stimulate cord blood IgA secretion in vitro. *Clin. Allergy* **14**: 259-267.
38. Prentice, A., 1987, Breast feeding increases concentrations of IgA in infants´ urine. *Arch. Dis.Childh.* **62**: 792-795.
39. Duchén, K., 1999, Humoral milk factors and atopy in early childhood. Thesis No 580, Linköping University, Sweden.
40. Hattevig, G., Kjellman, B., Sigurs, N., Björkstén, B., and Kjellman, N.-I.M., 1989, Effect of maternal avoidance of eggs, cow's milk and fish during lactation upon allergic manifestations in infants. *Clin. Exp. Allergy* **19**: 27-32.
41. Sigurs, N., Hattevig, G., and Kjellman, B., 1992, Maternal avoidance of eggs, cow's milk, and fish during lactation: effect on allergic manifestations, skin-prick tests, and specific IgE antibodies in children at age 4 years. *Pediatrics* **89**: 735-739.
42. Machtinger, S., and Moss, R., 1986, Cow's milk allergy in breast-fed infants: The role of allergen and maternal secretory IgA antibody. *J. Allergy Clin. Immunol.* **77**: 341-47.
43. Savilahti, E., Tainio, V.M., Salmenpera, L., Arjomaa, P., Kallio, M., Perheentupa, J., and Siimes, M.A., 1991, Low colostral IgA associated with cow's milk allergy. *Acta Paediatr. Scand.* **80**: 1207-13.
44. Fälth-Magnusson, K., and Kjellman, N.-I. M., 1992, Allergy prevention by maternal elimination diet during late pregnancy-a 5-year follow-up of a randomized study. *J.Allergy Clin. Immunol.* **89**: 709-13.
45. Yu, G., Duchén, K., and Björkstén, B., 1998, Fatty acid composition in colostrum and mature milk from atopic and non-atopic mothers during the first 6 months of lactation. *Acta Paediatr.* **87**: 729-736.
46. Duchén, K., Yu, G., and Björkstén, B., 1998, Atopic sensitisation during the first year of life in relation to long chain polyunsaturated fatty acid levels in human milk. *Ped. Res.*: **In press**.

47. Oldaeus, G., Anjou, K., Björkstén, B., Moran, J. R., and Kjellman, N.-I., 1997, Extensively and partially hydrolysed infant formulas for allergy prophylaxis.*Arch. Dis. Childh.***77**: 4-10.
48. Lilja, G., Dannæus, A., Foucard, T., Graff-Lonnevig, V., Johansson, S., and Öman, H., 1989, Effects of maternal diet during late pregnancy and lactaction on the development of atopic diseases in infants up to eighteen months of age - in vivo results. *Clin. Exp. Allergy* **19**: 473-479.
49. Zeiger, R., and Heller, S., 1995, The development and prediction of atopy in high risk children: Follow-up at age seven years in a prospective randomized study of combined maternal and infant food allergen avoidance. *J: Allergy Clin. Immunol.* **95**: 1179-90.
50. Halken, S., Høst, A., Nilsson, L., and Taudorf, E., 1995, Passive smoking as a risk factor for development of obstructive respiratory disease and allergic sensitization. *Allergy* **50**: 97-105.
51. Björkstén, B., and Kjellman, N.-I.M.,1998, Risk factors in the development of allergy. In: Asthma and Immunologic Diseases in Pregnancy and Early Infancy. *Lung Biology in Health and Disease,* Eds. M Schatz, Claman HM, Zeiger RN. Marcel Dekker Inc, New York, **vol 110**: 677-702
52. Hesselmar, B., Åberg, N., Åberg, B., Eriksson, B., and Björkstén, B., 1999, Does early exposure to cat or dog protect against later allergy development. *Clin. Exp. Allergy* **29**: 611-617.

10

BREAST-FEEDING AND THE DEVELOPMENT OF COWS' MILK PROTEIN ALLERGY

[1]K.M. Saarinen, M.D., [1]K. Juntunen-Backman, M.D., [2]A-L. Järvenpää , M.D., [3]P. Klemetti, M.D., [4]P. Kuitunen, M.D., [4]L. Lope, M.D., [5]M. Renlund , M.D., [6]M. Siivola, PhD., [3]O. Vaarala, M.D. and [1]E. Savilahti, M.D.

[1]*Hospital for Children and Adolescents, University of Helsinki;* [2]*Helsinki City Maternity Hospital;* [3]*National Public Health Institute, Helsinki;* [4]*Jorvi Hospital, Espoo;* [5]*Deptartment of Obstetrics, Helsinki University Central Hospital;* [6]*Department of Public Health, University of Helsinki; Helsinki and Espoo, Finland*

Key words: Cow milk, colostrum, breast-feeding, food allergy, infant, IgE, transforming growth factor-$\beta1$

Abstract: Early feeding with cows' milk (CM) may cause cows' milk allergy (CMA). Breast milk contains many immune factors which compensate for the undeveloped defence mechanisms of the gut of the newborn infant. We studied the effect of supplementary CM feeding at the maternity hospital on the subsequent incidence of CMA, the effects of formula and breast feeding on the subsequent immunologic types of CMA, and the importance of immune factors present in colostrum in the immune responses of infants with CMA. In a cohort of 6209 infants, 824 were exclusively breast-fed and 87% required supplementary milk while in the maternity hospital: 1789 received CM formula, 1859 pasteurized human milk, and 1737 whey hydrolysate formula. The cumulative incidence of CMA, verified by a CM elimination-challenge test, was 2.4% in the CM, 1.7% in the pasteurized human milk and 1.5% in the whey hydrolysate group. Among these infants, exposure to CM at hospital and a positive atopic heredity increased the risk of CMA. Of the exclusively breast-fed infants, 2.1% had CMA. Risk factors for the development of IgE-mediated CMA were: exposure to CM at hospital, breast-feeding during the first 8 weeks at home either exclusively or combined with infrequent exposure to small amounts of CM and long breast-feeding. The content of transforming growth factor-$\beta1$ (TGF-$\beta1$) in colostrum from mothers of infants with IgE-mediated CMA was lower than from mothers of infants with non-IgE-mediated CMA. In infants with CMA, TGF-$\beta1$ in colostrum negatively correlated with the result of skin prick test and the stimulation of peripheral

Short and Long Term Effects of Breast Feeding on Child Health
Edited by Berthold Koletzko *et al.*, Kluwer Academic/Plenum Publishers, 2000

121

blood mononuclear cells to CM, but positively with infants' IgA and IgG antibodies to CM proteins. Feeding of CM formula at maternity hospital increases the risk of CMA, but exclusive breast-feeding does not eliminate the risk. Prolonged breast-feeding exclusively or combined with infrequent exposure to small amounts of CM during the first 8 weeks induces the development of IgE-mediated CMA. Colostral TGF-β1 may inhibit IgE- and cell mediated reactions and promote IgG-IgA antibody production to CM in infants prone to developing CMA

1.   INTRODUCTION

Food allergies, particularly cows' milk allergy (CMA), develop during the first months of life in infants in whom both the non-specific and specific defence mechanisms of the gastrointestinal tract are undeveloped. A positive atopic heredity is a known risk factor for food allergies,[1] but very little is know about the other factors predisposing to CMA.

1.1   Breast-feeding and the development of CMA

Breast milk contains many immunologic and nonspecific defence factors which compensate for the underdeveloped defences of the gut of the newborn infant.[2,3] Low levels of secretory IgA or cows' milk (CM) specific IgA in colostrum have been associated with the development of CMA.[4,5] On the other hand, exclusively breast-fed infants are shown to be sensitised to food antigens present breast milk[6,7] and the symptoms of atopic eczema have alleviated after cessation of breast-feeding.[8] Breast milk also contains soluble immunoregulatory factors.[3,9-11] However, the effects of these factors on the infants' immune responses are unknown.

1.2   Early exposure to food antigens

The first exposure to food antigens provokes an immune reaction in an infant, the type of which depends on the age at introduction and the quantity and frequency of doses.[12] In one study,[13] the exclusively breast-fed infants with symptoms of CMA were all exposed to CM at maternity hospital, whereas in another study,[14] early exposure to CM reduced the emergence of allergic diseases during the first 18 months. Infrequent exposure to small amounts of food antigen has been associated with the development of specific IgE-response.[15,16]

2.   OBJECTIVE

We sought to study prospectively:

(1)   Whether feeding newborn infants CM formula at maternity hospital increases the risk of CMA and could the risk be reduced by feeding them pasteurized human milk or extensively hydorolyzed formula.[17]

(2)   The effects of breast- and formula feeding on the subsequent type of CMA classified by the presence or absence of CM-specific IgE antibodies.[18]

(3)   The importance of immune factors present in breast milk on the development of CMA and on the immune responses of allergic infants to the proteins in CM.[19]

3.   METHODS

3.1   Patients

We followed prospectively 6209 healthy, full-term infants, whose mothers volunteered to participate to the study immediately after delivery.[17] Although breast-feeding was strongly encouraged in the 3 hospitals, 5385 (87%) of the infants required supplementary milk at hospital. According to the month of birth and delivery hospital, these infants were randomly assigned to receive blindly one of 3 study supplements: liquid CM formula (Tutteli; Valio, Finland); pasteurized human milk (a mixture of milk from multiple donors expressed 1 to 6 months after delivery); and extensively hydrolysed whey formula (Pepti-Junior®, Nutricia, The Netherlands). The comparison group comprised 824 exclusively breast-fed infants. The infants were kept in the hospital for a mean of 4 days. When at home, the mothers recorded the infant-feeding regimen daily during the first 8 weeks. They were advised to supplement breast-feeding with CM formula when required and start solid foods at 4 to 6 months of ages. Data on infant feeding were recorded also at the ages of 6 and 12 months. The mothers were given written information about symptoms suggestive of CMA and advised to call on of the authors (KMS) if an infant had any of such symptoms. The diagnosis of CMA was based on typical symptoms (urticaria, exanthema, atopic dermatitis, vomiting, diarrhoea, wheezing, or allergic rhinitis), their disappearance after CM elimination and a recurrence in a challenge test with CM at hospital. Of the 247 challenges performed, 118 (48%) were positive. In addition to these, CMA was diagnosed elsewhere in 81 infants. These infants are, however, excluded from the following analyses due to possible heterogeneity in diagnostic criteria. The data on atopic heredity was recorded at maternity hospital. Obvious atopy was defined as asthma or symptoms from 2 different organs in 1 or both parents.

3.2   Immune responses of infants with CMA

Before the CM challenge test, a skin prick test with liquid CM formula was performed and a blood sample drawn.[18] Serum total and CM-specific IgE were measured by the Pharmacia CAP system (Pharmacia & Upjohn Diagnostics, Uppsala, Sweden). For classification as IgE-mediated reactions, a weal diameter $\geq$ 3 mm in skin prick test or values of CM-specific IgE $\geq$ 0.7 kU/L were taken as positive responses. Serum IgA was measured by an immunoturbidometric method, IgG and IgA antibodies to whole CM, β-lactoglobulin and α-casein by means of an ELISA.[19,20] Proliferation tests of peripheral blood mononuclear cells with CM antigens were performed randomly on 54 infants with CMA as described earlier.[21] Proliferation was expressed as a stimulation index (SI): median counts per minute incorporated in the presence of the antigen divided by median counts per minute incorporated in the absence of the antigen.

3.3   Breast milk samples

We had a sample of colostrum from 108 mothers of the 118 infants with CMA, 207 control samples were randomly selected from mothers of infants without CMA. Total IgA was measured by an immunoturbidometric method. An ELISA assay was used to measure the concentrations of CM-specific IgA, interferon-gamma (IFN-γ), interleukin-6 (IL-6) and transforming growth factor-beta1 (TGF-β1).[19] The detection level of the assay for IFN-γ was 150 pg/mL, for IL-6 50 pg/mL and for TGF-β1 60 pg/mL.

3.4   Statistical analyses

The data are presented with mean and 95% confidence intervals (CI) or range. The data with skewed distribution were analysed after logarithmic transformation. Pearson's chi square test, Student's *t* test and ANOVA were used in statistical comparisons. Multivariate logistic regression model was used to analyse the independent contribution of factors to the events studied and presented with odds ratios (OR) and 95% CI. Correlations were calculated by using the Spearman's rank correlation test.

4. RESULTS

The CM challenge was positive in 118 infants at a mean (range) age of 6.7 (2.8-12.7) months giving a cumulative incidence of 1.9 % in the present cohort. In the whey hydrolysate group fewer infants developed CMA than in the CM group (Table 1). In the pasteurized human milk group there was a similar trend. The exclusively breast-fed infants and those exposed to CM were at similar risk.

Table 1. Cumulative Incidence of CMA and ORs for the Risk of CMA according to Feeding Group at Maternity Hospital
Infants with CMA

Feeding Group (N tot)	N (%)	OR (95% CI)
CM formula (1758)	43 (2.4)	1.0
Pasteurized human milk (1844)	32 (1.7)	0.70 (0.44-1.12)
Whey hydrolysate formula (1715)	26 (1.5)	0.61 (0.38-1.00)
Own mother's milk (811)	17 (2.1)	0.85 (0.48-1.51)

During the first 8 weeks of life, 54% of the allergic infants and 55% of the tolerant infants in the randomised groups had been exposed to CM at home compared with only 6% and 20% in the comparison group, respectively. The percentage of allergic infants with a history of obvious parental atopy was almost double that of tolerant infants: 36% vs 19%. In the 4 groups of allergic infants the prevalence was similar: 33%, 38%, 35%, 47% in the CM, pasteurized human milk, whey hydrolysate and comparison groups, respectively. Among the tolerant infants respective figures were: 18%, 19%, 20% and 19%. Among the infants given supplementary feedings at hospital, significant risk factors for CMA were exposure to CM at hospital (OR 1.54, 1.04-2.30) and a positive atopic heredity (OR 2.32, 1.53-3.52).

At challenge, 75 (64%) infants showed IgE-mediated and 43 (36%) non-IgE-mediated response to CM. Of the IgE-positive infants, 68% reacted within 2 hours compared with 16% in the non-IgE-mediated group. The IgE-positive infants had more often urticaria (76% vs 9%), but less frequently atopic dermatitis (28% vs 72%), vomiting (9% vs 30%), diarrhoea (0% vs 23%) and wheezing (1% vs 14%) than those with non-IgE-mediated reaction. During the first 8 weeks at home, the infants with IgE-mediated reaction were exposed to CM less frequently and those who were exposed were given smaller amounts of CM during a shorter period (Table 2). They were breast-fed longer, and greater percentage of them had symptoms suggestive of CMA during exclusive breast-feeding. Of the 50 infants showing symptoms during exclusive breast-feeding, 18 were given CM at hospital. Thus 32 infants were sensitised during exclusive breast-feeding.

Table 2. Infant Formula and Breast-feeding Patterns in the IgE-Positive and IgE–Negative Groups
CMA

Feeding Pattern	IgE-mediated	Non-IgE-mediated
CM formula exposure at maternity hospital	41%	28%
CM formula exposure at home <8 weeks of age	40%	61%*
-duration of exposure (wk)	1.3 (0.8-2.0)	4.0 (2.9-5.5)**
- daily dose / infant (mL)	40 (30-70)	150 (100-240)**
- total volume/infant (mL)	400 (210-770)	4280 (2100-8750)**
Symptoms during exclusive breast-feeding	49%	30%*
Total breast-feeding (mo)	8.4 (7.8-9.1)	4.5 (3.5-5.7)**

*p<0.05 **p<0.001

Significant risk factors for the development of IgE-mediated CMA were: exposure to CM at hospital (OR 3.5, 1.2-10.1), breast-feeding during the first 8 weeks at home either exclusively (OR 5.1, 1.6-16.4) or combined with infrequent exposure to small amounts of CM (OR 5.7, 1.5-21.6), and long breast-feeding (OR 3.9, 1.6-9.8). The prevalence of parental atopy was similar in the IgE-positive and IgE-negative groups: 33% and 42%, respectively.

The mean concentrations of IgA and milk-specific IgA were similar in colostrum samples from mothers of infants with IgE-mediated and non-IgE-mediated CMA and also from control subjects (Table 3). IFN-γ could be measured only in 27% and IL-6 only in 48% of samples. For both IFN-γ and IL-6, the mean levels of samples with values above the detection level were similar in the study groups and the CIs for these samples were wide (data not shown). The mean concentration of TGF-β1 in colostrum of mothers of infants with IgE-mediated CMA was significantly lower than in samples from mothers of infants with non-IgE-mediated CMA (t=2.57, p=0.012; Table 3). The level of TGF-β1 in control samples was between the 2 groups of allergic infants and did not differ from either group.

Table 3. Mean (95% CI) Concentrations of IgA, Milk-Specific IgA and TGF-β1 in Colostrum Samples of Mothers of Infants with CMA and From Control Mothers [Number of samples]

Mothers of infants with	IgA, g/L	IgA CM antibodies, AU*	TGF-β1, pg/mL**
IgE-mediated CMA	2.4 (2.3-2.4) [69]	188 (103-342) [68]	589 (413-840) [65]
Non-IgE-mediated CMA	2.0 (1.5-2.8) [39]	114 (50-261) [38]	1162 (881-1531) [37]
Control subjects	2.1 (1.9-2.4) [207]	207 (160-269) [203]	807 (677-963) [126]

*AU = Arbitrary units. **p = 0.015, ANOVA.

The concentration of TGF-β1 in colostrum significantly correlated with the serum antibody levels of IgA to β-lactoglobulin (r=0.204, p=0.04), IgG to α-casein (r=0.237, p=0.02), IgG to CM (r=0.240, p=0.02), diameters of the skin prick test responses with CM (r=-0.228, p=0.02) and SI's to α-casein (r=-0.282, p=0.04) and β-lactoglobulin (r=-0.347, p=0.01) measured from infants with CMA at the time of the challenge. Of the 315 mothers, 19% had obvious atopy. Maternal atopy had no influence on any of the parameters measured from colostrum

5.   CONCLUSIONS

In this prospective study we show that in an unselected group of 6209 healthy, full-term infants exposure to CM while in the maternity hospital increases the risk of subsequent CMA, but exclusive breast-feeding did not reduce it.[17] The adverse effects of early exposure to CM may derive from the higher permeability of the immature gastrointestinal tract of newborn infants to macromolecules.[22] As suggested earlier, a positive atopic heredity was another significant risk factor for CMA.[1] More surprisingly, the exclusively breast-fed infants were at similar risk than those exposed to CM. Similarly, in a recent study newborn infants exposed to CM or placebo in addition to breast-feeding during the first 3 days had similar percentage of allergic diseases at 0 to 2 years. In contrast, in an earlier study, none of the 210 infants who were exclusively breast-fed at hospital developed CMA.[13] In the present study, all but one of the allergic infants in the comparison group were exclusively breast-fed for at least the first 8 weeks. The non-randomised comparison group was formed on the basis of mother's ability to fully breast-fed her infant while in hospital. They were more often non-smokers and multiparous (data not shown), factors associated with reduced risk of atopic diseases.[1,23] However, a know risk factor, a positive atopic heredity, was not more prevalent in the comparison group. The small amounts of food antigen present in breast milk may elicit a specific IgE-response in exclusively breast-fed infants,[7] and the emergence of food allergies was reduced when both the nursing mother and her infant avoided CM.[24]

Feeding of whey hydrolysate formula at hospital reduced the risk of CMA. In earlier studies on infants at high risk for atopic diseases feeding with extensively hydrolysed formula for several months after birth has reduced the incidence of food allergies.[24-26] Our study shows that the extensively hydrolysed formula was at least as good in preventing CMA as pasteurized human milk.

We also found that differences in infant feeding patterns modulate the subsequent immune response to CM in infants prone to CMA.[18] Breast-feeding exclusively or combined with infrequent exposure to small amounts of CM during the first 8 weeks of life was associated with the development of specific IgE-response, whereas the infants with non-IgE-mediated CMA had been given larger volumes of CM more frequently. Similar effect of antigen load on the milk-specific IgE response has been described.[15] Also, in animal studies small oral doses of food antigen stimulated IgE production,[16] whereas the specific IgE response was the more suppressed the larger the antigen dose.[27] Of the 50 infants having their first symptoms during exclusive breast-feeding, 18 had been exposed to CM at hospital. Thus, 32 infants were probably sensitised to CM proteins present in breast milk.[6] Our results suggest that CM proteins in breast milk are capable of both sensitising and triggering the allergic immune reaction to CM.

This is the first study to show that TGF-β1 in colostrum may have a significant effect on CM-specific immune responses in infants with CMA.[19] Low content of TGF-β1 was associated with more vigorous IgE-response and proliferation of lymphocytes to CM proteins. On the other hand, TGF-β1 in colostrum positively correlated with the antibody levels of IgA to β-lactoglobulin and IgG to α-casein and CM measured from the sera of the infants with CMA. The function of TGF-β1 in human milk is still vague. Homozygous TGF-β1 null mice die of devastating autoimmune disease soon after weaning, probably having been rescued until that age by transfer of maternal TGF-β1 across the placenta and in the mothers' milk.[28] TGF-β1 strongly inhibits the proliferation of T cells.[29] This is also suggested by our findings of reduced proliferation of lymphocytes to CM proteins in infants with CMA of mothers having high concentration of TGF-β1 in colostrum. The level of TGF-β1 did not differ between patient groups and control subjects suggesting that low level of TGF-β1 is not the sole factor predisposing to CMA. We found that low content of TGF-β1 promotes the development of IgE-response, but at higher levels other types of abnormal immune reactions prevail. This is in accord with the role of TGF-β in the class switch of immunoglobulins; it directs switching to IgA[30] and inhibits IgE switching.[31]

In conclusion, early feeding with CM increases the risk of CMA, but exclusive breast-feeding does not reduce the risk. Differences in infant breast and CM formula feeding influence the subsequent type of CMA, and also, TGF-β1 in colostrum modulates the immune responses of infants prone to developing CMA.

REFERENCES

1. Zeiger RS 1990 Prevention of food allergy in infancy. Ann Allergy 65:430-42
2. Hanson LÅ, Ahlstedt S, Andersson B, Carlsson B, Fällström SP, Mellander L, et al. 1985 Protective factors in milk and the development of the immune system. Pediatrics 75:172-6
3. Eglinton BA, Roberton DM, Cummins AG. 1994 Phenotype of T cells, their soluble receptor levels, and cytokine profile of human breast milk. Immunol Cell Biol 72:306-13
4. Savilahti E, Tainio VM, Salmenperä L, Arjomaa P, Kallio M, Perheentupa J, et al. 1991 Low colostral IgA associated with cow's milk allergy. Acta Paediatr Scand 80:1207-13
5. Machtinger S, Moss R. 1986 Cow's milk allergy in breast-fed infants: The role of allergen and maternal secretory IgA antibody. J Allergy Clin Immunol 77:341-47
6. Axelsson I, Jakobsson I, Lindberg T, Benediktsson B. 1986 Bovine β-lactoglobulin in the human milk. A longitudinal study during the whole lactation period. Acta Paediatr Scand 75:702-7
7. Hattevig G, Kjellman B, Sigurs N, Grodzinsky E, Hed J, Björkstén B. 1990 The effect of maternal avoidance of eggs, cow's milk, and fish during lactation on the development of IgE, IgG, and IgA antibodies in infants. J Allergy Clin Immunol 85:108-15
8. Isolauri E, Tahvanainen A, Peltola T, Arvola T. 1999 Breast-feeding of allergic infants. J Pediatr 134:27-32
9. Hawkes JS, Bryan DL, James MJ, Gibson RA. 1999 Cytokines (IL-1 beta, IL-6, TNF-α, TGF-β1, and TGF-β2) and prostaglandin E-2 in human milk during the first three months postpartum. Pediatr Res 46:194-9
10. Saito S, Yoshida M, Ichijo M, Ishizaka S, Tsujii T. 1993 Transforming growth factor-beta (TGF-β) in human milk. Clin Exp Immunol 94:220-4
11. Srivastava MD, Srivastava A, Brouhard B, Saneto R, Groh-Wargo S, Kubit J. 1996 Cytokines in human milk. Res Commun Mol Pathol Pharmacol 93:263-87
12. Hanson LÅ, Dahlman-Höglund A, Lundin S, Karlsson M, Dahlgren U, Ahlstedt S, et al. 1996 The maturation of the immune system. Monogr Allergy 32:10-5
13. Hρst A, Husby S, Θsterballe O. 1988 A prospective study of cow's milk allergy in exclusively breast-fed infants. Acta Paediatr Scand 77:663-70
14. Lindfors A, Enocksson E. 1988 Development of atopic disease after early administration of cow milk formula. Allergy 43:11-6
15. Firer MA, Hosking CS, Hill DJ. 1981 Effect of antigen load on development of milk antibodies in infants allergic to milk. BMJ 283:693-6
16. Jarrett EE. Perinatal influences on IgE responses. 1984 Lancet 2:797-9
17. Saarinen KM, Juntunen-Backman K, Järvenpää A-L, Kuitunen P, Lope L, Renlund M, et al. 1999 Supplementary feeding in maternity hospitals and the risk of cow's milk allergy:A prospective study of 6209 infants. J Allergy Clin Immunol 104:457-61
18. Saarinen KM, Savilahti E. 2000 Infant feeding patterns affect the subsequent immunological features in cow's milk allergy. Clin Exp Allergy; *in press.*
19. Saarinen KM, Vaarala O, Klemetti P, Savilahti E. 1999 Transforming growth factor-β1 in mothers' colostrum and immune responses to cows' milk proteins in infants with cows' milk allergy. J Allergy Clin Immunol 104:1093-8
20. Savilahti E, Saukkonen T, Virtala E, Tuomilehto J, Åkerblom HK. 1993 Increased levels of cow's milk and β-lactoglobulin antibodies in young children with newly diagnosed IDDM. Diabetes Care 16:984-9
21. Vaarala O, Klemetti P, Savilahti E, Reijonen H, Ilonen J, Åkerblom HK. 1996 Cellular immune response to cow's milk β-lactoglobulin in patients with newly diagnosed IDDM. Diabetes 45:178-82

22. Kuitunen M, Savilahti E, Sarnesto A. 1994 Human α-lactalbumin and bovine β-lactoglobulin absorption in infants. Allergy 49:354-60
23. Strachan D. 1996 Socioeconomic factors and the development of allergy. Toxicol Lett 86:199-203
24. Zeiger RS, Heller S. 1995 The development and prediction of atopy in high-risk children: follow-up at age seven years in a prospective randomized study of combined maternal and infant food allergen avoidance. J Allergy Clin Immunol 95:1179-90
25. Chandra RK, Puri S, Hamed A. 1989 Influence of maternal diet during lactation and use of formula feeds on development of atopic eczema in high risk infants. BMJ 299:228-30
26. Halken S, Hρst A, Hansen LG, θsterballe O. 1992 Effect of an allergy prevention programme on incidence of atopic symptoms in infancy. A prospective study of 159 "high-risk" infants. Allergy 47:545-53
27. Fritsché R, Pahud JJ, Pecquet S, Pfeifer A. 1997 Induction of systemic immunologic tolerance to β-lactoglobulin by oral administration of a whey protein hydrolysate. J Allergy Clin Immunol 100:266-73
28. Letterio JJ, Geiser AG, Kulkarni AB, Roche NS, Sporn MB, Roberts AB. 1994 Maternal rescue of transforming growth factor-β1 null mice. Science 264:1936-8
29. Ahuja SS, Paliogianni F, Yamada H, Balow JE, Boumpas DT. 1993 Effect of transforming growth factor-β on early and late activation events in human T cells. J Immunol 150:3109-18
30. Ehrhardt RO, Strober W, Harriman GR. 1992 Effect of transforming growth factor (TGF)-β1 on IgA isotype expression. TGF-β1 induces a small increase in sIgA+ B cells regardless of the method of B cell activation. J Immunol 148:3830-6
31. Stavnezer J. 1995 Regulation of antibody production and class switching by TGF-β. J Immunol 155:1647-51

11

MATERIAL ASTHMA STATUS ALTERS RELATION OF INFANT FEEDING TO ASTHMA CHILDHOOD

[1,2] Anne L. Wright, PhD, [1,2] Catharine J. Holberg, PHD, [3]Lynn M. Taussig, M.D, and [1,2] Fernando Martinez, MD
1. Respiratory Sciences Center, University of Arizona, Tucson, AZ; 2. Department of Pediatrics and Steele Memorial Children's Research Center, University of Arizona, Tucson, AZ; 3. National Jewish Medical and Research Center, Denver CO

Key words: Asthma, breastfeeding, infant feeding practices, wheezing, childhood, epidemiology

Abstract: The relation of infant feeding to childhood asthma is controversial. This study tested the hypothesis that maternal asthma alters the relation of breastfeeding to childhood asthma. Questionnaires were completed at age 6, 9 or 11 years by parents of 1043 children enrolled at birth. Active MD asthma was defined as a physician diagnosis of asthma plus asthma symptoms reported on one of the questionnaires. Duration of exclusive breastfeeding, categorized as never, <4 months, or ≥4 months, was based on prospective physician reports or questionnaires completed at 18 months. The relationship between breastfeeding and asthma differed by maternal asthma status. For children with maternal asthma, the percent developing active MD asthma increased significantly with longer duration of exclusive breastfeeding. Odds of developing asthma among these children were significantly elevated (OR: 5.7,CI: 2.8-11.5), after adjusting for confounders. This association of longer exclusive breastfeeding with increased risk of reported asthma among children with asthmatic mothers may be biologically based, or may reflect reporting biases.

1. INTRODUCTION

It is well known that breastfeeding is associated with lower rates of wheezing illnesses in infancy and perhaps beyond.[1-3] However, the literature

Short and Long Term Effects of Breast Feeding on Child Health
Edited by Berthold Koletzko *et al.*, Kluwer Academic/Plenum Publishers, 2000

on the relation between infant feeding practices and the development of childhood asthma is conflicting.[4-6] Studies have assessed the association between feeding and asthma after adjusting for *parental* history of allergy, to control for confounders and to determine whether allergic predisposition might alter the relationship. However, given the well-documented individual variability in milk composition, it is plausible that the milk of asthmatic mothers may differ from that of nonasthmatic mothers. Thus, adjustment by *maternal* asthma might reveal differential effects of breastfeeding on the development of asthma.

2.   OBJECTIVE

This study tested the hypothesis that maternal asthma alters the relation of breastfeeding to childhood asthma.

3.   METHODS

3.1   Study Design

Data for this report came from the Tucson Children's Respiratory Study (CRS), a prospective longitudinal study of risk factors for the development of asthma in childhood. Healthy newborns (n=1246) and their families, not selected for allergy history, were enrolled at birth from 1980-1984.[7] Data on parental characteristics (ethnicity, education, physician diagnosed asthma, smoking) was obtained by questionnaire at enrollment. Infant feeding information was obtained prospectively, from forms completed by physicians at well child visits, and retrospectively, from parent completed questionnaires when the child was 1.6 years old. Prospective data were given priority. Children were categorized with regard to duration of <u>exclusive</u> breastfeeding (never breastfed, breastfed exclusively <4 months, breastfed exclusively ≥4 months).

3.2   Questionnaires and Analyses

Parents were asked by questionnaire at ages 6, 9, and 11 years whether a doctor had ever said that the child had asthma, and whether the child wheezed in the past year. Children were considered to have active MD asthma if the parents reported that a physician had diagnosed asthma in the child *and* that the child had asthma symptoms and/or wheezing on one or more of these questionnaires. Relations between feeding history and asthma in the child were assessed bivariately and then stratified by maternal asthma status. The chi square test for homogeneity of odds ratios was used to determine if the effect of feeding differed between maternal strata.[8] Logistic regression was used to assess whether the relation persisted, after adjusting for potential confounders.

4.   RESULTS

4.1   Active MD asthma and infant feeding status

There was no significant relationship between active MD asthma by age 11 and duration of exclusive breastfeeding, as seen in Table 1. However, the association between feeding and asthma differed by maternal asthma status. For children with non-asthmatic mothers, the percent with active MD asthma by age 11 was unrelated to duration of breastfeeding. In contrast, among children with maternal asthma, there was a direct relation between duration of breastfeeding and asthma, with 9%, 36%, and 57% developing asthma, for those starting formula at birth (n=11), in the first 3 months of life (n=53), and after 4 months (n=37, trend $\chi^2 = 8.9$, p<.005), respectively. The association of breastfeeding and asthma in the child differed significantly by maternal asthma status (χ^2 for homogeneity 4.9, p<.01), indicating effect modification by maternal asthma. Presence of asthma in the father did not similarly alter the relation between breastfeeding and asthma. These relationships did not appear to be confounded by the severity of maternal asthma, since breastfed children in all maternal asthma groups appear to have more asthma.

Table 1. Percent (n) with active MD asthma at age 6, 9 or 11 by duration of exclusive breastfeeding, and stratified by maternal and paternal asthma status

	Total	Never BF	Exclusive BF <4mo.	Exclusive BF ≥4 mo.
Total group	20.8%(904)	17.6%(142)	20.4%(441)	22.7%(321)
Maternal asthma*	40.6%(101)	9.1% (11)	35.8% (53)	56.8% (37)
No maternal asthma	18.3%(792)	17.3%(127)	18.5%(384)	18.5% (281)

| Paternal asthma | 30.3%(109) | 26.1% (23) | 26.5% (49) | 37.8% (37) |
| No paternal asthma | 19.5%(704) | 16.4%(110) | 19.2%(364) | 21.1%(270) |

(*p<.01, trend chi square p<.005)

4.2   Multivariate analyses

The relations between feeding and active MD asthma were further analyzed using logistic regression (n=875;177 asthmatics). Since maternal asthma altered the relationships shown, feeding status was entered into the logistic model in interaction terms with maternal asthma. Odds of active MD asthma were calculated for three groups of children (see below) compared to children not exclusively breastfed $\geq$4 months whose mothers did not have asthma. Maternal education, maternal smoking in the first year of life, gender, and ethnicity were also included as possible confounders. Odds of developing MD asthma were: 5.7 [2.8 – 11.5, p<0.001] for those exclusively breastfed $\geq$4 mos. with asthmatic mothers; 2.0 [1.1 – 3.6, p<.05] for those exclusively breastfed $\geq$4 mos. by non-asthmatic mothers; and 1.0 [0.7 – 1.5] for those not exclusively breastfed $\geq$4 mos.

5.   CONCLUSIONS

This analysis suggests that maternal asthma status alters the relation of breastfeeding to the development of asthma in childhood. Among children of asthmatic mothers, longer exclusive breastfeeding was found to be associated with a higher risk of asthma; asthma was unrelated to feeding status for children who lacked maternal asthma.

Whether breastfeeding protects against asthma has been long debated.[9] Most studies which find an apparent protective effect of breastfeeding assessed "asthma" in early childhood.[4] Thus, these studies only validate the well-documented protective effect of breastfeeding against early wheezing illnesses. [1,2,10]   Other studies which found a protective effect failed to adjust for confounders,[9] and most lack objective confirmation of asthma such as IgE levels, making it difficult to minimize the effect of recall bias. Further, non-breastfed infants in earlier studies often received cows' milk, meats and other foods in the first months of life,[11] which might have increased their allergic symptoms. Larger population based studies[5,6] find no relation between breastfeeding and asthma, but results were not adjusted by maternal asthma status.

The finding of a different relation of breastfeeding to asthma in the child depending on maternal asthma status is consistent with our observations reported elsewhere[12] that the association between breastfeeding and total serum IgE in the child depends on maternal IgE level: IgE was elevated in children of mothers with high IgE *only* if they are breastfed, whereas IgE was lower in children of mothers with lower IgE *only* if they were breastfed.

If the association reported here is biologically based, as suggested by the IgE relationships, it may be explained in two ways.   First, the milk of allergic mothers may differ from milk of nonallergic mothers in ways that affect subsequent allergic susceptibility. The presence of allergens or allergen-specific antigens, as well as cytokine profiles, may differ by maternal atopic status, but this has not, to our knowledge, been studied. Differences have been found[13] in the levels of long chain polyunsaturated fatty acid levels in the milk of atopic vs. nonatopic mothers. *In vitro* experiments by Allardyce and Wilson[14] showed that cord blood lymphocytes stimulated with supernatants from milk of atopic mothers were significantly more likely to produce IgE than were lymphocytes stimulated with supernatants from nonatopic mothers. It is unknown, however, what components of milk were responsible for the observed effect.

The second speculation is that breastfeeding alters some other outcome in the infant, which in turn affects susceptibility to asthma.   It has been hypothesized[15] that one cause of the worldwide increase in asthma may be a decline in infectious illness through improved sanitation, and the use of antibiotics.   Breastfeeding is both protective against a wide range of infections,[2,16] and exclusively breastfed infants have lower levels of gram negative enterobacteria in their gastrointestinal tract.[17] While beneficial with regard to infant illness, these consequences of breastfeeding may reduce the stimulus for maturation of dendritic cells, thereby attenuating or delaying the Th1 response,[18] particularly among infants genetically predisposed to asthma.

However, it is also possible that the relationship between breastfeeding and asthma in children of asthmatic mothers results from reporting bias. Asthmatic mothers who breastfeed may behave differently from asthmatic mothers who do not in ways which affect their child's risk of reported asthma. For example, they may be more likely to seek medical attention for wheeze in their child, they may be more likely to remember a diagnosis of asthma, or they may differ with regard to use of asthma medications during pregnancy. It is also impossible to differentiate shared exposures between breastfed infants and their mothers, from potential differences in milk. The observation of a similar pattern with IgE suggests a biological base, and analyses adjusted for potential confounders.   Nevertheless, it is possible that either unmeasured confounders or some reporting bias may account for the current findings, particularly given the relatively small number of asthmatic mothers in this population who never breastfed.

From the public health standpoint, it is important to put the finding of lower rates of asthma associated with formula feeding for children with asthmatic mothers into perspective. First, these observations do not apply to the vast majority of mothers who do not have asthma. If the relation of breastfeeding to asthma in children of asthmatic mothers is substantiated by other studies, those effects would need to be weighed against the many other health benefits[19] associated with breastfeeding, including optimal nutrition, protection against infection, long term benefits and potential cognitive advantages, as well as benefits for maternal health.

6.   ACKNOWLEDGMENTS

The authors are indebted to the study nurses, Marilyn Smith, RN and Lydia De La Ossa, RN; to Bruce Saul MS and Debra Stern, MS, for technical assistance.   This study was funded through NHLBI grants HL14136 and RO1 HL56177.

REFERENCES

1. Wright A.L., Holberg C.J., Martinez F.D., et al.   1989.   Breastfeeding and lower respiratory tract illness in the first year of life. *Br Med J*; **229**:946-949.
2. Howie P.W., Forsyth J.S., Ogston S.A., et al. 1990. Protective effect of breastfeeding against infection. *Br Med J*;**300**:11-16.
3. Wright A.L., Holberg C.J., Taussig L.M., et al. 1995. Relationship of infant feeding to recurrent wheezing at age six. *Arch Pediatr Adolesc Med*;**149**:758-763.
4. Arita M., Mikawa H., Shirataka M., et al. 1997. Epidemiological research on incidence of atopic disease in infants and children in relation to their nutrition in infancy; English abstract. *Arerugi-Japanese Journal Allergology*;**46**:354-69.
5. Wjst M., Dold S., Reitmeier P., et al. 1992. Does breast feeding prevent asthma and allergies?   Results of the Munich asthma and allergy study.   *Monatsschrift Kinderheilkunde*;**140**:769-74.
6. Lewis S., Butland B., Strachan D., et al. 1996. Study of the aetiology of wheezing illnesses at age 16 in two national British birth cohorts. *Thorax*;**51**:670-676.
7. Taussig L.M., Wright A.L., Harrison H.R., et al.   1989.   The Tucson Children's Respiratory Study (I): Design and implementation of a prospective study of acute and chronic respiratory illness in children. *Am J Epidemiol*;**129**:1219-1231.
8.   Rosner, B. 1994. *Fundamentals of biostatistics.* 4th ed. Duxbury Press, Boston.
9. Kramer, M.S. 1988. Does breast feeding help protect against atopic disease? Biology, methodology and a golden jubilee of controversy. *J Pediatr*;**112**:181-90.
10. Holberg C.J., Wright A.L., Martinez F.D., et al. 1991. Risk factors for respiratory syncytial virus associated LRIs in the first year of life. *Amer J Epidemiol*;**133**:1135-1151.

11. Gruskay, F.L. 1982. Comparison of breast, cow and soy feeding in the prevention of onset of allergic disease: a 15-year prospective study. *Clin Pediatr* 1982;**21**:486-491.
12. Wright A.L., Holberg C.J., Halonen M., et al. 1999. Breastfeeding, maternal IgE and total serum IgE in childhood. *J Allergy Clin Immunol*:104; 589-94.
13. Duchen K., Yu G., Bjorksten B. 1998. Atopic sensitization during the first year of life in relation to long chain polyunsaturated fatty acid levels in human milk. *PediatrRes*;**44**:478-484.
14. Allardyce R.A., Wilson A. 1984. Breast milk cell supernatants from atopic donors stimulate corb blood IgE secretion in vitro. *Clin Allergy*;**14**:259-267.
15. Martinez F.D. 1994. Role of viral infections in the inception of asthma and allergies during childhood: could they be protective? *Thorax*;**49**:1189-91.
16. Cunningham A.S., Jelliffe D.B., Jelliffe E.F.P. 1991. Breastfeeding and health in the 1980s: A global epidemiologic review. *Pediatr*;**118**:659-666.
17. Yoshioka H., Iseki K., Fujita K. 1983. Development and differences of intestinal flora in the neonatal period in breast-fed and bottle-fed infants. *Pediatr*; **72**:317-321.
18. Holt PG, Sly PD, Bjorksten B. Atopic versus infectious diseases in childhood: a question of balance? *Pediatr Allergy Immunol* 1997;**8**:53-58.
19. American Academy of Pediatrics Work Group on Breastfeeding. 1997. Breastfeeding and the use of human milk. *Pediatr*;**100**:1035-1039.

12

DOES BREAST-FEEDING AFFECT THE RISK FOR COELIAC DISEASE?

[a,b]Ivarsson A, [b]Persson LÅ and [a]Hernell O.
Affiliation [a] Department of Clinical Science, Paediatrics and [b] Department of Public Health and Clinical Medicine, Epidemiology, Umeå University, Umeå, Sweden.

Key words: Breast-feeding, Coeliac disease, Epidemiology, Gluten, Prevention

Abstract: Coeliac disease, or permanent gluten sensitive enteropathy, has emerged as a widespread health problem. It is considered an immunological disease, possibly of autoimmune type, albeit strictly dependent on the presence in the diet of wheat gluten and similar proteins from rye and barley. There are reasons to believe that the aetiology of coeliac disease is multifactorial, i.e. that other environmental exposures than the mere presence in the diet of gluten affect the disease process. Our studies have shown that prolonged breast-feeding, or perhaps even more important, ongoing breast-feeding during the period when gluten-containing foods are introduced into the diet, reduce the risk for coeliac disease. The amount of gluten consumed is also of importance in as much as larger amounts of gluten-containing foods increase the risk for coeliac disease, while it still is uncertain if the age for introducing gluten into the diet of infants is important. Thus, a challenging possibility, that need to be further explored, is if the coeliac enteropathy can be postponed, or possibly even prevented for the entire life span, by favourable dietary habits early in life.

1.   INTRODUCTION

Coeliac disease, or permanent gluten sensitive enteropathy, is now recognised as a widespread health problem.[1, 2] This is certainly of concern, because in many countries gluten-containing cereals are an important constituent of the daily diet. Further, if not treated the disease is associated with a number of complications related to malabsorption, e.g. diarrhoea and growth retardation in infancy, and depression, osteoporosis and malignancies later in life. The wide spectrum of symptoms contributes to diagnostic difficulties, and in many countries screening studies have unveiled the fact that the majority of cases are undiagnosed.[3-10] The diagnosis is ascertained by a small intestinal biopsy revealing an enteropathy, which, however, resolves with gluten-free diet.[11] Thus, effective treatment is available.

The aetiology of coeliac disease is not fully understood.[12] Genetic susceptibility is a prerequisite, although the genes involved have not yet been identified. Further, it is considered an immunological disease, possibly of autoimmune type, albeit strictly dependent on wheat gluten and similar proteins from rye and barley. According to one view the disease has a multifactorial aetiology, with additional environmental exposures of importance.[13-15] Such exposures on which research has thus far focused relate to infant feeding, i.e. breast-feeding duration and mode of introducing dietary gluten with respect to age of the infant and amounts given. However, according to another view such environmental exposures merely affect the clinical expression of the disease and not the immunological process resulting in the small intestinal coeliac lesion.[16]

2.   IS COELIAC DISEASE PREVENTABLE?

In the evolution of mankind, cultivation of cereals is a rather recent practice,[17] although cereals have become an important part of the diet. Generally abandoning the use of gluten-containing cereals is therefore unrealistic, even if this would effectively prevent onset of coeliac disease. If environmental exposures, except for the mere consumption of gluten, e.g. infant dietary patterns, do influence development of the small intestinal coeliac lesion, a change in these patterns might have a preventive effect. However, if such exposures only affect the clinical expression of the disease, then except for genetic modification of wheat, rye and barley, secondary prevention is what remains, i.e. treatment with a gluten-free diet after the disease has been diagnosed.

It has been suggested that there is a strong genetic influence in coeliac disease as compared with other immunological diseases such as insulin-dependent diabetes mellitus.[12] This is supported by a considerably increased risk for disease among relatives compared to the general population, e.g. a prevalence for first-degree relatives of 5-10% and a concordance rate of 70% in monozygotic twins. However, usually family members share not only genes but also have a common environment. This is especially true for dietary habits. Therefore, when using the family level to study the potentially causal role of such exposures there is a risk of overestimating the impact of genetics at the expense of environmental exposures.

Mäki et al have demonstrated that there may well be a latency between introduction of gluten into the diet of a genetically susceptible individual and the development of the small intestinal coeliac lesion.[18] They identified individuals, both children and adults, who on a gluten-containing diet had a normal small intestinal mucosa that, with a delay of years, became pathological. This observation may support the view that the disease is precipitated by environmental exposures besides mere presence of gluten in the diet.

Further, abrupt changes in incidence in genetically stable populations, indicate the importance of a change in environmental exposures over time. Recently Sweden experienced a quite unique epidemic of symptomatic childhood coeliac disease.[19-21] From 1985 to 1987 the annual incidence rate in children below two years of age increased fourfold to 198 cases (95% CI 186-210) per 100 000 person years, followed from 1995 and onward by a sharp decline to 51 cases (95% CI 36-70) per 100 000 person years in 1997, i.e. back to the level preceding the increase.[21] Interestingly, in the 1970s a decline in incidence of coeliac disease was observed in England, Scotland and Ireland, and according to some of these studies it was also preceded by a rise.[22-24] However, as these studies are based on symptomatic cases, they do, of course, not constitute definite proof of a change in incidence of the coeliac enteropathy.

In the 1970s Finland experienced a decreased incidence of symptomatic coeliac disease in children below two years of age, which was counteracted by an increased incidence among school children, who had more vague symptoms.[25] In Sweden the decline in incidence in children below two years of age has thus far not been counteracted by any increase in older children, but the observation time is too short to exclude that this will occur. It is noteworthy, however, that during the peak of the Swedish epidemic the cumulative incidence reached 5.0 per 1000 births by four years of age,[21] as compared to Finland with a cumulative incidence of 1.0 per 1000 births and Denmark with 0.14 per 1000 births at sixteen years of age.[25, 26] This could possibly be explained by differences between the populations with regard to genetic predisposition or case ascertainment. However, it might also be an effect of differences in environmental exposures, and if this is so, the proportion of children with possibly preventable disease is larger in Sweden than in neighbouring countries.

In many countries screening studies have revealed that the majority of coeliac disease cases are undiagnosed,[3-10] with a study in Estonia as an exception.[27] Further, the prevalences reported for different countries were surprisingly similar, which is an argument for a strong genetic influence in disease aetiology. However, with the exception of the Italian study,[4] a problem with all these studies is that the prevalence estimates are imprecise, as illustrated by broad confidence limits. Thus, larger studies are needed to exclude - or confirm - differences in prevalence between populations. Interestingly, a recent screening of Saharawi children in Algeria suggested a prevalence of 56 per 1000 (95% CI 42-71),[28] which is considerably higher than all earlier studies. The extent to which this is a result of genetic susceptibility or environmental exposures, respectively, is so far merely a matter of speculation.

3.   BREAST-FEEDING DURATION

Based on observations of coeliac disease patients it was suggested as early as the 1950s that breast-feeding delays onset of the disease,[29] a view later supported by other similar studies.[30, 31]

National ecological studies comparing changes in exposure and disease occurrence over time in groups of individuals considered to be representative of the country's population at large have resulted in contradictory findings. An increase in breast-feeding was suggested as a possible contributing factor in the decline in incidence in England, Scotland and Ireland in the early 1970s.[22-24] In the Netherlands, however, an increase in breast-feeding paralleled a recent increase in incidence.[32] Furthermore, a four-fold increase in incidence in Sweden in the 1980s was paralleled by unchanged breast-feeding habits.[21]

Italian case-referent studies concluded that increased duration of breast-feeding was associated with decreased risk for coeliac symptoms.[33, 34] A protective effect of prolonged breast-feeding was also demonstrated in Swedish case-referent studies by Ivarsson *et al* [14] and Fälth-Magnusson *et al*,[35] but not in a study by Ascher *et al*.[36]

4.   INFANT FORMULAS

A question is whether breast-feeding is protective or if it is early introduction of infant formula that increases the risk for coeliac disease. However, the protective effect of prolonged breast-feeding was also demonstrated in the Swedish setting, where infants were often breast-fed past six months of age.[14, 35]

It has been suggested that a change in infant formulas, from diluted cow's milk to modern, adapted formulas more similar to human milk with regard to protein content and composition, has reduced the risk for coeliac disease. This was suggested with respect to the decline in incidence of childhood coeliac disease in Ireland,[24] and the decrease in incidence of symptomatic disease in young children in Finland.[25] In Sweden no decline in incidence followed the change to adapted formulas.[37]

5. BREAST-FEEDING AND GLUTEN INTRODUCTION

A major finding in the two larger Swedish case-referent studies was the significant protective effect of introducing gluten containing foods while breast-feeding was still ongoing,[14, 35] and in the former study this effect remained after adjustment both for age at introduction of dietary gluten and for quantity of gluten consumed during this period (to be published). In the Swedish family study based on silent disease this was not confirmed.[36] However, the latter study was small (8 cases) and the referents were siblings of the cases, with the risk of matching for dietary habits.

Furthermore, taking our increased knowledge about the immunological impact of breast-milk into account,[38] it is biologically plausible that introduction of dietary gluten while the child is still breast-fed might increase the possibility of developing oral tolerance to gluten.

6. AGE AT INTRODUCTION OF GLUTEN

In the 1950s Dicke *et al* showed that presence of gluten in the diet is a prerequisite for developing coeliac disease.[39] It has been discussed if the age at introduction of gluten into the diet affects the age at which the coeliac enteropathy develops, and, more importantly, if it has an impact on the overall risk of contracting the disease.

Comparing English coeliac disease patients in the 1950s and 1960s, respectively, it was suggested that earlier introduction of dietary gluten resulted in earlier presentation of the disease.[40] However, in clinical studies which also took differences in breast-feeding duration into account, no relation was found between age at introduction of dietary gluten and presentation of disease.[30, 31]

Based on a national ecological approach it was suggested that a later introduction of gluten into the diet of infants may have contributed to the decline in incidence in England, Scotland and Ireland in the 1970s.[22-24] In contrast, postponed introduction of gluten into the diet of infants preceded the increase in incidence in Sweden in the 1980s.[19-21]

Several case-referent studies have reported age at introduction of dietary gluten as a factor of no importance.[33-36] However, our incident case-referent study indicates that introduction of gluten into the diet at five to six months of age may be associated with an increased risk compared to both earlier and later introduction (to be published).

7.   QUANTITY OF DIETARY GLUTEN

Quantity of dietary gluten during infancy as a risk factor for coeliac disease has mainly been investigated by means of international ecological studies. Thus, several countries have been compared with respect to estimated gluten intake in healthy infants and the incidence of the disease.[41-43] A higher intake of wheat gluten was reported for infants in Sweden and Italy, compared to Finland, Denmark and Estonia. Further, the first mentioned countries reported a higher occurrence of coeliac disease than the latter. A report from the Netherlands contradicted this; in spite of a comparatively high intake of dietary gluten the incidence of symptomatic coeliac disease was low.[44] However, a recent screening study revealed that the disease is much more common than previously recognised.[10] Thus, it seems that the Netherlands can also be included among those countries in which a comparison using an ecological approach supports the importance of a larger quantity of dietary gluten as a risk factor for coeliac disease.

The Swedish case-referent study by Fälth-Magnusson *et al* found that the cases were introduced to gluten-containing food by bottle more often than the referents, which presumably contributed a larger amount of gluten.[35] Further, the findings in our case-referent study also support larger amounts of gluten as a risk factor for the disease, irrespective of type of food, i.e. gluten-containing follow-on formula or other foods (to be published).

Moreover, clinical experimental design has also been used as an approach to this question by giving individuals a certain amount of dietary gluten and following the possible effect on the small intestinal mucosa. This has been done in adult volunteers, patients with dermatitis herpetiformis,[45] and in children with diagnosed coeliac disease and treated with a gluten free diet.[46] All these studies reported a dose-related effect on the small intestinal mucosa.

8. WHAT CAN BE LEARNT FROM THE SWEDISH EPIDEMIC?

During the epidemic of symptomatic coeliac disease in children below two years of age the incidence reached levels higher than reported from any other country, and the decline that followed was amazingly abrupt.[21] These conspicuous changes in incidence is indicative of an abrupt increase and decrease, respectively, of one or a few environmental factors influencing a large proportion of Swedish infants.

We analysed this further using an ecological study design, and explored any temporal relationships between changes in early feeding patterns and changes in disease occurrence (Figure). The period of rapidly increasing incidence was preceded by *i)* about half the infants being breast-fed at six months of age, *ii)* a twofold increase in the average daily consumption of the total amount of wheat, rye and barley provided by follow-on formula, and *iii)* a new national recommendation at the end of 1982 to postpone introduction of gluten from four until six months of age. The rapid decline in incidence rate started in 1995, and the period of interest with respect to exposure was characterised by *i)* a continuous increase from 54% to 76% in the proportion of infants still breast-fed at six months of age, *ii)* the average daily consumption of the total amount of wheat, rye and barley from follow-on formula decreasing, starting in 1995, by one third, and *iii)* a change in the national recommendation in the autumn of 1996 to introduction of dietary gluten in smaller amounts from four months of age, preferably while the child is still being breast-fed.

Results based on this ecological approach must, of course, be interpreted with caution, as they are not based on exposure data and disease risk on an individual level. The findings are, however, compatible with the epidemic being a result, at least in part, of a change in and interplay between age at introduction of gluten, amount of gluten given, and whether breast-feeding was ongoing or not when gluten was introduced. Other factor(s) may also have contributed, and the search for these should be encouraged.

9. CONCLUSIONS

Coeliac disease has emerged as a widespread health problem. Genetic susceptibility and presence of gluten in the diet are prerequisites for developing the disease. However, there are some evidence to suggest that the aetiology is multifactorial, with additional environmental exposure of importance.

The search for such exposures has focused on infant dietary patterns. Prolonged breast-feeding, or perhaps even more important, ongoing breast-feeding during the period when gluten-containing foods are introduced into the diet, seems to reduce the risk for coeliac disease. Larger amounts of gluten-containing foods most likely increase the risk for coeliac disease, while it still is uncertain if the age for introducing gluten into the diet of infants is important.

Bringing together knowledge from clinical, epidemiological and experimental studies it seems likely that infant dietary patterns, also besides presence of gluten in the diet, interact with the genetic endowment, resulting in an immunological process which may, or may not, lead to the small intestinal coeliac lesion. Thus, a challenging possibility, that need to be further explored, is if the coeliac enteropathy can be postponed, or possibly even prevented for the entire life span, by favourable dietary habits early in life.

ACKNOWLEDGMENTS

We thank Susanne Walther, administrative assistant, Epidemiology, Department of Public Health and Clinical Medicine, Umeå University. Financial support from the Swedish Council for Forestry and Agricultural Research, the Swedish Foundation for Health Care Sciences and Allergy Research, the Swedish Foundation for Research on Asthma and Allergy, and the Västerbotten County Council is gratefully acknowledged.

REFERENCES

1.   Mäki M, Collin P. Coeliac disease. Lancet 1997; 349: 1755-9.

2.   Murray JA. The widening spectrum of celiac disease. Am. J. Clin. Nutr. 1999; 69: 354-65.

3.   Grodzinsky E, Franzen L, Hed J, Ström M. High prevalence of celiac disease in healthy adults revealed by antigliadin antibodies. Ann. Allergy 1992; 69: 66-70.

4.   Catassi C, Fabiani E, Rätsch IM, Coppa GV, Giorgi PL, Pierdomenico R, Alessandrini S, Iwanejko G. The coeliac iceberg in Italy. A multicentre antigliadin antibodies screening for coeliac disease in school-age subjects. Acta Paediatr. 1996; Suppl 412: 29-35.

5.   Weile B, Grodzinsky E, Skogh T, Jordal R, Cavell B, Krasilnikoff PA. Screening Danish blood donors for antigliadin and antiendomysium antibodies. Acta Paediatr. 1996; Suppl 412: 46.

6. Corazza GR, Andreani ML, Biagi F, Corrao G, Pretolani S, Giulianelli G, Ghironzi G, Gasbarrini G. The smaller size of the "Coeliac Iceberg" in adults. Scand. J. Gastroenterol. 1997; 32: 917-9.

7. Johnston SD, Watson RGP, McMillan SA, Sloan J, Love AHG. Coeliac disease detected by screening is not silent--simply unrecognized. QJM 1998; 91: 853-60.

8. Not T, Horvath K, Hill ID, Partanen J, Hammed A, Magazzu G, Fasano A. Celiac disease risk in the USA: High prevalence of antiendomysium antibodies in healthy blood donors. Scand. J. Gastroenterol. 1998; 33: 494-8.

9. Ivarsson A, Persson LA, Juto P, Peltonen M, Suhr O, Hernell O. High prevalence of undiagnosed coeliac disease in adults: a Swedish population-based study. J. Intern. Med. 1999; 245: 63-8.

10. Csizmadia CGDS, Mearin ML, von Blomberg BME, Brand R, Verloove-Vanhorick SP. An iceberg of childhood coeliac disease in the Netherlands [letter]. Lancet 1999; 353: 813-4.

11. Walker-Smith JA, Guandalini S, Schmitz J, Shmerling DH, Visakorpi JK. Revised criteria for diagnosis of coeliac disease. Report of Working Group of European Society of Paediatric Gastroenterology and Nutrition. Arch. Dis. Child. 1990; 65: 909-11.

12. Sollid LM. Molecular basis of celiac disease. Annu. Rev. Immunol. 2000; 18: 53-81.

13. Logan RFA. Epidemiology of coeliac disease. In: Coeliac disease, editor. Marsh MN. Oxford: Blackwell Scientific Publications; 1992: 192-214.

14. Ivarsson A, Persson LÅ, Hernell O. Risk factors for coeliac disease in childhood: a report from the Swedish multicenter study [ESPGAN abstracts]. J. Pediatr. Gastroenterol. Nutr. 1995; 20: 475.

15. Ferguson A. New perspectives of the pathogenesis of coeliac disease: evolution of a working clinical definition [editorial]. J. Intern. Med. 1996; 240: 315-8.

16. Ascher H, Kristiansson B. The highest incidence of celiac disease in Europe: The Swedish experience. J. Pediatr. Gastroenterol. Nutr. 1997; 24: 3-6.

17. Greco L. Epidemiology of coeliac disease. In: Coeliac disease: Proceedings of the seventh international symposium on coeliac disease, 1996, Tampere, Finland, editor. Mäki M, Collin P, Visakorpi JK. Tampere: Coeliac Disease Study Group; 1997: 9-14.

18. Mäki M, Holm K, Koskimies S, Hällström O, Visakorpi JK. Normal small bowel biopsy followed by coeliac disease. Arch. Dis. Child. 1990; 65: 1137-41.

19. Ascher H, Krantz I, Kristiansson B. Increasing incidence of coeliac disease in Sweden. Arch. Dis. Child. 1991; 66: 608-11.

20. Cavell B, Stenhammar L, Ascher H, Danielsson L, Dannaeus A, Lindberg T, Lindquist B. Increasing incidence of childhood coeliac disease in Sweden. Results of a national study. Acta Paediatr. 1992; 81: 589-92.

21. Ivarsson A, Persson LÅ, Nyström L, Ascher H, Cavell B, Danielsson L, Dannaeus A, Lindberg T, Lindquist B, Stenhammar L, Hernell O. The epidemic of coeliac disease in Swedish children. Acta Paediatr. [In press].

22.   Kelly DA, Phillips AD, Elliott EJ, Dias JA, Walker-Smith JA. Rise and fall of coeliac disease 1960-85. Arch. Dis. Child. 1989; 64: 1157-60.

23.   Logan RFA, Rifkind EA, Busuttil A, Gilmour HM, Ferguson A. Prevalence and "incidence" of celiac disease in Edinburgh and the Lothian region of Scotland. Gastroenterology 1986; 90: 334-42.

24.   Stevens FM, Egan-Mitchell B, Cryan E, McCarthy CF, McNicholl B. Decreasing incidence of coeliac disease. Arch. Dis. Child. 1987; 62: 465-8.

25.   Mäki M, Holm K. Incidence and prevalence of coeliac disease in Tampere: Coeliac disease is not disappearing. Acta Paediatr. Scand. 1990; 79: 980-2.

26.   Weile B, Krasilnikoff PA. Low incidence rates by birth of symptomatic coeliac disease in a Danish population of children. Acta Paediatr. 1992; 81: 394-8.

27.   Uibo O, Uibo R, Kleimola V, Jogi T, Mäki M. Serum IgA anti-gliadin antibodies in an adult population sample. High prevalence without celiac disease. Dig. Dis. Sci. 1993; 38: 2034-7.

28.   Catassi C, Rätsch IM, Gandolfi L, Pratesi R, Fabiani E, El Asmar R, Frijia M, Bearzi I, Vizzoni L. Why is coeliac disease endemic in the people of the Sahara? [letter]. Lancet 1999; 354: 647-8.

29.   Andersen DH, Di Sant'Agnese PA. Idiopathic celiac disease: I. Mode of onset and diagnosis. Pediatrics 1953; 11: 207-22.

30.   Greco L, Mayer M, Grimaldi M, Follo D, De Ritis G, Auricchio S. The effect of early feeding on the onset of symptoms in celiac disease. J. Pediatr. Gastroenterol. Nutr. 1985; 4: 52-5.

31.   Mäki M, Kallonen K, Lähdeaho ML, Visakorpi JK. Changing pattern of childhood coeliac disease in Finland. Acta Paediatr. Scand. 1988; 77: 408-12.

32.   George EK, Mearin ML, Franken HCM, Houwen RHJ, Hirasing RA, Vandenbroucke JP. Twenty years of childhood coeliac disease in the Netherlands: a rapidly increasing incidence? Gut 1997; 40: 61-6.

33.   Auricchio S, Follo D, De Ritis G, Giunta A, Marzorati D, Prampolini L, Ansaldi N, Levi P, Dall'Olio D, Bossi A, Cortinovis I, Marubini E. Does breast feeding protect against the development of clinical symptoms of celiac disease in children? J. Pediatr. Gastroenterol. Nutr. 1983; 2: 428-33.

34.   Greco L, Auricchio S, Mayer M, Grimaldi M. Case control study on nutritional risk factors in celiac disease. J. Pediatr. Gastroenterol. Nutr. 1988; 7: 395-9.

35.   Fälth-Magnusson K, Franzén L, Jansson G, Laurin P, Stenhammar L. Infant feeding history shows distinct differences between Swedish celiac and reference children. Pediatr. Allergy Immunol. 1996; 7: 1-5.

36.   Ascher H, Krantz I, Rydberg L, Nordin P, Kristiansson B. Influence of infant feeding and gluten intake on coeliac disease. Arch. Dis. Child. 1997; 76: 113-7.

37.   Stenhammar L, Ansved P, Jansson G, Jansson U. The incidence of childhood celiac disease in Sweden. J. Pediatr. Gastroenterol. Nutr. 1987; 6: 707-9.

38.   Hanson LA. Breastfeeding provides passive and likely long-lasting active immunity. Ann. Allergy Asthma Immunol. 1998; 81: 523-33.

39. Dicke WK, Weijers HA, Kamer JH. The presence in wheat of a factor having a deleterious effect in cases of coeliac disease. Acta Paediatr. 1953; 42: 34-42.

40. Anderson CM, Gracey M, Burke V. Coeliac disease. Some still controversial aspects. Arch. Dis. Child. 1972; 47: 292-8.

41. Mäki M, Holm K, Ascher H, Greco L. Factors affecting clinical presentation of coeliac disease: Role of type and amount of gluten-containing cereals in the diet. In: Common food intolerances 1: Epidemiology of coeliac disease, editor. Auricchio S, Visakorpi JK. Basel: Karger; 1992: 2: 76-82.

42. Weile B, Cavell B, Nivenius K, Krasilnikoff PA. Striking differences in the incidence of childhood celiac disease between Denmark and Sweden: A plausible explanation. J. Pediatr. Gastroenterol. Nutr. 1995; 21: 64-8.

43. Mitt K, Uibo O. Low cereal intake in Estonian infants: the possible explanation for the low frequency of coeliac disease in Estonia. Eur. J. Clin. Nutr. 1998; 52: 85-8.

44. George EK, Mearin ML, Van der Velde EA, Houwen RHJ, Bouquet J, Gijsbers CFM, Vandenbroucke JP. Low incidence of childhood celiac disease in the Netherlands. Pediatr. Res. 1995; 37: 213-8.

45. Ferguson A, Blackwell JN, Barnetson RS. Effects of additional dietary gluten on the small intestinal mucosa of volunteers and of patients with dermatitis   herpetiformis. Scand. J. Gastroenterol. 1987; 22: 543-9.

46. Catassi C, Rossini M, Ratsch IM, Bearzi I, Santinelli A, Castagnani R, Pisani E, Coppa GV, Giorgi PL. Dose dependent effects of protracted ingestion of small amounts of gliadin in coeliac disease children: a clinical and jejunal morphometric study. Gut 1993; 34: 1515-9

13

BREASTFEEDING AND GROWTH IN RURAL KENYAN TODDLERS

Adelheid Werimo Onyango

Department of Nutrition, World Health Organization, Geneva, Switzerland

Key words: child growth, breastfeeding, complementary feeding, second year, prospective
cohort study

Abstract: Research has not provided unequivocal support for the recommendation to
continue breastfeeding until children reach at least age 24 months. In many
circumstances, breastfeeding duration is chosen or conditioned by factors other
than scientific evidence and recommendations. Even in communities where
breastfeeding into the second year is the norm, a significant number of toddlers
are weaned before the recommended age. The research reported here was
conducted in a rural community of western Kenya. We prospectively followed
a cohort of 264 children for 6 months (mean age at baseline, 14.1 ± 2.4
months) to examine the effect of variable breastfeeding duration on length and
weight gain. We found that breastfeeding was positively associated with
growth in a manner that we inferred to be causal, the effect being stronger on
linear growth than on weight gain. This was despite the fact that in a cohort
where 95% were breastfeeding at baseline, the prevalence of stunting (height-
for-age below −2 standard deviations of the WHO-NCHS reference) was
already 48%. The present paper examines the socioeconomic characteristics,
sanitation, morbidity, and complementary feeding practices that define the
context of this apparently contradictory relationship. The population was poor,
no household had running water, and malaria is endemic in the study area.
Complementary feeding was initiated for 93% of the cohort before age 3
months. The weaning diet was bulky (77% energy from carbohydrate), and
high in phytate content ([phytate]:[zinc] molar ratio, 28). Diet quality, judged
by diversity and animal source food intake, was low. Several micronutrient
intakes were below current recommendations, including riboflavin (63%),
niacin equivalents (64%), calcium (72%), iron (74%) and zinc (33%). Based
on a locally defined socioeconomic status scale, children in higher SES
households were breastfed for a shorter duration than were children from
poorer households. Sanitation and water consumption modified the effect of
breastfeeding duration on growth: the effect was stronger in the absence of a
pit latrine and at low water consumption. Our results support the

recommendation to sustain breastfeeding in the second year, particularly in economically depressed environments with inadequate sanitation and water supplies

1.   INTRODUCTION

Traditional norms rather than scientific recommendations are responsible for the universal initiation of breastfeeding at birth in Marachi Central Location, Busia District in western Kenya. As is the case in the rest of sub-Saharan Africa[1] over 90% of children continue breastfeeding beyond infancy. For a variety of reasons, however, only half of those who survive to their second birthday are likely to be breastfed for the recommended minimum 24 months.[2] Because of the controversy surrounding the cross-sectional association between prolonged breastfeeding and child nutrition,[3-6] we used a prospective cohort design to more rigorously examine the relationship between continued breastfeeding and growth in the second year. If continued breastfeeding negatively influenced growth, then 90% of this young population would be at risk of growth failure through continued breastfeeding. If, on the other hand, it were good for growth throughout the second year, this would need to be established to support the recommendation on prolonged breastfeeding. But whatever the influence might be, other factors that jointly or interactively with breastfeeding affect growth would need to be established for more comprehensive understanding and management of child nutrition in the second year.

2.   METHODS

Children born between 1 May 1994 and 31 January 1995 were identified in a door-to door survey throughout the location. Twins, children who had a congenital malformation, or whose mother intended to leave the study location within the next six months, was mentally unstable or deceased were excluded. Out of 296 children enrolled into the study in November 1995 (baseline), 264 were followed up successfully till May 1996 (final assessment).

Anthropometry was measured at baseline and final assessment to estimate growth in weight and length. Morbidity data were collected by recall in weekly cycles. Food intake data were collected using 24-hour dietary recall interviews administered every three weeks during the study. Demographic and other descriptive information about the household, mother and child was collected in face-to-face interviews at baseline and final assessment. Among the specific factors described were water use, sanitation facilities and socio-economic status. Breastfeeding status was monitored throughout the study. Breast milk intake in a single 24-hour period was estimated in a sample of 50. Observed intakes were regressed on the child's age (months) to estimate the age effect on breast milk consumption. For average breast milk intake in the sample, the regression equation was applied using each child's midpoint age over the period that he/she was breastfeeding. The result was weighted by duration of breastfeeding as percent of time follow-up to estimate average breast milk intake during the observation period. Energy and nutrients in breast milk were estimated on the basis of mature milk composition data from sub-Saharan Africa and India.[7]

Statistical analyses were carried out using SPSS for Windows 95. Multiple linear regression and general linear models were used for multivariate analyses.

3.   RESULTS

3.1   Basic child characteristics and growth

Mean age at baseline was 14.1 months (range, 9-18 mo). Only 14 children (5%) in the final sample (n=264) had been weaned (i.e., stopped breastfeeding) before enrolment into the study and 77 others (29%) were weaned before final assessment. Reported reasons for weaning were pregnancy (30%), to make the child eat other foods (23%), unexplained refusal by the child (13%), maternal or child illness (12%), insufficient milk production (8%), the child considered to be old enough (5%), prolonged separation (5%) and maternal employment (3%).

Based on the WHO-NCHS reference, 48% of children were stunted at baseline with no observed improvement during the follow-up period. The prevalence of underweight (weight-for-age z-score below -2 SD) fell from 37% to 23%, while wasting (below -2 SD weight-for-length) was prevalent in 6% of the sample at baseline and in 3% at final assessment. The average duration of follow-up was 5.6 months, during which children gained an average of 5 cm and 1.3 kg. There was a positive association between the duration of breastfeeding and both weight and length gain.

Table 1. Attained growth and malnutrition prevalence at baseline and final assessment

	Baseline (n=264)	Follow-up (n=264)
Age (months)	14.1 ± 2.4	19.7 ± 2.4
Length (cm)	71.8 ± 3.6	76.7 ± 3.9
Weight (kg)	8.5 ± 1.3	9.9 ± 1.3
Stunting (<-2 LA z-score)	48%	48%
Underweight (<-2 WA z-score)	37%	23%
Wasting (<-2 WH z-score)	6%	3%

3.2   Child morbidity

With free treatment available throughout the study period, the reported incidence and duration of infections may not reflect usual patterns in the population. According to the weekly morbidity recalls, fever was reported for 19% of the observation period. Malaria is endemic in the study area and was the infection for which treatment was most frequently sought at the clinic. Two non-specific signs of infection, namely, reduced activity and reduced food intake due to illness, were reported for 12% and 15% of the observation period, respectively. Upper respiratory infections (mild-moderate cough and nasal discharge, with or without fever) were present 11% of the time, while lower respiratory infections (severe cough or difficulty breathing with or without fever) were reported for a mean 3% of the observation period. Diarrhoea was present 5% of the time and bloody diarrhoea for less than 1%. There was no evidence of significantly increased morbidity when breastfeeding was curtailed, and none of the recorded measures of infection were significantly associated with growth in the sample.

3.3   Child feeding

3.3.1   Complementary feeding

Recall information on the weaning process showed that exclusive breastfeeding was short-lived. Almost 50% of mothers gave their newborns water within the first three days postpartum, and by the end of the first month, over 80% of infants had begun to receive water. The introduction of complementary foods followed a similar pattern (Fig 1). Over two-thirds of children were placed on semisolids within the first month, and by the end of the second month, 85% were receiving complementary food. Less than 3% of the sample maintained exclusive breastfeeding for the recommended minimum four months.

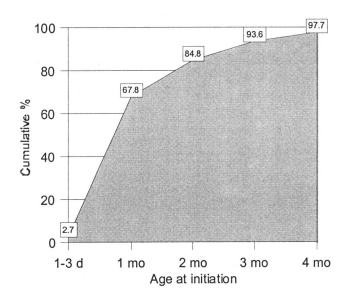

Figure 1. Age at initiation of complementary feeding

Complementary food selection patterns initiated in infancy did not change significantly through the second year. The first complement chosen by more than half the sample (n=149; 56%) was cereal-based gruel. A few mothers (27%) added milk, beans, dried fish, or leguminous seeds to the basic gruel recipe to improve its nutritive value. Other first weaning foods were cow's milk (39%) and fruit (3%). For more than 90% of the sample, gruel was an important component of the daily diet throughout the study. The household staple, *ugali* (a stiff porridge served with meat/vegetables) gained prominence over the observation period, consumed daily by 73% at the start, and by 94% at the end of the study.

Average diversity in children's diets increased only minimally from 6 unique food items (from 4 food groups) at baseline to 7 food items (from 5 food groups) at final assessment. Specific information was collected on the consumption of foods that are indicative of high quality diet. Meat and its animal origin substitutes were regularly consumed by an average 40% of the sample. Fruit was consumed by small but generally increasing proportions of the sample through the study period, from 22% at baseline to 34% at final assessment.

Mean dietary energy intake over the observation period was 718 kcal/d, of which 96 kcal (13%) was obtained from foods of animal origin. Total protein intake averaged 21 g/d while fat and carbohydrate intakes were 11 g/d and 139 g/d, respectively. More than three-quarters (77%) of total dietary energy came from carbohydrate, 14% from fat, and 10% from protein.

Considering the complementary diet alone, percent energy from foods of animal origin and vitamin B_2 intake were each positively associated with linear growth, while increased fat intake was associated positively with both length and weight gain.

3.3.2   Energy and nutrient intakes from breast milk and complementary foods

Estimated energy and nutrient intakes from breast milk and complementary foods were pooled to assess total and per kg body weight consumption. Energy requirements for 1-2 year-old toddlers have been estimated to be 86 kcal/kg/d or 1092 kcal/d,[8] while estimated protein requirements were 160 mg N/kg/d for age 1-1.5 y and 151 mg N/kg/d for 1.5-2 y.[9]

At average energy intake (112 kcal/kg/day), these children were receiving 130% of average daily energy requirements, although per day intake was 93% of the estimated requirement for children in the second year. Average protein intake (308 mg N/kg/d) was also above the upper limit (average requirement + 2 SD) of nitrogen per kg body weight (197%). Other nutrients whose average daily intake was above the estimated requirements were vitamins B_1, B_{12}, and C, folic acid and phosphorus. Nutrients whose mean intakes were below the lower limit of the recommended range were calcium (72%), iron (74%), vitamin A (80%), vitamin B_2 (63%), niacin (64%), and zinc (33%).[10,11]

In multiple regression analyses, energy intake was significantly associated with both measures of growth. It was estimated that at average energy intake (1018 kcal/d), children gained 0.5 cm and 280 g more than those consuming 822 kcal/d, or 1 SD below the sample mean. Neither protein nor carbohydrate intake were significantly associated with growth. On the other hand, fat intake was positively associated with both length and weight gain. Children whose daily fat intake was 1 SD (6.9 g) below the mean gained 0.6 cm and 207 g less than those with mean intakes equal to the sample's daily average. The model with fat explained 18.5% variation in length gain and 13.4% in weight gain, while the one including a measure of average energy intake explained 10.3% and 9.6% variation in length and weight gains, respectively. Vitamin B_2 intake was positively associated with linear growth but not with weight gain, and no other micronutrient was significantly associated with either measure of growth.

3.4 Household water consumption and sanitation

Less than 2% of the study households had piped water. The two most important water sources were hydraulic pumps and natural springs. Most households drank the water without further processing or treatment (n=195, 74%). Those who did strained it with a cloth or sieve (n=39, 15%), boiled (n=20, 8%), or let the water sit in the sun for a few hours before storing it (n=10, 4%). Average household consumption was equivalent to 62 L/d (range, 20-240 L/d) and per capita consumption 10 L/d. Total household water consumption was positively associated with both measures of growth, but when replaced with per capita consumption, these associations were no longer statistically significant.

Three-quarters of households had access to a pit latrine, which had a non-significant positive association with linear growth (β=0.51 cm) in a multiple regression model adjusting for child age, sex and the duration of follow-up. On the other hand, its average relationship with weight gain was negative (β=-150 g). Neither per capita water consumption nor access to a pit latrine was correlated with the duration of breastfeeding. However, in the absence of a latrine, breastfeeding duration had a stronger positive association with linear growth than in opposite conditions. A similar interaction was observed with per capita water use, where the positive association between breastfeeding duration and linear growth was more evident in households with per capita water consumption below 10L/d.

3.5   Socio-economic status

Household income was not measured, but 40% of fathers and 1% of mothers were reported as having paid employment. The majority of the sample depended on petty trade and farming for cash incomes. Of six variables considered to be sensitive markers of wealth in the study population, nearly half of the households owned a bicycle (n=127, 48%); 117 (44%) possessed a radio; and 108 (41%) purchased meat in the week prior to final assessment. Less than one-third of the sample (n=73, 28%) owned a portable stove, 48 mothers owned a watch, and only 41 (16%) used a hurricane lantern for household lighting. These variables were summed to create a socio-economic status (SES) score. The median household in the sample had a score of 2 (range, 0-6).

Children from households with a higher SES score were weaned earlier than those from lower SES households. Each of the six items in the score was examined individually for its relationship with growth. The only factor that had a significant association with a measure of growth was the possession of a bicycle. Children whose parents owned a bicycle gained 0.5 cm more than the comparison group. The other factors individually had non-significant associations with growth. The summated score obtained from all six items was strongly associated with improved linear growth (β=0.20 cm for each additional point on the scale), but not with weight gain (β=10 g) in multivariate analyses. For example, in households with a socio-economic status score 5, average length gain was 1 cm more than the length gained over an equivalent period by children of the same age and gender in households with a score of 0.

4.   DISCUSSION

Despite the fact that 95% of the cohort was breastfeeding, the prevalence of stunting at baseline was 48% and that of underweight 37%. If this were a correlational study, it might be concluded that prolonged breastfeeding was negatively correlated with growth. Multivariate analyses that adjusted for confounding factors showed, however, that continued breastfeeding in the second year was positively associated with length and weight gain in the sample.

One recalls that the recommendation is to breastfeed *exclusively* for at least four months, followed by safe and nutritious foods to complement breast milk from about age six months onwards. More than 90% of children in our sample were placed on complementary foods before they were 3 months old. The nutritional implications of premature initiation of complementary fluids and solid foods in locations like Marachi Central have been reviewed.[12,13] Exposure to infections is increased because of poor sanitation and water supplies, breast milk is replaced by low-quality foods, and it is possible that micronutrient-chelating agents in the complementary foods reduce the bioavailability of iron and zinc in breast milk beginning at this early age. A previous study in this population found a link between stunting and the introduction of cereal-based gruel before age 4 months.[14]

A study in Embu, eastern Kenya, also reported a high prevalence of stunting in the second year with onset dating back to infancy.[15] Apart from low energy density, the typical diets in Embu and Marachi Central had a [phytate]:[zinc] molar ratio of 28.[16] Breast milk intake in our sample reduced this ratio to 24, which is still above the level (15) at which improvement in zinc bioavailability would be expected.[17] Moreover, total zinc intake was only one-third of estimated requirements, and breast milk, being low in zinc at that stage of lactation, could not adequately compensate for the deficiency in the diet.

The weaning diet in Marachi Central had other characteristics that have been associated with reduced growth, such as low intake of animal foods.[18] Low dietary fat intake has been linked with reduced linear growth elsewhere.[19] In our sample, estimated daily energy intake was not severely restricted despite the fact that the proportion of dietary energy obtained from fat was only 14%. Apart from increasing energy density, fat intake may be a marker for an overall higher quality diet, which has also been associated with improved growth.[20] Breast milk in our sample accounted for 61% of overall fat intake.

Low birth size and infections during infancy may also have contributed to the observed levels of malnutrition. However, in the absence of data on either factor, it is impossible to estimate the extent of their influence on the observed rate of malnutrition. Malaria is endemic in the study area and was the problem for which medical care was most frequently sought at the project clinic during the study. Its control may have played a part in improving weight-for-length and weight-for-age during the period of follow-up. Infection was not associated with growth in our study, but others have observed reduced infection with continued breastfeeding in the second year.[21] Other benefits of breastfeeding during acute infections have also been reported.[22-25]

Sanitation and water consumption modified the association between breastfeeding duration and linear growth. Similar effect modification has been reported in the association between breastfeeding and infant mortality.[26] In populations where the water supply is inadequate and basic sanitation lacking, early weaning will very likely compromise growth. It has been shown that increased water usage and improved sanitation have synergistic positive influences on child growth.[27] Apart from making a direct contribution to hygiene, increased water consumption has been associated with frequent meal preparation.[28] If this in turn implies more frequent child feeding, it might explain why increased water consumption was particularly important for children who had stopped breastfeeding.

Socio-economic status was a negative confounder of the association between breastfeeding and linear growth. Children from poorer households had lower weight-for-height and were also breastfed longer than those from higher SES households. Rather than poor malnutrition causing prolonged breastfeeding, it is more likely, as was observed in the Sudan,[29] that economic wellbeing facilitates the choice to stop breastfeeding and also provides for at least close to adequate replacements for breast milk.

5.   CONCLUSION

Given the quality of the typical weaning diet in Marachi Central, neither the high prevalence of malnutrition (underweight and stunting) nor the positive association between breastfeeding and growth is surprising. The list of wealth markers in the community and the low average score on the chosen index suggest that the majority of families could not be expected to afford a nutritious weaning diet to replace breast milk in the second year. On the other hand, interactions between breastfeeding and sanitation suggest that when the former must be curtailed, care should be taken to improve sanitation if the potential negative impact of interrupted breastfeeding is to be attenuated.

ACKNOWLEDGMENTS

This research was supported by grants from the International Development Research Centre (IDRC), Canada, and The Rockefeller Foundation.

REFERENCES

1. Caulfield LE, Bentley ME, Ahmed S. Is prolonged breastfeeding associated with malnutrition? Evidence from nineteen Demographic and Health Surveys. *Int J Epidemiol* 1996;25:693-703.
2. World Health Organization. The World Health Organization's infant feeding recommendation. *Wkly Epidemiol Rec* 1995;70:119-120.

3. Victora CG, Vaughan JP, Martines JC, Barcelos LB. Is prolonged breast feeding associated with malnutrition? *Am J Clin Nutr* 1984;39:307-314.

4. Ng'andu NH, Watts TEE. Child growth and duration of breast feeding in urban Zambia. *J Epidemiol Comm Hlth* 1990;44:281-285.

5. Taren D, Chen J. A positive association between extended breast feeding and nutritional status in rural Hubei Province, People's Republic of China. *Am J Clin Nutr* 1993;58:862-67.

6. Nube M, Asenso-Okyere WK. Large differences in nutritional status between fully weaned and partially breast fed children beyond the age of 12 months. *Euro J Clin Nutr* 1996;50:171-177.

7. Prentice A. Regional variations in the composition of human milk. In Jensen R. G. (Ed) *Handbook of Milk Composition*. New York: Academic Press, 1995.

8. Torun B, Davies PSW, Livingstone MBE, Paolisso M, Sackett R, Spurr GB. Energy requirements and dietary energy recommendations for children and adolescents 1 to 18 years old. *Euro J Clin Nutr*, 1996;50 (Suppl. 1) S37-S81.

9. Dewey KG, Beaton G, Fjeld C, Lonnerdal B, Reeds P. Protein requirements for infants and children. *Euro J Clin Nutr* 1996;50 (Suppl. 1) S119-S150.

10. FAO/WHO. Requirements of Vitamin A, Iron, Folate and Vitamin B_{12}. Report of a Joint FAO/WHO Expert Consultation. *FAO Food and Nutrition Series* No. 23. Rome: FAO, 1988.

11. World Health Organization. *Trace Elements in Human Nutrition*. Geneva: WHO, 1996.

12. Walker AF. The contribution of weaning foods to protein-energy malnutrition. *Nutr Res Rev* 1990;3:25-47.

13. Huffman SL, Martin LH. First feedings: optimal feeding of infants and toddlers. *Nutr Res* 1994;14:127-159.

14. Onyango A, Koski KG, Tucker KL. Food diversity versus breastfeeding choice in determining anthropometric status in rural Kenyan toddlers. *Int J Epidemiol* 1998;27:484-489

15. Neumann CG, Harrison GG. Onset and evolution of stunting in infants and children. Examples from the Human Nutrition Collaborative Research Support Program. Kenya and Egypt studies. *Euro J Clin Nutr* 1994;48 (Suppl. 1):S90-S102.

16. Murphy SP, Beaton GH, Calloway DH. Estimated mineral intakes of toddlers: predicted prevalence of inadequacy in village populations in Egypt, Kenya and Mexico. *Am J Clin Nutr* 1992;56:565-572.

17. Gibson RS. Zinc nutrition in developing countries. *Nutr Res Rev* 1994;7:151-173.

18. Marquis GS, Habicht J-P, Lanata CF, Black RE, Rasmussen KM. Breast milk or animal-product foods improve linear growth of Peruvian toddlers consuming marginal diets. *Am J Clin Nutr* 1997;66:1102-1109.

19. Kaplan RM, Toshima MT. Does a reduced fat diet cause retardation in child growth? *Preventive Medicine* 1992;21:33-52.

20. Allen LH, Backstrand JR, Stanek III EJ, Pelto GH, Chavez A, Molina E, *et al.* The interactive effects of dietary quality on the growth and attained size of young Mexican children. *Am J Clin Nutr* 1992;56:353-364.

21. Molbak K, Jakobsen M, Sodemann M, Aaby P. Is malnutrition associated with prolonged breastfeeding? *Int J Epidemiol* 1997;26:458-59.

22. Hoyle B, Yunus MD, Chen LC. Breast feeding and food intake among children with acute diarrhoeal disease. *Am J Clin Nutr* 1980;33:2365-71.

23. Brown KH, Stallings RY, Creed de Kanashiro H., Lopez de Romana G. & Black R. Effects of common illnesses on infants' energy intakes from breast milk and other foods during longitudinal community-based studies in Huascar (Lima), Peru. *Am J Clin Nutr* 1990;52:1005-13.

24. Launer LJ, Habicht J-P, Kardjati S. Breast feeding protects infants in Indonesia against illness and weight loss due to illness. *Am J Epidemiol* 1990;131:322-31.

25. Dickin KL, Brown K, Fagbule D, *et al.* Effect of diarrhoea on dietary intake by infants and young children in rural villages of Kwara State, Nigeria. *Euro J Clin Nutr* 1990;44:307-17.

26. Butz WP, Habicht J-P, DaVanzo J. Environmental factors in the relationship between breastfeeding and infant mortality: The role of sanitation and water in Malaysia. *Am J Epidemiol* 1984;119:516-525.

27. Esrey SA, Habicht J-P, Casella G. The complementary effect of latrines and increased water usage on the growth of infants in rural Lesotho. *Am J Epidemiol* 1992:135:659-66.

28. Cairncross S, Cliff JL. Water use and health in Mueda, Mozambique. *Trans R Soc Trop Med and Hyg* 1987;81:51-54.

29. Fawzi WW, Herrera MG, Nestel P, Amin A, Mohamed KA. A longitudinal study of prolonged breastfeeding in relation to child undernutrition. *Int J Epidemiol* 1998, 27:255-260.

14

BREASTFEEDING AND STUNTING AMONG TODDLERS IN PERU

[1]Grace S. Marquis, Ph. D. and [2]Jean-Pierre Habicht
[1]*Department of Food Science and Human Nutrition, Iowa State University, Ames, IA;* [2]*Division of Nutritional Sciences, Cornell University, Ithaca, NY*

Key words: breastfeeding, stunting, child-feeding, linear growth, reverse causality, complementary feeding

1.   INTRODUCTION

At least as early as 1977, prevalence studies have demonstrated a negative association between children's growth and breastfeeding beyond 12 months[1-3]. Over this past decade, health professionals have struggled to understand this apparent negative relationship while increasing their efforts to promote breastfeeding in accordance with the World Health Organization's recommendation to breastfeed for at least two years[4]. Given the well-known health benefits of breastfeeding during the first year of life, a negative relationship with later growth is surprising.

One proposed explanation of this enigma is that lengthy breastfeeding results in poor total dietary intake; however, results from recent studies do not support this explanation. First, in an analysis of data from Peruvian toddlers 12-14 mo of age, previous 3-mo breastfeeding practice was not a predictor of low intakes of complementary foods; only per person food expenditure had a significant (positive) association with intake ($p=0.03$;

Short and Long Term Effects of Breast Feeding on Child Health
Edited by Berthold Koletzko *et al.*, Kluwer Academic/Plenum Publishers, 2000   163

Marquis, unpublished data). Second, studies in Guinea-Bissau, Peru, Sudan, and Senegal have analyzed growth and breastfeeding data and have provided clear evidence that the negative association reflects maternal decisions to continue to breastfeed those children in poorest health (that is, the negative relationship is due to reverse causality)[5-8]. For example, in Sudan, Fawzi et al.[7] found a 50 percent reduction in weaning over a 6-mo interval for children who were stunted at the beginning of the interval. Finally, breastfeeding was predicted by low growth, previous low dietary intakes, and increase in diarrheal morbidity in Peruvian children 12-15 mo of age.[6]

This paper ascertains whether this reverse causality continued beyond the 15th month of life. Two questions that have arisen from review of the recent studies will be addressed. First, how does the association between prolonged breastfeeding and growth change over the second year of life? Second, if the association does change with age, does reverse causality continue to be the explanation of the negative association between breastfeeding and growth? These questions will be examined through the analysis of data from a poor urban community in Peru.

2.   METHODS

The study site is an arid valley, just 20 minutes from the center of Lima, Peru. Although many families had lived in the community for years, at the time of the study few people had the resources to complete a permanent structure for their home. Poor hygiene conditions, with no piped water or sewage, was the norm. Most families were nuclear with a father living in the home; however, incomes were unstable, relying on daily wages. The majority of women did not work outside of the home.

This analysis was based on data from 677 children 0 to 36 months of age who were participants of a diarrheal surveillance study between 1985 and 1987[9]. The children were chosen for the surveillance study through an initial random selection of 400 households. This analysis included only 279 children who were between 12 and 24 mo of age, had anthropometric measurements at the beginning and end of at least one of the 3-mo periods of interest (12-14; 15-17; 18-20; and 21-23 completed months), and had dietary and diarrheal morbidity information from previous study periods. Table 1 demonstrates the number of children with complete data and those who breastfed in each study period. Data from children who breastfed at the beginning of each period were used in the analysis of risk of weaning analysis.

Principal factors of interest included children's anthropometric measurements, complementary food intakes, breastfeeding behaviors, and diarrheal morbidity. Weights and recumbent lengths were measured monthly. The breastfeeding variable was the 3-mo average of the monthly reports of breastfeeding frequency. A monthly food frequency questionnaire documented intakes of 27 categories of common foods and liquids. The complementary food intake variable was the 3-mo average value of the reported number of food categories consumed by the child two or more times per week and correlated with total energy intake[10]. Diarrheal morbidity was determined through twice-weekly home visits to document symptoms of diarrhea, defined as three or more liquid or semi-liquid stools in a 24-h period.

3.   STUDY CHARACTERISTICS

By twelve months of age, almost one-fifth of the children were stunted and/or underweight (Table 1). The rates of underweight dropped sharply after 14 mo of age, however, the proportion of children who were stunted almost doubled by 18 months and remained high through 24 months.

The median duration of breastfeeding was 19.5 mo. Seventy percent of children breastfed between 12-15 mo, dropping to 41.3% between 21-23 mo. Among those toddlers who continued to breastfeed, the feeding frequency was about two feeds/day lower at 21-23 months then during the 12-14 mo period.

Children's diets became more varied at older ages, as demonstrated by an increased number of complementary foods reported to be eaten. However, at 15 months, diets were still limited; only 60% of mothers reported that their children regularly drank milk or ate meat and one-fifth did not eat eggs.

Diarrheal disease rates and number of days ill remained high throughout the second year. The median number of days ill showed a small, nonsignificant decline with age.

Table 1. Characteristics of study children, by study period (mo)

	12-14 (n=174)	15-17 (n=169)	18-20 (n=164)	21-24 (n=160)
Stunted (%)	20.1	33.7	37.8	37.5
Underweight (%)	19.0	14.8	12.2	13.1
Breastfed (n {%})	123 (70.7)	110 (65.1)	90 (54.9)	66 (41.3)
Dietary intake (# foods)	14.1±2.2[1]	14.6±2.0	14.7±2.5	14.7±2.1
Diarrheal incidence (# episodes)	2.2±1.8	2.3±2.1	2.3±2.1	2.1±1.9

[1]Mean±SD

4.   HOW DOES THE ASSOCIATION BETWEEN BREASTFEEDING AND LINEAR GROWTH VARY OVER THE SECOND YEAR OF LIFE?

Breastfeeding had a complicated relationship with linear growth. When 12-24 mo data were analyzed together, diet and morbidity jointly modified the association between breastfeeding and growth (p=0.02). Increased breastfeeding was associated with lower linear growth only in children with low complementary food intakes and high morbidity. For example, when these children were breastfed at the 75th percentile value (5.7 breastfeeds/d), they had slightly lower length gain (-0.23 cm/3 mo) than their weaned contemporaries. For all other children without the combination of low intakes and high illness, breastfeeding was associated with a slight increase in linear growth; thus, the rest of this article will focus on the comparison between children with low complementary foods and high morbidity and all other children.

We developed a categorical variable to represent the combined effect of low (below the mean) complementary food intake and high (equal or above the mean) incidence of diarrhea, assuming that those children with this combination (LDHM) were the children who had the worse health conditions.

Throughout the second year, when complementary food intakes were above the mean or when food intake was low but diarrheal morbidity was also low (thus representing the non-LDHM group), there was at best a very slight increase in linear growth in breastfeed as compared to weaned children (Figure 1).

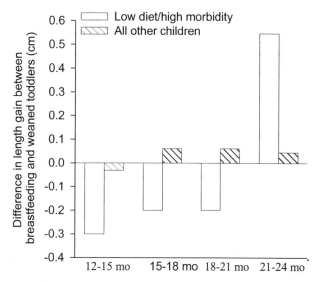

Fig. 1: Difference in linear growth bertween breastfed and weaned children, by complementary food and diarrhea. A negative value reflects lower growth in breastfed children.

The negative association between breastfeeding and growth was noted only in the LDHM group. Between 12 and 14 mo, there was a decrease of 0.44 cm/3 mo in linear growth associated with breastfeeding. LDHM breastfed children continued to have lower 3-mo length gains than weaned children through 20 months of age. Between 21-23 mo, the situation reversed itself and the average breastfed child had a 0.54 cm increase in 3-mo length gain as compared to a weaned child. We tested whether the slopes for the interaction term for breastfeeding and LDHM were significantly different across the four study periods. The slopes for 15-17 and 18-20 mo periods were not significantly different than that for 12-14 mo; however, the slope for 21-23 mo was significantly different. Therefore, age modulated the interactive effect of breastfeeding, diet, and diarrhea on linear growth.

In summary, the Peruvian data provide an example of where the relationship between breastfeeding and linear growth is not constant over the second year of life. There is a negative association from 12 through 20 months of age. However, the relationship reverses itself and is positive at the end of the year. Even with the change in the direction of the association, complementary food intakes and diarrheal morbidity continue to modify the effect of breastfeeding on growth. Only those children who had the poorest conditions demonstrated a negative association between breastfeeding and linear growth early on and had increased growth related to the continued presence of human milk in their diet at the end of the year.

4.1   Other supporting evidence

There is recent evidence from other longitudinal research studies to support the Peruvian results. Fawzi et al.[7] analyzed length and weight gains in Sudanese children 6 to 36 mo of age. The reduction in length and weight gains in breastfed as compared to weaned children was amplified for those who were poor as compared to their relatively affluent contemporaries.

Mulder-Sibanda and Sibanda-Mulder[11] provided similar results from Bangladesh but with diarrhea as the outcome. Bangladeshi children who breastfed for over 24 months had increased risk of diarrhea, however, this effect was only seen in the poorest children, as was case in the Sudanese and Peruvian studies.

Finally, in a cross-sectional study of prevalence of malnutrition in Uganda children, there was a dramatic increase in the odds ratio of being stunted for children breastfed 18-24 mo (OR=6.69) as compared to children breastfed for less than 12 months[12]. However, this was reversed for children who breastfed for over 24 months (OR=0.06), demonstrating a similar change in the direction of the association between breastfeeding and growth as seen in the Peru data.

The results from Peru, Bangladesh, Sudan, and Uganda lend support to the conclusion that the association of breastfeeding with growth often is modulated by factors that are proxies of dietary intakes and illness (such as those used in these studies, access to health facilities, income). The influence of these factors on the breastfeeding-growth relationship may change with age.

5.   IF CHANGE OCCURS, DOES REVERSE CAUSALITY CONTINUE TO BE THE EXPLANATION FOR A NEGATIVE ASSOCIATION BETWEEN BREASTFEEDING AND GROWTH DURING THE SECOND YEAR OF LIFE?

Analysis of cross-sectional data of breastfeeding and growth cannot determine the direction of causality because the sequential direction of events cannot be clearly delineated. If poor growth were a determinant of maternal breastfeeding decisions and, therefore, were the reason for a negative association between growth and breastfeeding (i.e., reverse causality), then one would expect to find delayed weaning in those children who initially had the poorest health. We analyzed the Peruvian data using linear logistic regression to predict the probability of weaning across the second year. An earlier analysis focused on risk of weaning during the 14th mo of life[6]. We repeated the analysis for the risk of weaning during the 12-23 months, using the same categorization of age (12-20 and 21-23 mo) as we had used in the analysis of growth. The sample for these analyses included only those children who still were breastfeeding at the beginning of the period and, therefore, were at risk of being weaned.

The determinants of weaning were weight-for-age at the beginning of the risk period, mean complementary food intake during the three previous months, and change in mean incidence of diarrhea over the previous six months (that is, incidence for the last quarter minus incidence for the previous quarter) (Table 2). For risk of weaning at 14 mo, 12-mo weight for age, 9-11 mo dietary intake, and the change of incidence of diarrhea from 9-14 mo had been used. The probability of weaning for the 25th (low) and 75th (high) percentile values of the three determinants were calculated and compared.

Table 2. Logistic regression equations for the risk of weaning, by study period (n=415)

	beta	SE	t	p
Constant	-0.406	0.431	-0.941	0.346
Initial WA (z-score)	0.334	0.354	0.942	0.346
Low diet/high morbidity=LDHM (0=no;1=yes)	-1.363	1.178	-1.157	0.247
Age (0=21-23; 1=12-20)	-0.760	0.480	-1.582	0.114
WA*LDHM	-1.786	0.942	-1.897	0.058
WA*Age	-0.419	0.385	-1.089	0.276
LDHM*Age	2.115	1.236	1.711	0.087
WA*LDHM*Age	2.349	0.988	2.377	0.017

From 12-21 months, when children's complementary food intakes were low and diarrheal morbidity was high,mothers made different weaning decisions depending on the child's nutritional status. When the W/A was also low, mothers decreased the probability of weaning by almost one-half. No change in the probability of weaning was noted in those children who were not part of the LDHM group.

Similar results were not seen at 21-23 months. Poor nutritional status accompanying poor dietary intakes and frequent illness did not alter the risk of weaning. In contrast, mothers weaned more frequently when the child had better dietary intakes and W/A and less illness. Mothers may view these children as not at any risk and able to be weaned without problem.

In summary, data on risk of weaning support the conclusion that the negative association between growth and breastfeeding is due to reverse causality through the first nine months of the second year. Over the months that the negative asssociation is detected, mothers reduce the probability of weaning when multiple health concerns are present. By the end of the year, when a positive effect of breastfeeding on growth is observed, poor health no longer delays weaning.

5.1   Other supporting evidence

There are a few studies that have examined the role of child health on risk of weaning. Simondon and Simondon have published results from Senegal demonstrating that low (<-2.0) HA at 9-10 mo was related to a 2.3 mo prolongation of breastfeeding duration as compared to mean HA[8]. Molbak and collaborators[5] followed a cohort of children in a longitudinal study in semi-urban district in Guinea-Bissau. The relative risk of weaning for children with a WA <-2.5 Z scores was 0.6, that is, poorly nourished children had a 40% reduction in risk of weaning as compared to children with z-score WA > -2.5. The data from Senegal and Guinea-Bissau both support the Peruvian results demonstrating that maternal child-feeding decisions are influenced by child health.

6.   CONCLUSIONS AND IMPLICATIONS

The relationship between breastfeeding and linear growth in the Peruvian context is complex and fluid. The observed lower growth rate in breastfed children from 12-20 mo can be explained by reverse causality. Mothers purposefully continue to breastfeed children with the poorest health conditions and wean those who are healthier. At the end of the second year, child health has a reduced influence on weaning decisions. At this older age, a strong positive effect of breastfeeding can be noted in those children who have the poorest health. It is not surprising that the negative association indicating reverse causality disappears at the end of the second year in the Peruvian data. We have reported elsewhere that, by 24 months, maternal breastfeeding decisions are more closely tied to maternal needs rather than child needs.[14]

There is now sufficient evidence from the Peruvian study and other published studies, to accept reverse causality as the explanation for a negative relationship between growth and prolonged breastfeeding in poor, disadvantaged communities. Breastfeeding did not place the Peruvian children at risk of poor diets; dietary intakes were only predicted by families' ability to purchase food. Given the growth benefits noted in children with diets poor in quality and quantity, reduction in morbidity and mortality associatied with continued breastfeeding, health professionals should promote the World Health Organization's recommendation to breastfeed for two years or beyond in addition to promoting optimal complementary feeding at an affordable price.

ACKNOWLEDGMENTS

We thank Drs. Robert E. Black and Claudio F. Lanata who provided the data for this analysis and the staff at the Instituto de Investigacion Nutritional, Lima, Peru for their excellent field work and analytical support.

REFERENCES

1. Central Bureau of Statistics. The rural Kenyan nutrition survey. February-March 1977. 1977;2:1-19.

2. Victora CG, Vaughan JP, Martines JC, Barcelos LB. Is prolonged breast-feeding associated with malnutrition? Am J Clin Nutr 1984;39:307-314.

3. Jansen GR. The nutritional status of preschool children in Egypt. World Rev Nutr Diet 1985;45:42-67.

4. Saadeh RJ, Labbok MH, Cooney KA, Koniz-Booher P (eds). Breast-feeding: The technical basis and recommendations for action. Doc WHO/NUT/MCH/93.1. Geneva: World Health Organization. 1993.

5. Molbak K, Gottschau A, Aaby P, Hojlyng N, Ingholt L, da Silva APJ. Prolonged breast feeding, diarrhoeal disease, and survival of children in Guinea-Bissau. BMJ 1994;308:1403-6.

6. Marquis GS, Habicht J-P, Lanata CF, Black RE, Rasmussen KM. Association of breastfeeding and stunting in Peruvian toddlers: An example of reverse causality. Int J Epidemiol 1997a;26:349-56.

7. Fawzi WW, Herrera MG, Nestel P, Amin AE, Mohammed. A longitudinal study of prolonged breastfeeding in relation to child undernutrition. Int J Epidemiol 1998;27:255-60.

8 . Simondon KB, Simondon R. Mothers prolong breastfeeding of undernourished children in rural Senegal. Int J Epidemiol 1998;27.

9. Lanata C, Black RE, Gilman RH, Lazo R, Del Aguila R. Epidemiologic, clinical, and laboratory characteistics of acute vs. persistent diarrhea in peri-urban Lima, Peru. J Pediatr Gastroenterol Nutr 1991;12:82-88.

10. Marquis GS, Habicht J-P, Lanata CF, Black RE, Rasmussen KM. Human milk or animal protein foods improve linear growth of Peruvian toddlers on marginal diets. Am J Clin Nutr 1997b;66:1102-9.

11. Mulder-Sibanda M, Sibanda-Mulder FS. Prolonged breastfeeding in Bangladesh: indicators of inadequate feeding practices or mothers' response to children's poor health? Public Health 1999;113:65-8.

12. Kikafunda JK, Walker AF, Collett D, Tumwine JK. Risk factors for early childhood malnutrition in Uganda. Pediatrics 1998;102:1-8.

13. Marquis GS, Díaz J, Bartolini R, Creed de Kanashiro H, Rasmussen KM. Recognizing the reversible nature of child-feeding decisions. Breastfeeding, weaning, and relactation patterns in a shanty town community of Lima, Peru. Social Sci Med 1998;47:645-56.

15

BREASTFEEDING AND GROWTH IN RURAL SENEGALESE TODDLERS

[1]Kirsten B. Simondon, [2]Aldiouma Diallo and [1]François Simondon
Research Institute for Development (IRD), [1]Montpellier, France and [2]Dakar, Senegal

Key words: weaning, length, weight, stunting, malnutrition, reverse causality, West Africa

1.   INTRODUCTION

While the benefits of breastfeeding during infancy have been well described for developing countries in terms of health and survival,[1,2] its positive effects have been questioned for older children. From 12 to 36 months of age, the continuation of breastfeeding has frequently been associated with a low nutritional status, in terms of either weight-for-age, as in Botswana,[3] Bangladesh[4] and Guinea-Bissau,[5] height-for-age, as in Nepal,[6] Senegal,[7] Ghana,[8,9] People's Republic of Congo,[10] Brazil,[11] and Uganda[12], or weight-for-height.[7,9,12,13] A recent review of demographic and health surveys (DHS) found a significant, negative association between the persistence of breastfeeding and height-for-age in 5 out of 11 Sub-Saharan African countries and in 9 out of 11 countries from North Africa or other continents.[14] A positive association has been decribed for a few settings only, such as China (with height-for-age and weight-for-height)[15] and Bangladesh (with left upper arm circumference).[16]

Since the negative relationships do not seem to be explained by confounding by poverty or other factors,[9,11,14] several reviews have suggested that it might be explained by "reverse causality", that is, the mother lets the decision of weaning depend on the child's nutritional status, health, growth or appetite.[14,17-19]

Some evidence for reverse causality in Africa was provided for over 30 years ago from rural Nigeria. Duration of breastfeeding was two months longer for children with a low weight-for-age during infancy (median duration was 25 months vs. 23 months for children with a good weight-for-age).[20] Similarly, in rural Guatemala, children weaned early (at 12-29 months of age) had been larger in the first year of life compared to those weaned at 30-47 months of age.[21]

More recent evidence comes from studies conducted in Guinea-Bissau, Peru and Sudan. In periurban Guinea-Bissau, 59 children with a very low weight-for-age (<-2.5 z-scores) at 10-17 months of age were breastfed for 1.8 months longer than the remaining 295 children (24.1 vs. 22.3 months).[5] The lower relative risk of weaning of children with very low weight-for-age remained significant in a Cox model including child's sex and maternal age, ethnic group and education. In periurban Peru, children who had simultaneous low weight-for-age, low dietary intake and increased diarrheal incidence at about 1 year of age tended to be less often weaned by 15 months.[22] In a large longitudinal study in Northern Sudan, the risk of being weaned over the following six months was 50% lower for stunted children, compared to normally nourished children, in a logistic regression model which also included age, sex, morbidity, maternal education and economic level.[23] There was no relationship between wasting and risk of weaning.

In this report, we describe the results of a study on the relationship between prolonged breastfeeding and growth in a poor African context.

2.   STUDY AREA AND POPULATION

The studies were conducted in a rural area of Senegal in Sahelian West Africa. The nearly 30 000 inhabitants are of the Sereer ethnic group, over 90% are farmers and grow millet, for their own consumption, and groundnuts, mainly for sell, during the rainy season from June to October. Electricity and indoor piped water are not available. Only the larger villages have outdoor piped water, while the others use wells. Less than 20% of the compounds have pit latrines. Main declared religions are Islam (75%) and Christianism (20%), but these have been adopted during the last 30 years and traditional animistic beliefs and practices are still strong. The social organization consists of extended families and polygamic marriages.

Both mortality and fertility are high. From 1994 to 1996, the infant mortality rate and the child mortality rate were 77 and 182 per thousand, respectively, while the total fertility rate was 7.1 live-born children per woman.[24] Morbidity and nutrition, in particular transmission of malaria and wasting in preschool children, are very dependent on season. They peak at the end of the rainy season in October-November and are at their lowest level during the dry season.

The area has been under demographic and epidemiological surveillance since the sixties. From 1987 to 1997, information about all births, deaths, migrations and weaning events was collected weekly by highly trained fieldworkers, while bi-monthly rounds were used from 1997 to 1999. Several studies on pertussis vaccines included organization of monthly vaccination sessions according to the Senegalese Expanded Program of Immunization (EPI), from 1989 to 1997.[25] A high level of participation (about 80% of infants) was obtained by systematic call of eligible infants during home visits by field workers the week before the session and by transport services. Anthropometric measurements (length measured to the nearest mm and weight measured to the nearest 10 g) were taken routinely.

3.   BREASTFEEDING AND GROWTH

According to a study of the relationship between nutritional status, growth and mortality risk in a sample of more than 5000 children aged 0-5 years, conducted in the Niakhar study area from 1983 to 1985, breastfed children had significantly lower height-for-age and weight-for-height than weaned children from 18 to 36 months of age.[7] Traditional midwives, field workers and mothers of underfives in the area consistently stated that this association between malnutrition and breastfeeding did not surprise them, but that it was due to later weaning of malnourished children (K. Simondon, unpublished observations). In order to test this statement, a retrospective analysis of factors associated with age at weaning was conducted in a sample of 4515 children, who were born from 1989 to 1995 and had attended vaccination sessions from 1990 to 1996.[26] Duration of breastfeeding was analyzed using Cox's proportional hazards models, because about 20% of the sample was right-censored, i.e. date of weaning was not available either because the child had died or out-migrated before weaning or because the child was still breastfed when follow-up was stopped. Median duration of breastfeeding was 23.7 months and half of the children were weaned between the ages of 21.7 and 25.9 months. Main factors related to duration of breastfeeding were maternal age and parity (greater values were associated with longer durations), height (greater values were associated with shorter durations), education and occupation (if any: shorter durations), and season (longer durations for children born at the end of the rainy season and shortest durations for those born at the onset of the rainy season). The child's height-for-age and weight-for-height at the time of the last vaccination (at 9-10 months of age) were both very significantly associated with age at weaning. Infants with a height-for-age below -2 z-scores at 9-10 months of age were weaned 2.3 months later on average than children with a z-score above 0 (25.0 vs. 22.7 months), while differences were somewhat smaller for weight-for-height (24.2 vs. 23.2 months). These differences remained very significant when all variables linked to duration of breastfeeding were entered into a multivariate Cox model. Although these differences in median duration of breastfeeding seemed quite modest, great differences in prevalence of malnutrition existed during late infancy when four groups of increasing age of weaning were compared (Table 1).

Since the high levels of stunting and wasting among children weaned late existed already during infancy, at an age at which all children were still breastfed, prolonged breastfeeding could not be the reason of their poor nutritional status. Our study thus proved that prolonged breastfeeding not necessarily impairs growth, even in communities where breastfed children are more malnourished.

Table 1. Prevalence of stunting and wasting at 9-10 months of age with 95% confidence intervals (CI), by duration of breastfeeding

Age at weaning (months)	Stunting (%)	95% CI	Wasting (%)	95% CI
<18	6.4	2.4 - 10.3	7.7	3.4 - 12.0
18-23.9	9.5	8.1 - 10.8	9.2	7.8 - 10.6
24-30	17.6	15.6 - 19.6	11.9	10.2 - 13.6
>30	26.6	18.7 - 34.5	14.5	8.2 - 20.8

From[26]

However, since no indicator of economic status was available in the database, these results did not prove that mothers **consciously** prolonged breastfeeding in response to a poor nutritional status of their child. It was still possible that richer mothers *per se* had less malnourished children and breastfed for shorter durations. Furthermore, the existence of other, unknown confounding factors could not be excluded.

Published studies on the relationship between breastfeeding and growth have given conflicting results. Marquis *et al* found that breastfeeding was associated with faster growth in length (from 12 to 15 months).[27] The dependent variable was intensity of breastfeeding, measured as the mean number of feeds per day (from 0-15.3). Thirty-one children were weaned by 12 months and 15 more were weaned during the interval, within the sample of 107. Second, part of the initial sample (27 out of 134 children) was excluded from the analysis because these children with a high diarrheal incidence and low dietary intake from non-breast milk foods were at significantly lower risk of weaning and thus showed evidence of reverse causality, as described above. Since the relationship between breastfeeding intensity and linear growth was negative for these children, no significant relationship between breastfeeding intensity and linear growth existed before their exclusion.[22] Even after their exclusion from the analysis, the main effect of breastfeeding intensity on linear growth was not significant in a multiple linear regression analysis. However, the interaction between breastfeeding intensity and intake of animal-product foods was significant, which meant that breastfeeding intensity was positively associated with linear growth for children with low intake of animal products only. Growth in weight was not analyzed in this study.

A prospective, community-based study of 1116 children from periurban Guinea-Bissau used random effect models to assess the effect of weaning on weight or length, while adjusting for previous weight or length, age, sex, season and previous diarrheal prevalence.[28] Weaning was associated with a significant, relative decrease in weight but not in length. The negative effect was strongest during infancy, but remained significant during the second year of life.

A prospective study of the effects of vitamin A supplementation on health and survival in Sudan was used to assess the relationship between breastfeeding and growth in length and weight in a sample of 28,753 children.[23] From 12 to 24 months of age, breastfed children had 2 cm lower length increments and 50-100 g lower weight increments, compared to weaned children. These differences remained in all subgroups when the sample was stratified by economic level and maternal literacy. However, as stated by the authors themselves, it was difficult to exclude the possibility of additional confounding.

4. MATERNAL REASONS FOR WEANING

Although reverse causality seems to exist in a variety of settings, more knowledge is needed about the reasons for the relationship between the child's nutritional status, health and duration of breastfeeding. Is weaning child-driven or mother-driven? Are child characteristics more or less important than mother's characteristics, and which child characteristics are important for mothers' weaning decisions?

In rural Nigeria, children were weaned when they were considered "sturdy and healthy".[20] In an rural area of Ivory Coast, mothers were reported to use developmental milestones (mainly independent walking) in their decision of weaning, and children were weaned at about 18-24 months of age.[29] In urban Egypt, both child-centered reasons, such as developmental milestones (walking, complete dentition) and good appetite for family food, and mother-centered reasons, such as illness, Islamic fasting during Ramadan and desire for a new pregnancy, seemed important.[30] However, in periurban Guinea-Bissau, the effect of illness on the duration of breastfeeding was ambigious.[31] Most children were weaned because they were healthy or "old enough" (67.6%; N=945), while a few were weaned because of child illness (7.3%) or maternal illness (9.0%). The last two groups were weaned significantly earlier than the former (medians of 19 and 18 months, respectively, vs. 23 months for the healthy children). It is difficult to know why both health and illness were reported as reasons to wean in this area. Weaning because of child's illness may be explained by so different reasons as hospitalization of the child without the mother,[30] or mother's belief that her breastmilk caused the illness. In many settings, diarrhea of the breastfed toddlers, while the mother is pregnant, systematically leads to weaning because of a widespread belief that a pregnant mother's milk can harm the child.[31-34]

Brazilian mothers stated that they did not adapt duration of breastfeeding to their child's state,[11] while in an rural area of Kenya, reasons for weaning among 98 toddlers did not include either the child's nutritional status, growth health or motor development, but rather maternal pregnancy (54%), child's refusal or inability to continue (13%) and parents' preference for weaning (11%).[35] A low appetite for family food may have been a reason for weaning in this society, since some mothers weaned in order to "get the child to eat other foods" (9%). A low appetite for non-breast milk foods, especially when associated with malnutrition, was also reported as a reason for weaning in urban Mali, West Africa.[36] These mothers practices are thus exactly the opposite to those of Egyptian mothers who weaned in response to a good appetite for non-breastmilk foods.[30]

In periurban Peru, mothers stated to wean mainly in order to protect maternal health but a "big" child was also mentioned as a reason for weaning, while prolonging of breastfeeding was often due to illness of the child.[34] The later weaning of children with high diarrheal morbidity in this community was confirmed by survival analysis as mentioned above.

Thus, review of the literature suggests that reverse causality might be inexisting in some settings, or even that ill or poorly growing children may be weaned earlier than others, such as in developed or emerging countries where non-breast milk foods of high nutritional and hygienic value are available. Conversely, especially in poor societies, breastmilk may be considered better than other existing foods, and in these settings, poor child health, nutritional status or growth are more likely to incite the mother to prolong breastfeeding. In some traditional West African communities, height seems to be important and this factor will of course have a major influence on differences in the prevalence of stunting between breastfed and weaned children. In areas such as urban Peru where morbidity seems the most important factor of reverse causality, differences in height between groups are likely to be more subtle.

5. CONCLUSION

In his textbook entitled 'Pediatrics in Developing Countries', published in 1973, Morley concluded from his experience in rural Nigeria: "Mothers cease breastfeeding when the child is healthy and sturdy"…"Since malnourished children are breastfed longer, some physicians have, falsely, concluded that undernutrition was caused by the long duration of breastfeeding.[37] This statement is also valid for rural Senegal and probably for many other areas in Africa south of Sahara.

To conclude from cross-sectional differences in nutritional status between breastfed and weaned toddlers that prolonged breastfeeding impairs growth is to neglect mothers' knowledge and optimal use of very limited resources. To recommend weaning of malnourished African children by 12 months of age, as has been done in the literature,[8] would be extremely dangerous in settings where mothers trust "experts", but would only discredit nutritional education with mothers in traditional, rural settings where the benefits of breastfeeding are well-known.

ACKNOWLEDGMENTS

During the study period, the Niakhar Population and Health Project was supported by Pasteur-Mérieux Sérums et Vaccins, Paris. The authors thank Laurence Chabirand and Agnès Gartner for logistic support. Adama Marra helped with management of data files, and Eric Bénéfice made helpful comments on the manuscript.

REFERENCES

1. Feachem, R. G., and Koblinsky, M. A., 1984, Interventions for the control of diarrhoeal diseases among young children: promotion of breastfeeding. *Bull. World Health Org.* 62: 271-291.
2. Victora, C. G., Vaughan, J. P., Lombardi, C., Fuchs, S. M. C., Gigante, L. P., Smith, P. G., Nobre, L. C., Teixera, A. M. B., Moreira, L. B., and Barros, F. C., 1987, Evidence for protection by breast-feeding against infant deaths from infectious diseases in Brazil. *Lancet* 2: 319-322.
3. Michaelsen, K.F., 1988, Value of prolonged breastfeeding. *Lancet* ii: 788-789.

4. Briend, A. and Bari, A., 1989, Breastfeeding improves survival, but not nutritional status, of 12-35 months old children in rural Bangladesh. *Eur. J. Clin. Nutr.* 43: 603-608.

5. Mølbak, K., Gottschau, A., Aaby, P., Højlyng, N., Ingholt, L., and da Silva, A.P.J., 1994, Prolonged breastfeeding, diarrhoeal disease, and survival of children in Guinea-Bissau. *Br.Med. J.* 308: 1403-1406.

6. Martorell, R., Leslie, J., and Moock, P.R., 1984, Characteristics and determinants of child nutritional status in Nepal. *Am. J. Clin. Nutr.* 39: 74-86.

7. Garenne, M., Maire, B., Fontaine, O., Dieng, K., and Briend, A., 1987, *Risques de Décès Associés à Différents Etats Nutritionnels chez l'Enfant d'Age Préscolaire [Mortality Risks Associated with Different Nutritional States in Preschool Children].* ORSTOM, Dakar.

8. Brakohiapa, L.A., Bille, A., Quansah, E., Kishi, K., Yartey, J., Harrison, E., Armar, M.A., and Yamamoto, S., 1988, Does prolonged breastfeeding adversely affect a child's nutritional status? *Lancet* ii: 416-418.

9. Nubé, M. and Asenso-Okyere, W.K., 1996, Large differences in nutritional status between fully weaned and partially breastfed children beyond the age of 12 months. *Eur. J. Clin. Nutr.* 50: 171-177.

10. Cornu, A., Simondon, F., Olivola, D., Goma, I., Massamba, J.-P., Tchibindat, F., and Delpeuch, F., 1991, Allaitement Maternel Prolongé et Malnutrition [Prolonged Breast Feeding and Malnutrition]. In *Alimentation et Nutrition dans les Pays en Développement [Food and Nutrition in Developing Countries]*, (D. Lemonnier, Y. Ingenbleek and P. Hennart, eds.), ACCT-AUPELF-KARTHALA, Paris, pp. 225-232.

11. Victora, C. G., Huttly, S. R. A., Barros, F. C., Martines, J. C., and Vaughan, J. P., 1991, Prolonged breastfeeding and malnutrition: confounding and effect modification in a Brazilian cohort study. *Epidemiology* 2: 175-181.

12. Vella, V., Tomkins, A., Borghesi, A., Migliori, G.B., Adriko, B.C., and Crevatin, E., 1992, Determinants of child nutrition and mortality in north-west Uganda. *Bull.World Health Org.* 70: 637-643.

13. Victora, C. G., Vaughan, J. P., Martines, J. C., Barcelos, L. B., 1984, Is prolonged breast-feeding associated with malnutrition? *Am. J. Clin. Nutr.* 39: 307-314.

14. Caulfield, L.E., Bentley, M.E., and Ahmed, S., 1996, Is prolonged breastfeeding associated with malnutrition? evidence from nineteen demographic and health surveys. *Int. J. Epidemiol.* 25: 693-703.

15. Taren, D., and Chen, J., 1993, A positive association between extended breast-feeding and nutritional status in rural Hubei Province, People's Republic of China. *Am. J. Clin. Nutr.* 58: 862-867.

16. Briend, A., Wojtyniak, B., and Rowland, M. G. M., 1988, Breast feeding, nutritional state, and child survival in rural Bangladesh. *Br. Med. J.* 296: 879-882.

17. Prentice, A., 1991, Breast feeding and the older infant. *Acta Paediat. Scand.*, Suppl 374: 78-88.

18. Grummer-Strawn, L.M., 1993, Does prolonged breast-feeding impair child growth? A critical review. *Pediatrics* 91: 766-771.

19. Simondon, K.B. and Simondon, F., 1997, Prolonged breastfeeding and malnutrition. *Int. J. Epidemiol.* 26: 677.

20. Morley, D., Bicknell, J., and Woodland, M., 1968, Factors influencing the growth and nutritional status of infants and young children in a Nigerian village. *Trans. R. Trop. Med. Hyg.* 62: 164-195.

21. Mata, L. J., Kronmal, R. A., Garcia, B., Butler, W., Urrutia, J. J., and Murillo, S., 1976. Breast-feeding, weaning and the diarrheal syndrom in a Guatemalan Indian village. In *Acute Diarrhea in Childhood* (C. Elliot and J. Knight, eds.), Elsevier, Amsterdam, pp. 311-338.

22. Marquis, G.S., Habicht, J.P., Lanata, C., Black, R.E., and Rasmussen, K.M., 1997, Association of breastfeeding and stunting in Peruvian toddlers: an example of reverse causality. *Int. J. Epidemiol.* 26: 349-356.

23. Fawzi, W. W., Herrera, M. G., Nestel, P., El Amin, A., and Mohamed, K. A., 1998, A longitudinal study of prolonged breastfeeding in relation to child undernutrition. *Int. J. Epidemiol.* 27: 255-260.

24. Delaunay, V., 1998, *La Situation Démographique et Epidémiologique dans la Zone de Niakhar au Sénégal, 1984-1996. [The Demographic and Epidemiological Situation of the Niakhar Study Area in Senegal, 1984-1996].* ORSTOM, Dakar.

25. Simondon, F., Préziosi, M.-P., Yam, A., Kane, C. T., Chabirand, L., Iteman, I., Sanden, G., Mboup, S., Hoffenbach, A., Knudsen, K., Guiso, N., Wassilak, S., and Cadoz, M., 1997, A randomized double-blind trial comparing a two-component acellular to a whole-cell pertussis vaccine in Senegal. *Vaccine* 15: 1606-1612.

26. Simondon, K.B. and Simondon, F., 1998, Mothers prolong breastfeeding of undernourished children in rural Senegal. *Int. J. Epidemiol.* 27: 490-494.

27. Marquis, G.S., Habicht, J.P., Lanata, C.F., Black, R.E., and Rasmussen, K.M., 1997, Breast milk or animal-product foods improve linear growth of Peruvian toddlers consuming marginal diets. *Am. J. Clin. Nut.* 66: 1102-1109.

28. Mølbak, K., Jakobsen, M., Sodemann, M., and Aaby, P., 1997, Is malnutrition associated with prolonged breastfeeding? *Int. J. Epidemiol.* 26: 458-459.

29. Lauber, E. and Reinhardt, M., 1981, Prolonged lactation performance in a rural community of the Ivory Coast. *J. Trop. Pediatr.* 27: 47-77.

30. Harrison, G.G., Zaghloul, S.S., Galal, O.M., and Bagr, A., 1993, Breastfeeding and weaning in a poor urban neighbourhood in Cairo, Egypt: maternal beliefs and perceptions. *Soc. Sci. Med.* 36:1063-1069.

31. Jakobsen, M.S., Sodemann, M., Mølbak, K., and Aaby, P., 1996, Reason for terminating breastfeeding and the length of breastfeeding. *Int. J. Epidemiol.* 25: 115-121.

32. Almedon, A. M., 1991, Infant feeding in urban low-income households in Ethiopia: II. Determinants of weaning. *Ecol.Food Nutr.* 25: 111-121.

33. Bøhler, E., and Ingstad, B., 1996, The struggle of weaning: factors determining breastfeeding duration in east Bhutan. *Soc. Sci. Med.* 43: 1805-1815.

34. Marquis, G.S., Diaz, J., Bartolini, R., Creed de Kanashiro, H., and Rasmussen, K.M., 1998, Recognizing the reversible nature of child-feeding decisions: breastfeeding, weaning, and relactation patterns in a shanty town community of Lima, Peru. *Soc. Sci. Med.* 47: 645-656.

35. Onyango, A., Koski, K.G., and Tucker, K.L., 1998, Food diversity versus breastfeeding choice in determining anthropometric status in rural Kenyan toddlers. *Int. J. Epidemiol.* 27: 484-489.

36. Dettwyler, K. A., 1987, Breastfeeding and weaning in Mali: cultural context and hard data. *Soc. Sci Med.* 24: 633-644.

37. Morley, D., 1973, *Pediatrics in Developing Countries.* Butterworth and Co, London.

16

DURATION OF BREAST-FEEDING AND LINEAR GROWTH

Kim Fleischer Michaelsen[1]; Erik Lykke Mortensen[2,3]; June Machover Reinisch[2]

[1]*Research Department of Human Nutrition and LMC Centre for Advanced Food Studies, The Royal Veterinary and Agricultural University, Rolighedsvej 30, 1958 Frederiksberg C, Denmark,* [2]*Institute of Preventive Medicine and* [3]*Department of Health Psychology, University of Copenhagen*

Key words: Breast-feeding, linear growth

1. INTRODUCTION

Many studies from both industrialized and developing countries have shown significant differences in growth between breastfed and formula fed infants. Most of the studies found that during the last half of infancy breastfed infants weigh less than formula fed infants. In developing countries it has been convincingly shown that this is often due to reverse causation. Mothers with small and weak infants tend to breast-feed their infants longer as they know from tradition that breast-feeding protects a weak infant. This is described in detail in the three chapters of this book which analyse the association between breastfeeding and growth among infants from Senegal (Simondon et al.), Kenya (Onyango), and Peru (Marquis et al.). Thus, breastfeeding *per se* is not likely to cause the slower weight gain among breastfed infants in these populations. The reason for the significant association between duration of breast-feeding and weight gain in industrialized countries is less clear.

Data on the association between duration of breast-feeding and linear growth in industrialized countries are conflicting, as will be discussed below.

Some studies show the same kind of association as for weight, while others show no significant association between breastfeeding and linear growth.

The aim of the present publication is to review studies from industrialized countries which have analysed the association between duration of breast feeding and linear growth, to present previously unpublished data on breast-feeding and growth from a large Danish study and to discuss possible mechanisms that could explain the difference in linear growth between breastfed and formula fed infants and possible long term consequences for growth.

2. STUDIES FROM INDUSTRIALISED COUNTRIES

In a study from Finland, the linear growth velocities of exclusively breastfed infants were compared to a group of infants breast-fed for less than 3.5 months[1]. The number of exclusively breast-fed infants studied were 116 at 6 months, 36 at 9 months, and 7 at 12 months. Linear growth velocity was slower in breast-fed infants at 3 to 6 months, 6 to 9 months, and 9 to 12 months. It is interesting that linear growth was different already during the 3-6 months period, but not surprising that exclusive breast-feeding beyond 6 months is associated with reduced growth velocity. There is now agreement that breastfed infants should start complementary feeding not later than six months, as prolonged exclusive breastfeeding is likely to result in suboptimal nutritional status, especially regarding zinc, iron and protein. Indeed there were signs of protein deficiency, with lower prealbumin values among breast-fed infants in the Finnish study, and a few of the infants showed catch-up after complementary feeding was started.

In a pooled analysis of data from seven longitudinal studies from North America and Europe, Dewey and coworkers analysed growth of breastfed infants[2]. Growth data were compared to the NCHS/WHO growth reference. In the group breast-fed for 12 months or more there was a decline with age in length-for-age SD (Z) scores, but it was less than the decline seen in weight-for-age. The mean SD score at 12 months was -0.29 equivalent to about 7 mm below the reference. Three of the seven studies included data up to the age of 24 months. It is remarkable that there was a considerable difference between the data from the Darling study which had z-scores above zero for almost the whole age period and the two studies by Krebs and Whitehead from the US and the UK, which had values resembling each other, at a level which from 12 to 24 months was close to -0.6 SD-scores. The Darling study recruited infants from a university town with a high socioeconomic status, and had also birth weights well above the other studies. Among infants with data at both 12 and 24 months; there was no increase in SD-score from 12 to 24 months ($p=0.55$).

Preliminary data from the Euro-growth Study[3], which includes data from 22 European centres found that length gain from 0-12 months was negatively influenced by duration of breast-feeding (p<0.001). Duration of breast-feeding did not influence length gain from 0-36 months, but the sample followed until 3 years was considerably smaller.

In the Darling study from California, a group of 41 formula fed infants was compared with a group of 46 infants breastfed up to the age of 18 months[4]. The weight of the breastfed infants was significantly below the formula fed group between 6 and 18 months, while there was no difference in length and head circumference. There was, however, a significant lower cumulative length gain from birth to 12 months in breastfed boys compared to formula fed boys (23.8 cm *vs* 25.4 cm, p<0.05), while there was no difference in girls.

In a study from Italy, growth during the first year of life was compared in three groups: 56 formula fed infants, 48 infants breast-fed for 4-11 months and only 13 infants breastfed for 12 months or more[5]. Growth was analysed by comparing NCHS/WHO SD-scores among the three groups. There was a highly significant (p=0.001) difference in weightgain from 0-12 months between the feeding groups with the formula group gaining most. The same tendency was seen for length-for-age, but the difference was not significant (p=0.21). The formula fed infants increased by 0.26 SD-scores, while those who were breast-fed for 4-11 months gained 0.08 SD-scores and those breast-fed for 12 months or more lost 0.09 SD-scores. The difference in length gain between the two outer groups (0.35 SD-score) is equivalent to approximately 0.8 cm.

Two previous, independent studies from Denmark have examined the association between breastfeeding and growth. Both found a significant negative association between longterm breastfeeding and linear growth.

In a pooled analysis of data from two longitudinal growth studies from the Copenhagen area, where infants were followed from birth to 12 months, the association between duration of breastfeeding and growth was analysed[6]. At 12 months infants breast-fed for 9 months or more weighed 400 g less (95% CI: 70-740 g) and were 1.0 cm shorter (95% CI: 0.3-1.8 cm) than infants breastfed for a shorter duration.

In another Danish study[7], the association between breastfeeding and growth from 5-10 months was examined in a random sample of Danish infants. A food questionnaire and a questionnaire on breastfeeding duration and on weight and length gain based on measurements from the child welfare clinics were returned with complete data by 339 families. In a multiple regression analysis controlling for mid-parental height, birth weight and protein intake, infants breast-fed for 7 months or more were gaining 198 g less in weight (p<0.01) and 7 mm less in length (p<0.01) than those breastfed for less than 7 months. Interestingly, those breastfed for 7 months or more received less meat (p=0.05) and less cow's milk (p=0.01) at the age of 10 months.

3. MATERIAL AND METHODS

The Copenhagen Perinatal Cohort consists of about 9000 infants born 1959-61 at Rigshospitalet, the main university hospital in Copenhagen. Data on length, weight and head circumference were collected at birth and at 12 months[8,9]. All measurements were done by paediatricians at the hospital. Furthermore, duration of breastfeeding (total duration) was recorded at the one year examination. Personal identification numbers have made it possible to collect data from several Danish public registers. Among these data is draft information on all conscripts (only males) which include data on adult height (and IQ). Thus, it will be possible to examine if an influence of breast-feeding on growth during infancy has any effect on adult stature. Data on the relation between linear growth and relevant background variables in males will be published elsewhere. Here we present data on the relation between linear growth during the first year of life and background variables in females from the cohort.

Table 1. Background variables included in the analysis

Maternal height	Gestational age
Maternal age	Birth weight
Parity	Social class
Pregnancy weight gain	Marital status
Smoking in pregnancy	

1250 girls had a complete data set and were included in the analysis. Analysis of variance was used to examine the relation between breastfeeding and linear growth. The variables in table 1 were included as covariates in analyses adjusting the relation between breastfeeding and linear growth for background variables.

4. RESULTS

The mean values of the raw data according to breastfeeding group is given in table 2. Interestingly, there was a significant positive association between breastfeeding and birth length with a gradual increase in length with increasing duration of breastfeeding. Despite this, length at 12 months showed the opposite association with a gradual decrease with increasing duration of breastfeeding. The difference in length gain from birth to 12 months was highly significant with infants being breast-fed for less than 1 month growing 2.7 cm more than those breastfed for more than 9 months.

Table 2. Birth length, length at 12 months and length gain according to duration of breastfeeding

Duration of breastfeeding	Birth length (cm)	Length 12 months (cm)	Length gain 0-12 months (cm)
1-4 weeks (n=349)	50.5	76.2	25.6
1-4 months (n= 602)	50.8	75.6	24.8
5-9 months (n=268)	51.1	75.3	24.2
> 9 months (n=31)	51.2	74.3	22.9
ANOVA (p value)	0.02	0.009	<0.0001

Table 3. Birth length, length at 12 months and length gain according to duration of breastfeeding. The means have been adjusted for the background variables in table 1 (birth weight was not included as a covariate in the analysis of birth length)

Duration of breastfeeding	Birth length (cm)	Length 12 months (cm)	Length gain 0-12 months (cm)
1- 4 weeks (n= 349)	50.7	76.2	25.2
1-4 months (n=602)	50.8	75.5	24.7
5-9 months (n=268)	50.8	75.4	24.5
> 9 months (n=31)	51.0	74.6	23.2
ANOVA (p value)	0.8	0.006	0.002

After controlling for the variables in table 1, the difference in birth length between the breast-feeding groups disappeared. However, there were still highly significant differences in length at 12 months and length gain from 0-

12 months between the feeding groups. The difference between the two
outer breastfeeding groups decreased to 2.0 cm.

In the analysis, the following factors were positively associated with birth
   length: Maternal height, pregnancy weight gain, gestational age and social
   status (borderline significant, p=0.07), while there was a negative
   association with smoking during pregnancy. Length at 12 months was
   positively associated with maternal height and birth weight and negatively
   with being offspring of a single mother. Length gain was positively
   associated with maternal height and gestational age and negatively with
   birth weight and being offspring of a single mother.

Data on weight and head circumference in the same group of infants have
   been analysed in the same way. Weight data showed the same pattern and
   the same level of significance as data for length while there were no
   significant associations between head circumference and duration of
   breastfeeding (data not shown).

5. DISCUSSION

In the present study and in two previous studies from Denmark, duration
of breast-feeding was significantly and negatively associated with linear
growth. The data suggest that the effect is strongest during the second half of
infancy. Other studies found the same association and among those which
did not find a significant effect, several found a trend towards the same
association.

It is not likely that the association is caused by a high number of infants
being breastfed exclusively beyond 6 months, as in the Finnish study[1]. In the
two previous studies from Denmark, only a few infants were exclusively
breastfed beyond 6 months and none beyond 7 months[6,7]. In the present
study, only 7% of the infants were breastfed exclusively beyond 6 months
and only 1% beyond 9 months (data not shown).

Analysis of the association between breastfeeding and growth should
take into account the complicated and strong associations between these two
factors and other biological and social factors. The present study
demonstrates the importance of adjusting for background variables. Both
birth size and growth from birth to 12 months are influenced by variables
which are also strongly associated with duration of breast-feeding, like social
status and smoking. Social status is positively associated with both growth
and breastfeeding in most populations in industrialized countries Smoking
has a negative effect on birth size and duration of breast-feeding as in the
present study (data not shown), while smoking might have a positive effect
on growth velocity during infancy due to catch-up after intrauterine growth

retardation. Interestingly, birth length was positively associated with duration of breastfeeding. The most likely explanation for this association is that mothers with a healthier life style (and a higher social class?) are also the mothers who decide to breastfeed for a longer period.

What are the possible mechanisms responsible for the association between breastfeeding and linear growth? Could it be reverse causation which seems to be the case in developing countries. We find it unlikely in our society as we would rather expect the opposite; that mothers with a small infant would tend to stop breastfeeding earlier, because she and those advising her would feel that breastfeeding might not be sufficient.

It could also be that mothers who decide to breastfeed for a longer period give complementary food that is different from what mothers who have stopped breastfeeding earlier give their infants. In one of the studies from Denmark[7], mothers who breastfed for a longer period gave their infants less meat and, not surprisingly, less cow's milk at the age of 10 months. Thus, these infants received less animal protein and less of the micronutrients associated with animal protein. In a previous study, we found indications of zinc deficiency at the age of 9 months in a group of Danish infants[10], but in another of our studies in which we randomised infants to a diet with low or high meat intake during the age period from 8 to 10 months, there was no effect of meat on growth[11]. However, these infants were not breastfed.

Protein intake is generally significantly lower in breastfed infants than in infants who are weaned, also during late infancy[12], but breastfed infants are usually receiving sufficient protein to cover their requirements. However, it has been suggested that a protein intake above the requirements can stimulate growth[13], perhaps through an effect of certain aminoacids on insulin secretion. Furthermore, it has been suggested that a high protein intake has a direct effect on IGF-1 secretion and thereby possibly on growth[14]. Breast milk also contains many hormones, growth factors and bioactive peptides that could have an effect on appetite or more directly on growth, perhaps through an endocrine modulation.

Is there an effect on long term growth and adult stature? Several studies have suggested that growth during infancy has a long-term effect on later growth. According to the growth model suggested by Karlberg, growth during the infancy period is regulated differently from growth during the childhood period[15]. Applying this model on growth data from Pakistan he suggested that a growth deficit accumulated during the infancy period was not picked up later[16]. These data are in accordance with the growth pattern seen in many developing countries where the average growth curve of a population typically has a pattern with adequate growth or even catch-up growth from birth to 6 months, a marked faltering from 6 to 18 months and thereafter a growth curve which is parallel to the reference curve, indicating that growth velocity after this age is close to the growth velocity in the reference population. However, the situation in developing countries is very different from the situation in most industrialized countries, and there are no data available to show if the slower growth in breast-fed infants have any effects on later growth and adult stature. If there is an effect on adult stature it could potentially have an effect on health as well, either positively or negatively. Adult stature is strongly negatively associated with the risk of death from cardiovascular disease, and positively associated with the risk of death from endocrine cancers like prostata cancer and mammae cancer[17].

In conclusion, infants who are breastfed well into the second half of infancy have a slower linear growth than infants who are weaned earlier, at least in some populations in industrialized countries. The mechanism behind this association is not known and it is not known if there are long term effects on linear growth. With the increasing focus on early programming or imprinting, and thereby also growth during infancy it is of interest to understand the mechanisms responsible for the association between breastfeeding and linear growth. Furthermore, it is important to know if there are any positive or negative long term effects on growth and health. In the meantime the results of studies showing a slower linear growth velocity in breast-fed infants should not be used to advocate against long term breastfeeding as we have no data suggesting any detrimental effects.

6. ACKNOWLEDGMENTS

Analysis of data from the Copenhagen Perinatal Cohort has been supported by the Danish Research Council grant 9700093 to EL Mortensen.

7. REFERENCES

1. Salmenperä L, Perheentupa J, Siimes MA. Exclusively breast-fed healthy infants grow slower than reference infants. Pediatric Research 1985;3:307-312.

2. Dewey KG, Peerson JM, Brown KH, Krebs NF, Michaelsen KF, Persson LA, Salmenperä L, Whitehead RG, Yeung DL, WHO Working Group on Infant Growth. Growth of breast-fed infants deviates from current reference data: A pooled analysis of US, Canadian, and European data sets. Pediatrics 1995;96:495-503.

3. Haschke F, Vant Hof MA, Euro-Growth Study Group. Influences of early nutrition on growth until 36 months of age. Journal of Pediatric Gastroenterology and Nutrition 1999;28:590.

4. Dewey KG, Heinig MJ, Nommsen LA, Peerson JM, Lönnerdal B. Growth of breast-fed and formula-fed infants from 0 to 18 months: The DARLING study. Pediatrics 1992;89:1035-1041.

5. Agostini C, Grandi F, Gianni ML, Silano M, Torcoletti M, Giovannini M, Riva E. Growth patterns of breast fed and formula fed infants in the first 12 months of life: an Italian study. Archives of Disease in Childhood 1999;81:395-399.

6. Michaelsen KF, Petersen S, Greisen G, Thomsen BL. Weight, length, head circumference, and growth velocity in a longitudinal study of Danish infants. Danish Medical Bulletin 1994;41:577-585.

7. Nielsen GA, Thomsen BL, Michaelsen KF. Influence of breastfeeding and complementary food on growth between 5 and 10 months. Acta Paediatrica 1998;87:911-917.

8. Zachau-Christiansen B, Ross EM. Babies: Human development during the first year. New York; John Wiley & Sons, 1975.

9. Mortensen EL. The Copenhagen Perinatal Cohort and the Prenatal Development Project. International Journal of Risk & Safety in Medicine 1997;10:199-202.

10. Michaelsen KF, Samuelson G, Graham TW, Lönnerdal B. Zinc intake, zinc status and growth in a longitudinal study of healthy Danish infants. Acta Paediatrica 1994;83:1115-1121.

11. Engelmann MDM, Sandström B, Michaelsen KF. Meat intake and iron status in late infancy: An intervention study. Journal of Pediatric Gastroenterology and Nutrition 1998;26:26-33.

12. Michaelsen KF. Nutrition and growth during infancy. The Copenhagen Cohort Study. Acta Paediatrica 1997:86(suppl 420):1-36.

13. Axelsson IE, Ivarsson SA, Räihä NC. Protein intake in early infancy: effects on plasma amino acid concentrations, insulin metabolism, and growth. Pediatric Research 1989;26.614-617.

14. Rolland-Cachera MF. Prediction of adult body composition from infant and child measurements. In: Davies PS, Cole T, eds. Body composition techniques in health and disease. Cambridge: Cambridge University Press, 1994.

15. Karlberg J, Jalil F, Lam B, Low L, Yeung CY. Linear growth retardation in relation to the three phases of growth. European Journal of Clinical Nutrition 1994;48(suppl 1):S25-43.

16. Karberg J, Jalil F, Lindblad BS. Longitudinal analysis of infantile growth in an urban area of Lahore, Pakistan. Acta Paediatrica Scandinavica 1988;77:392-401.

17. Barker DJP. Fetal and infant origins of adult disease. London: British Medical Journal Publishing Group, 1992.

17

THE ASSOCIATION BETWEEN PROLONGED BREASTFEEDING AND POOR GROWTH—
What are the implications?

Jean-Pierre Habicht, M.D.,Ph.D.,MPH
Division of Nutritional Sciences, Cornell University, Ithaca, NY 14853

Key words: Breast feeding, growth, reverse causality, confounding, complementary feeding:

Abstract: The smaller size of breast fed children in infancy and thereafter in malnourished and well-nourished populations has resulted in rushes to judgement that have been shown to be ill-advised. The reasons for the smaller size in malnourished populations is due to retaining the small and sickly child at the breast (reverse causality) and the consequent continuing sickliness of this breast fed child (negative confounding). Once the reverse causality and negative confounding have been taken into account breast feeding improves growth, at least through the second year of life. Thus prolonged breastfeeding should always be fostered, especially in malnourished populations. An exception remains when breast milk may transmit disease to the suckling child. In well-nourished populations the magnitude of the difference between breast fed and weaned children is much less than in malnourished populations, is observed to increase over the first year of life, but to have disappeared by the end of the second year. One may never-the-less be concerned that complimentary feeding practices are not adequate for these children.

1.   INTRODUCTION

The practical program and policy implication of the previous reports is that continued breastfeeding is good. The three studies from poor malnourished populations in Kenya, Senegal and Peru found (published here and in other reports) that the benefits of breastfeeding and suckling extend even into the third year of life in spite of the finding that sometimes babies

Short and Long Term Effects of Breast Feeding on Child Health
Edited by Berthold Koletzko *et al.*, Kluwer Academic/Plenum Publishers, 2000

who are partially breastfed beyond the age of six months are not as big as non-breast babies. When this occurred it was not that breastfeeding stunted growth but that small baby size and poor health determine continued breastfeeding.

While the studies from developing countries are clear, it is less clear why there is a negative association between infant size and continued breastfeeding in the latter half of infancy in the study from Denmark. However this study does not affect practical recommendations because there is no evidence that this decreased rate of growth is detrimental.

2.   EVOLUTION OF ISSUE

A review of the evolution in our thinking on the relationship between breastfeeding and size is instructive. The contribution by Simondon in this volume cites the various authors who have reported a negative association between breastfeeding and baby's size. Initially investigators who were known for their scientific rigor reported this negative association but were careful in their assessment of the implications for recommendations, awaiting further research to clarify the situation. However, a highly publicized report in 1988 (Brakohiapa et al. 1988 cited in Simondon) stated in their summary that , **"These results indicate that prolonged breastfeeding can reduce total food intake and thus predispose to malnutrition."** The possibility of reverse causality was not considered.

Reverse causality refers to the situation when the putative cause and effect relationship are reversed. This was, for instance, the reason for the extremely high association between not breastfeeding (putative cause) and infant mortality (effect) originally reported in the literature. The association was mostly due to the fact that children who died shortly after birth never breastfed and not because a lack of breastfeeding caused these deaths (Habicht et.al. 1986). In this case an important remaining component of the association was never-the-less causal, in that breast feeding did save lives.

The example of the breastfeeding-mortality association shows that after discarding the effect of reverse causality one must continue to search for and demonstrate causality. In other words, it is not enough to show reverse causality to negate causality. Analyses to determine causality and reverse causality require longitudinal data to establish a time sequence. The first study to do this in the examination of breast feeding and growth was in Africa but was reported in French in a source that was so obscure that it was unknown (Garrenne et al. 1987 cited in Simondon). This report was followed up shortly by a publication from Bangladesh, whose senior author was also

French (Briend and Bari, 1989 cited in Simondon), but published in the peer reviewed English literature. Since at least 1993 (review by Grummer-Strawn cited in Simondon) the possibility of reverse causality was well known, although it took some further time before it was established as the cause of the negative association between breastfeeding and growth, as reported in the three studies in this section. It is interesting that quantitative proof of reality comes for this issue, as for so many others, decades after anecdotal evidence is reported (e.g., Morley 1968 cited in Simondon) based upon facts that are well known to those working in the field.

In contrast to silence on the possibility of reverse causality, the methodological problem of confounding was considered as of the first reports about the negative association between breast feeding and child size. Confounding is the term used to refer to a situation in which the relationship between a putative determinant (e.g., breastfeeding) and an outcome (e.g., growth) is caused by a third factor (e.g., illness). The association of poor growth with breastfeeding would then be due to illness, or to poor complementary feeding, or to biased measurements and reporting, but not to breastfeeding. Longitudinal data do not help much in dealing with confounding. This issue must be addressed with imagination and persuasion to make a plausibility argument. Alternatively specially designed and difficult intervention trials can be used to make a statistical probability statement, which is stronger than a plausibility argument (Habicht et al.1999).

The position taken by a number of authors who have urged the abandonment of prolonged partial breastfeeding because of some biological anorexic properties is surprising, even without an understanding of the issue of reverse causality. Some of the authors who had looked for confounding and did not find evidence of it apparently were then led to the conclusion that it must be some unknown factor in breastmilk itself. But our understanding at the time of the advantages of breastfeeding in the kinds of populations in which it most occurs was solid. In particular the advantage of continuing breastfeeding when the complementary diet was poor in protein was often mentioned, and has since been shown to be the case in just these kinds of populations (Marquis et al 1997a).

The papers questioning the benefits of prolonged breastfeeding and those discussing these reports were not chary in inventing mechanisms to explain why breastfeeding stunted growth. Overwhelmingly they were biological and child- oriented in the sense that breastmilk was supposed to reduce appetite. None of these mechanisms were ever tested. The reverse causality mechanism, which is behavioral and under the control of the mother ("mother-oriented"), is easily testable. Why was it not invoked first?

We believe it is because quantitative research in breastfeeding is insufficiently informed about breastfeeding decisions and behaviors (such as those described Simondon's paper, in Dettwyller et al. (1987) and in Marquis et al (1997a) both cited in Simondon). This expertise and similar expertise about breast feeding in general (Pelto 1981) would be useful to our ISHM&L. It will require some recruiting to bring this scientific expertise to our society.

While inferring causality from statistical associations without other plausible evidence is a perennial problem, the scientific mill ultimately grinds finely enough to correct the mistake. However, the harm is not so quickly erased. In December, 1999 a graduate student approached me about investigating the anorectic properties of breast milk, in spite of having read all the pertinent literature! Apparently the idea was too beguiling. More serious than the effect on graduate students is the effect on programs and policy recommendations where such mistakes are not so benign, and continue to bedevil policy discussions long after the scientific mistake is corrected.

3.   SUMMARY OF THREE STUDIES IN DEVELOPING COUNTRIES

The reports at this meeting from rural Kenya, rural Senegal and a slum in Peru had a number of similarities and some differences. The similarities were that they were longitudinal, were of children who were more than a year old, and who were already markedly stunted. One can infer from the data presented that the mean stunting was in the range of −1.6 to −2.0 Z-score for children in their second year of life. This corresponds to the level of malnutrition usually seen in rural communities and slums around the world. Some countries, such as Guatemala and India, and the Sahel during famine periods have more severe levels (around −3.0 Z-scores). All the studies used linear OLS statistics with interactions. All three studies presented analyses that take into account confounding, either in this meeting's reports or in previous publications.

The major dissimilarities relate to the amount of information that was presented about each study in this book. The Senegal report reported a generally beneficial effect of breast feeding on growth up to 28 months of age. The Kenyan report mentioned that there was a positive association between the duration of breastfeeding and growth.. The Peruvian report followed the evolution of the negative association between breast feeding and growth through the second year of life – it did not present evidence of a beneficial effect of breast feeding as had the other two. However, that evidence had been presented in a previous publication (Marquis et al. 1997 b).

The Peruvian studies had ethnographic information, which showed the dynamics of decision making that led to reverse causality. Mothers are concerned that prolonged breast feeding weakens them so they stop when their child "no longer needs it". In Peru the information presented at this meeting showed that the strength of this preferential prolongation of breast-feeding for sickly children changes markedly over the second year of life. It was very strong at the beginning and had ceased by the end.

Reverse causality can be reinforced by confounding in that the children who continue to be breastfed are more sickly after their selection. This negative confounding has been described in the Peruvian study (Marquis et al 1997b). Of course, reverse causality and negative confounding biases are related in that children who are sickly and retained at the breast tend to remain sickly and continue to grow poorly.

Once reverse causality and negative confounding have been taken into account all three studies showed a beneficial effect of breast feeding on growth. At the meeting analyses of all three studies were discussed but not presented. Apparently the usual confounders that might explain this positive effect were investigated and found not to be reponsible. This increases the plausibility that the benefits on growth associated with breast feeding are causal and not artifactual. Plausibility is further increased if the conditions that potentiate this beneficial effect are those that would be expected given the biological benefits that are ascribed to breastfeeding. This was the case in these studies: the benefits were greater among children in environments with poor housing or hygienic conditions (verbally reported for Kenya and Senegal), and who have poor complementary diets (Peru in Marquis 1997a). Another finding in Peru confirms the mothers' perceptions about the special benefits of breast feeding for children who are not growing well (not "thriving"). These finding underscore the importance of recognizing and factoring in heterogeneity of response to nutritional activities when planning interventions and in analyzing study results. Testing for statistical interactions (synergisms and antagonisms) is important, but needs to be supported by thoughtful comparative analyses of subgroups to fully understand the relationships.

The practical implication of these studies is that in poor populations breast feeding improves growth and is most beneficial when other household circumstances are least propitious. This heterogeneity is not yet being taken into account adequately in the recommendations relative to breast feeding by HIV mothers. Neither are the heterogeneities in the likelihood of HIV transmission through breast milk being adequately considered. For instance the recent finding of much reduced transmission during exclusive breast feeding (Coutsoudis et al. 1999) may change the recommendations substantially for certain poor populations.

4.   THE COPENHAGEN STUDY

This study also found a negative association between breast feeding and growth. The longer the baby suckled the shorter it was at one year of age. This, and the above studies, were also comparable in that they were longitudinal, and they sought to take into account confounding and reverse causality. However, they were not comparable in age or in the level of poverty. In contrast to the other studies, this study collected data in infancy. The babies in the Copenhagen study lived in one of the most healthy and well-grown populations of the world, and were not stunted at the onset of the study, in contrast to the poverty-stricken, unhealthy and stunted children in the other studies. These differences are so profound that one might think that there is nothing to be learned from the other studies as relates to this study.

In fact the Copenhagen study is an important representative of many other studies that have shown that breastfeeding duration is associated with decreased growth in infancy in well off populations (WHO '95). This effect is presumed to be due to a biological effect of breast milk on child.appetite. It is a "child-oriented" mechanism in contrast to a behavioral mother-oriented mechanism. The Copenhagen study took into account biases due to self-selection and confounding. Once these were considered there was no difference in growth until after four months of age. Thereafter children who were breastfed were almost a centimeter shorter by nine months of age, and another centimeter for those who breast fed longer. One might conclude from this evidence that nothing more is needed to assert that this decreased growth is natural, and is a healthy consequence of prolonged breast feeding. This assertion is the basis of a world wide effort to establish growth standards for breast fed infants (De Onis et al. 1997). It is also the basis for the UNICEF recommendation to breastfeed exclusively to six months of age.

Aspects of the Copenhagen study, as well as studies in other countries, should give one some pause before concluding that no further research is needed on this subject. The magnitude of the growth effect associated with duration of breastfeeding is substantially different across all these studies. For instance the Copenhagen study found differences of two centimeters at one year of age in comparison to a half centimeter difference reported in WHO (1999). This variability across studies is not likely to be due to factors mediated only through breastfeeding.

In the Copenhagen study the proportion who breastfed to five months was 20%, and only 3% were breastfed beyond nine months. This very small proportion indicates that longer breastfeeding was not culturally normative in Copenhagen, and the small minority of mothers who did continue were likely to be different from the great majority who did not in multiple ways that affect growth. It is likely that child care and dietary patterns were different in this subgroup, and these differences need to be investigated before one can conclude that observed differences are due to breastfeeding. In the case of Denmark Dr. Michaelsen has pointed out that this seems to be particularly the case for those who breastfeed longest. Is this the reason for the much larger difference in length between the longest breast feeding group and the others? The possibility that other factors are responsible underscores the importance of further investigation, particularly because of concern about the adequacy of complementary feeding, even in wealthy families in developed countries.

On the other hand, scientific uncertainty about feeding in later infancy should not affect breastfeeding recommendations in wealthy countries, because the differences in growth between those who breast feed longer and those who receive breastmilk for a shorter period of time is usually small at one year of age and disappears thereafter.

However, it may well turn out that the effects on growth, especially among those who breast feed for longer periods of time, is due to inadequacies In complementary feeding. Our knowledge on this score is woefully lacking (Brown et al 1998), in contrast to our knowledge about the adequacy and benefits of human milk and breast-feeding. It is time that we turned our attention to this essential complementary element to breast-feeding.

ACKNOWLEDGMENT

I would like to thank Gretel Pelto for substantive discussions and critical comments.

REFERENCES

Brown,K., Dewey,K., and Allen,L., 1998, *Complementary Feeding of Young Children in Developing Countries*, World Health Organization, Geneva

Coutsoudis, A., Kubendran, P., Spooner, E., Kuhn, L., and Coovadia, H.M., 1999, Influence of infant-feeding patterns on early mother-to-child transmission of HIV-1 in Durban, South Africa: a prospective cohort study. *Lancet* 354:471-76.

de Onis, M., Garza, C., and Habicht, J-P., 1997,Time for a new growth reference. *Pediatrics*, 100: E8

Habicht, J-P., DaVanzo,J., and Butz,W.P., 1986, Does breastfeeding really save lives, or are apparent benefits due to biases? American Journal of Epidemiology 123: 279-290.

J. Habicht, J-P., Victora, C.G., and Vaughan, J.P., 1999, Evaluation designs for adequacy, plausibility and probability of public health programme performance and impact. *International Journal of Epidemiology.* 28:10-18.

Marquis, G.S., Habicht, J-P., Lanata, C.F., Black, R.E., and Rasmussen, K.M., 1997a, Breast milk or animal-product foods improve linear growth of Peruvian toddlers consuming marginal diets. American Journal of Clinical Nutrition 66: 1102-1109.

Marquis, G.S., Habicht, J-P., Lanata, C.F., Black, R. E., Rasmussen. K.M., 1997b, Association of breastfeeding and stunting in Peruvian toddlers: An example of reverse causality. International Journal of Epidemiology 26: 349-356.

Pelto, G.H., 1981, Perspectives on infant feeding: decision-making and ecology. *Food and Nutr. Bull.* 3:16-29.

WHO,1995, *Physical Status:The Use and Interpretation of Anthropometry.* Technical Report of a WHO Expert Committee, Geneva, World Health Organization, Geneva

18

BREASTFEEDING AND HIV-1 INFECTION
A review of current literature

Ruth Nduati
Department of Paediatrics, University of Nairobi, P.O. Box 19676, Nairobi, Kenya

1. PREVALENCE OF HIV-1 AMONG PREGNANT WOMEN IN SUB SAHARA AFRICA

HIV-1 infection is possibly the most common serious health problem facing pregnant women in Africa. The prevalence of HIV-1 among pregnant women ranges from 5-10% in West Africa, 10-30% in East and Central Africa and > 20% in Southern Africa. The prevalence of HIV is 4% in the Indian sub-continent and less than 2% elsewhere in the world (UNAIDS, 1998). Because there is mother-to-child transmission of HIV, the epidemic of HIV-1 among women of childbearing years is associated with a parallel epidemic in children. With the development of effective technologies to prevent MTCT, replacement feeding and anti-retroviral therapy, new paediatric infections are almost exclusively a problem of the developing world where there is limited capacity to rapidly adopt new strategies for prevention. It was estimated that in 1997 alone, ~ 600,000 children were infected with HIV-1 of whom 90% were in sub- Saharan Africa (UNAIDS, 1998).

Babies are at risk of HIV-1 infection while in utero, during delivery and postnatally through breastfeeding. In non-breastfed infants, most MTCT of HIV takes place during the intrapartum period. In breastfeeding populations, 30-50% of the overall transmission is attributable to breastfeeding (Van de

Short and Long Term Effects of Breast Feeding on Child Health
Edited by Berthold Koletzko *et al.*, Kluwer Academic/Plenum Publishers, 2000

Perre et al.1992a). This paper reviews what is currently known about breastmilk transmission of HIV.

2.   BREASTMILK TRANSMISSION OF HIV-1 AMONG WOMEN WITH NEW HIV INFECTIONS IN THE POSTNATAL PERIOD

A variety of studies utilizing different study designs have yielded evidence of breastmilk transmission of HIV-1. The initial evidence for breastmilk transmission was from case reports and case series of women who sero-converted in the postnatal period following transfusion with HIV-1 contaminated blood (Ziegler et al.1985, Colebunders et al.1988, Stiehm and Vink 1991, Palassanthiran et al. 1993). These were followed by cohort studies of HIV-1 uninfected women, where some sero-converted following heterosexual exposure to HIV while they were lactating (Hira etal. 1990, Van de Perre 1991b). Most of these studies had small sample sizes and marked variation in the estimate of risk. In order to provide a more accurate estimate of the risk of HIV-1 transmission a meta-analysis was carried out. The risk of breastmilk transmission of HIV-1 to infants of women who sero-convert in the postnatal period was estimated to be 29% (95% CI 16-42%) (Dunn et al. 1992).

3.   BREASTMILK TRANSMISSION OF HIV-1 AMONG WOMEN WITH ESTABLISHED INFECTION

Most babies who are exposed to HIV-1 are infants of women with established HIV-1 infection. Evidence for breastmilk transmission has been from birth cohort studies of infants of HIV-1 infected women. Within these cohorts, HIV infection rates have been higher in infants exposed to breastmilk compared to those who were formula fed (Ryder et al. 1991, European collaborative study 1992, Gabiano et al. 1992, Mayaux et al. 1995,).

Several problems have been experienced in determining the magnitude of breastmilk transmission of HIV. Following infection with HIV, there is a window period in which infection is undetectable using the currently available technology. Therefore it is technically impossible to isolate closely related exposure points, including very early breastfeeding, exposure from intra-partum and late pregnancy transmission of HIV. Published studies of MTCT of HIV-1 also have some fundamental differences. These include among others, differences in the techniques used to determine infant infection status with earlier studies using antibody-based tests and later studies using DNA PCR to document infant infection as well as differences in severity of disease in the study population (Ryder 1994). The studies also differed in the duration of follow-up as well as duration of exposure to breastmilk. Babies in developing countries breastfeeding into the second year of life while those in developed-countries breastfeeding for only a few weeks (European collaborative study 1992, Gabiano et al. 1992, Mayaux et al. 1995, Lepage et al. 1993, Datta et al. 1994). There were also differences in the nutritional status of women in the different cohorts with women from the developing countries having high levels of anemia and vitamin A deficiency (Semba et al. 1994, Nduati et al. 1995). The HIV-1 subtypes in the different regions differ with subtype B being the predominant one Europe, America and Australia while subtypes A, D, C predominate in sub-Saharan Africa. The role of these factors on breastmilk transmission of HIV have only been partially elucidated.

3.1 Magnitude of Transmission Among Women with Established Infections

In order to determine the magnitude of breastmilk transmission of HIV-1in women with established infections there is need to compare breastfeeding and formula feeding infants. In the early cohort studies, one mode of infant feeding predominated; breastfeeding in developing country cohorts and formula in developed country cohorts. In any one cohort there were few children having a different method of infant feeding to enable meaningful comparison. A meta-analysis of the published data estimated the additional risk of breastmilk transmission among infants of HIV-1 infected women to be 14% (95% CI 7%-22%) (Dunn et al. 1992). More recent cohort studies have included more even numbers of breastfeeding and formula feeding infants. These studies have found that breastfeeding doubles the risk of MTCT of HIV (Bobat et al 1997, Tess et al 1998).

The best estimate we have on the magnitude of breastmilk transmission of HIV-1 in the first month of life is from a randomized clinical trial of breastfeeding and formula feeding among infants of HIV-1 infected (Nduati et al. 1999). In this study where women and infants in the two study arms were comparable at baseline, differences in HIV-1 infection status in the two arms of the study could be attributed to breastfeeding. At the end of two years, the additional risk of HIV-1 infection in breastfeeding infants was found to be 16% (95% CI 6.5%-25.9%). In this study there was > 95% compliance in the breastfeeding arm of the study and 70% in the formula arm. Therefore, the estimates of breastmilk transmission of HIV-1 from this study was probably an underestimate of the true risk.

3.2   Timing of Breastmilk Transmission of HIV-1

Babies are at risk of HIV-1 infection as long as they are breastfeeding but the risk of breastmilk transmission of HIV-1 is highest in the first 6 months of life. In two breastfeeding cohorts studies that have presented data on the time to first positive HIV-1 PCR, a rapid increase in number of infected children in the first 6 months of life and relatively fewer sero-conversions after this period of time were observed as shown in table 1 (Simonon et al. 1994, Bertolli et al. 1996). The conclusions from these studies was that there was postnatal MTCT of HIV-1 among infants of women with established infection, babies were at risk as long as they were exposed to HIV-1 contaminated breastmilk, and the younger infant was more vulnerable. These studies could not separate late pregnancy, intrapartum and early breastmilk transmission and were therefore limited in determining the individual contribution of any of these time points to mother-to-child transmission of HIV.

Table 1. Timing of breastmilk transmission of HIV-1

Reference	In utero transmission	Intrapartum and early postpartum transmission	Late postnatal transmission
Simonon 1994	7.7%	12.7%*	4.9%
Bertolli 1996	6% (CI 4%-10%)	18 (CI 14%-24%)	4% (CI 2%-8%)

confidence intervals not given in the published paper, * calculated from data presented in the table.

An alternative approach has been to examine the risk of HIV-1 infection in babies who have been shown to be uninfected in the postnatal period. The term late-postnatal transmission is used to describe infection in infants who have had a period free of infection and subsequently become infected through exposure to breastmilk. Although this method has the advantage of isolating breastmilk transmission of HIV-1 from the late pregnancy, and intrapartum transmission, there is a drawback in that this method does not provide information on the risk of breastmilk transmission in the first few weeks of life. There is considerable variability in the estimated risk of late postnatal transmission of HIV. The earlier studies that used anti-body testing classified children to have late postnatal testing if they became infected after the 6 month of life or even later. With the current HIV PCR technology, HIV infection status of an infant can be determined as early as 2 months of life and thus the period of observation has been extended backward to begin from 2 months of life. The studies also vary in the duration of exposure to breastfeeding. In order to give an accurate estimate of the risk of postnatal transmission, a pooled analysis was carried out. The risk of late postnatal transmission was determined to be 5.4% (Leroy et al. 1998).

Estimation of the risk of early breastmilk transmission has continued to be a challenge. Three recent studies have examined this risk closely. In a study if central Africa, 19% (CI 8%,33%) breastfed infants of HIV-1 infected women who were PCR negative at 4 weeks of life and followed until 6 months seroconverted (Bequart et al. 1998). In the second study from Malawi examined the risk of postnatal transmission of HIV-1 in the first two years of life among babies who were PCR negative at 6 weeks of life. The HIV-1 infection rate was calculated to be 0.7% in the period 1-5 months of life, 0.6% /month in the 6-11 month period, 0.3%/month during 12-17 months of life and 0.2 in the 18-23 months of life (Miotti et al. 1999). This study suggests that after the first 6 weeks of life, the rate of breastmilk transmission is stable throughout the first year of life and thereafter declines significantly in the second year of life. This is probably due to declining amounts of milk consumed by the infant or through selection of genetically less vulnerable individuals.

The third approach has been to estimate the cumulative probability of infection in breastfed and formula fed infants and to determine the difference during the course of lactation. In the RCT of breastfeeding and formula feeding among infants of HIV-1 infected women described above, 63% of the risk difference in the two arms of the study had occurred by 6 weeks of life, and 75% by 6 months after delivery. These observations support the hypothesis that most breastmilk transmission takes place early during lactation(Nduati et al. 1999).

The fourth piece of evidence for continuing risk of HIV-1 infection in breastfed infants is from the studies that have evaluated the value of antenatal anti-retroviral therapy (ARV) as prophylaxis for prevention of MTCT of HIV in breastfeeding populations. In these studies there is declining efficacy of the ARV therapy with ongoing exposure to breasmilk (Dabis et al. 1999, Wiktor et al. 1999).

4. CORRELATES OF TRANSMISSION

The factors that correlate with breastmilk transmission of HIV-1 have not been exhaustively been investigated. These factors can be classified as viral factors, maternal factors, infectious and anti-infectious factors in breastmilk, and breast disease.

4.1   Maternal Plasma Viral Factors

Breastmilk transmission of HIV is associated with elevated maternal viral load (Semba et al. 1999, John et al. 1999). There is also preliminary evidence that subtype C is more easily transmitted postnatally compared to other subtypes(John et al. 1999).

4.2   Maternal Disease Status

The role of maternal immunosupression independent of maternal viral load is not well evaluated in the context of breastmilk transmission of HIV. A trend to wards increased postnatal transmission among women with CD4/CD8 ration < 0.5 has been reported(Van de Perre et al. 1993).

4.3   Breastmilk HIV

Several studies have demonstrated the presence of cell associated and cell free HIV-1 in breastmilk (Nduati et al. 1995, Van de Perre et al. 1993, Ruff et al. 1994, Guay et al. 1996, Lewis et al. 1998). Two studies have documented an association between breastmilk HIV and infant HIV infection. In the earlier Rwandan study, HIV-1 DNA in day 15 milk was associated with a five fold increased risk of infection in the infant (Van de Perre et al. 1993). A recent study in Malawi, women who transmitted HIV-1 through breastfeeding to their infants had significantly higher plasma and breastmilk viral load (Semba et al. 1999). In this study women who transmitted HIV-1 through breastmilk had a median breastmilk viral load of 700copies/ml compared to < 200 copies/ml among women who did not transmit.

4.4   Breast Disease

A number of studies have reported on the association between mastitis and breastfeeding ((Semba et al. 1999, John et al. 1999, Van de Perre et al. 1992, Ekpini et al. 1997). Most of the early studies did not have enough cases to allow for a meaningful analysis. In the Malawian study described earlier, mastitis was diagnosed in two ways, obvious clinical mastitis, and sub clinical mastitis based on biochemical estimation of elevated sodium in breastmilk. Both clinical and sub-clinical mastitis was associated with significantly increased risk breastmilk transmission. The probability of transmitting HIV-1 among women who experienced clinical mastitis was OR, 9.69 (955 CI 3.49-26.8, p < 0.0001) ((Semba et al. 1999). Women with elevated breastmilk sodium in week 6 breastmilk samples had higher median plasma viral load, and lower CD4 counts. The median breastmilk HIV-1 was 900 copies/ml among women with elevated breastmilk sodium compared to undetectable levels in those with normal levels. At 1 year the HIV-1 infection rate was 50.9% (28/55) among infants of women with elevated breastmilk sodium compared to 26% (71/273) among babies of women without elevated breastmilk sodium. Maternal plasma viral load, elevated breastmilk sodium and low maternal CD4/CD8 ratios were independent predictors of postnatal transmission of HIV ((Semba et al. 1999).

4.5   Infant Factors

There is data to suggest that breastmilk transmission of HIV is more efficient in the early months of life. Some studies have reported the association between oral thrush and infant sero-conversion (Ekpini et al. 1997, Njenga et al. 1997). It is not clear whether this is a causal relationship or oral thrush is as result of the profound transient immunosuppression associated with primary HIV-1 infection. The method of infant feeding also appears to have a role in determining the magnitude of postnatal transmission. One study has reported that babies who are exclusively breastfed in the first 3 months of life appear to have a lower risk of HIV infection compared to babies on mixed breast and formula (Coutsoudis 1999).

5.   ANTI-INFECTIVE PROPERTIES OF BREASTMILK

Breastmilk has many cellular and soluble anti-infection factors. The observation that the majority of infants exposed to breastmilk contaminated by HIV do not become infected suggest that some of these factors may mitigate against infection. HIV specific IgG, IGA and IGM have been found in breastmilk of HIV infected women(Van de Perre et al 1993, Belec et al, 1990). Persistence of HIV-1 specific IgM up to 18 postnatal months is associated with a 90% reduced risk of transmission. In vitro studies have demonstrated that there are soluble factors in breastmilk that have anti-HIV properties. There is need to carry out further research to determine how these properties of breastmilk could be enhanced to minimize breastmilk transmission of HIV.

6.   CONCLUSIONS

Breastmilk transmission of HIV presents major dilemmas in the provision of adequate nutrition and protection from infections for children living in resource poor settings. There is an urgent need to explore various strategies for minimizing or completely preventing breastmilk transmission of HIV while at the same time enabling the infant to breast feed. Anti-retroviral drugs that have been shown to reduce transmission during pregnancy and delivery need to be further evaluated for their possible role in pre- and post-exposure prophylaxis during lactation.

REFERENCES

Becquart P, Garin B, Sepou A et al. High incidence of early postnatal transmission of human immunodeficiency virus type 1 in Bangui, Central African Republic. J infect Dis. 1998;177:1770-1.

Belec L, Bouquety JC, Georges AJ, Siopathis MR, Martin PMV et al. Antibodies to human immunodeficiency virus in breast milk of healthy, seropositive women. Pediatrics 1990;85:1022-1026.

Bertolli J, St. Louis, Simonds RJ, et al. Estimating the timing of mother-to-child transmission of human immunodeficiency virus in a breastfeeding population in Kinshasa, Zaire. Journal of Infectious Diseases 1996;174:722-726.

Bobat R, Moodley D, Coutsoudis, Coovadia H. Breastfeeding by HIV-1 infected women and outcome in their infants: a cohort study from Durban, South Africa. AIDS 1997;11:1627-1633.

Colebunders R, Kapita B, Nekwei W, et al. Breastfeeding and transmission of HIV. Lancet 1988;2:1487.

Coutsoudis A, Pillay K, Spooner E et al. Influence of infant feeding patterns on early mother-to-child transmission of HIV-1 in Durban, South Africa. Lancet

Dabis F, Msellatu P, Meda N et al. 6-month efficacy, tolerance, and acceptability of a short regimen of oral zidovudine to reduce vertical transmission of HIV in breastfed children in Cote d'Ivoire and Burkina Faso: a double blind placebo-controlled multicentre trial. Lancet 1999;353:786-92.

Datta P, Embree JE, Kreiss JK, et al. Mother-to-child transmission of human immunodeficiency virus type 1 report from the Nairobi study. Journal of Infectious Diseases 1994;170:1134-1140.

Dunn DT, Newell ML, Ades AE, Peckham C. Risk of human immunodeficiency virus type 1 transmission through breastfeeding. Lancet 1992;340:585-588.

Ekpini E, Wiktor SZ, Satten GA, et al. Late postnatal transmission of HIV-1 in Abidjan, Cote d'Ivoire. Lancet 1997;349:1054-1059.

European Collaborative Study. Risk factors for mother-to-child transmission of HIV-1. Lancet 1992;339:1007-1012.

Gabiano C, Tovo PA, Martino M et al. Mother-to-child transmission of human immunodeficiency virus type 1: risk of infection and correlates of transmission Paediatrics 1992;90:369-374.

Guay LA, Hom DL, Mmiro F et al. Detection of human immune deficiency virus type 1 (HIV-1) DNA and p24 antigen in breastmilk of Hiv-1 infected Ugandan women and vertical transmission Pediatrics 1996;98:438-444.

Hira SK, Mangrola UG, Mwale C, et al. Apparent vertical transmission of human immunodeficiency virus type 1 by breastfeeding in Zambia. Journal of Pediatrics 1990; 117: 421-424.

John G, Nduati R, Ngacha D, et al. Correlates of perinatal transmission in the Kenyan breastfeeding study. In: Proceedings of the XI International conference on AIDS and STDS in Africa 12-16 September, 1999, Lusaka, Zambia Abstract 13ET5-1

Lepage P, Van de Perre, Msellati P, et al. Mother-to-child transmission of human immunodeficiency virus type (HIV-1) and its determinants: a cohort study from Kigali, Rwanda. American Journal of Epidemiology 1993;137:589-599.

Leroy V, Newell ML, Dabis F. International multicentre pooled analysis of late postnatal mother-to-child transmission of HIV infection. Lancet 1998;352:597-600.

Lewis P, Nduati R, kreiss JK et al. Cell-free human immunodeficiency virus type 1 in breastmilk. J Infect Dis. 1998;177:68-73.

Mayaux MJ, Blanche S, Rouzioux C et al. Maternal factors associated with perinatal HIV-1 transmission: the French cohort study: 7 years of follow-up observation. J of Acquired Immune defic Syndrome and Human retrovirology 1995;8:188-194.

Miotti PG, Taha TET, Kumwenda NI, et al. HIV Transmission through breastfeeding, a study in Malawi. JAMA 1999;282:744-749.

Nduati R, John G, Richardson B, et al. Human immunodeficiency virus type-1 infected cells in breast milk: Association with immunosupression and vitamin A deficiency. Journal of Infectious Disease 1995;172:1461-1468.

Nduati R, John G, Mbori-Ngacha D et al. Breastfeeding transmission of HIV-1: A randomized clinical trial. In: Proceedings of the XI International conference on AIDS and STDS in Africa 12-16 September, 1999, Lusaka, Zambia Abstract No. 13ET5-2.

Njenga S, Embree JE, Ndinya-Achola, et al. Risk factors for postnatal mother-to-child transmission of HIV in Nairobi. Conference on Global Strategies for Prevention of HIV Transmission from Mothers to Infants, September 1997, Washington DC.

Palasanthiran P, Ziegler JB, Stewart GJ, et al. Breastfeeding during primary maternal immunodeficiency virus infection and risk of transmission from mother to infant. Journal of Infectious Disease 1993;167:441-444.

Ryder RW, Manzila T, Baende E, et al. Evidence from Zaire that breastfeeding by HIV seropositive mothers is not a major route for perinatal HIV-1 transmission but does decrease morbidity. AIDS 1991; 5:709-714.

Ryder RW, Behets F. Reasons for wide variation in reported rates of mother-to-child transmission of HIV-1. AIDS 1994;8:1495-1497.

Ruff A, Coberly J, Halsey N, et al, Prevalence of HIV-1 DNA and P24 antigen in breast milk and correlation with maternal factors. Journal of Acquired Immune Deficiency Syndrome 1994;7:68-72.

Semba RD, Miotti PG, Chiphangwi JD, et al. Maternal vitamin A deficiency and mother-to-child transmission of HIV-1. Lancet 1994;343:1593-1597.

Semba RD, Kumwenda N, Hoover DR et al. Human immunodeficiency virus load in breast milk, mastitis, and mother-to-child transmission on human immunodeficiency virus type 1. J Infect Dis 1999;180:93-8.

Simonon A, Lepage P, Karita E, et al. An assessment of the timing of mother-to-child transmission of human immunodeficiency virus type 1 by means of polymerase chain reaction. Journal of Acquired Immune Deficiency Syndromes 1994;7:952-957.

Stiehm R, Vink P. Transmission of human immunodeficiency virus infection by breastfeeding. Journal of Pediatrics 1991;118:410-12.

Tess BH, Rodrigues LC, Newell M-L et al. Breastfeeding, genetic, obstetric and other risk factors associated with mother-to-child transmission of HIV-1 in Sao Paulo state, Brazil. AIDS 1998;12:513-520.

UNAIDS Report on the global HIV/AIDS epidemic June 1998. UNAIDS/98.10 – WHO/EMC/VIR/98.2 – WHO/ASD/98.2

Van de Perre P, Lepage P, Homsy J, Dabis F. Mother-to-infant transmission of human immunodeficiency virus by breastmilk: presumed innocent or presumed guilty. Clinical Infect Dis 1992;15:502-7.

Van de Perre, Simonon A, Msellati P et al. Postnatal transmission of human immunodeficiency virus type 1 from mother to infant; a prospective cohort study in Kigali, Rwanda. N Engl J Med 1991;325:593-8.

Van de Perre P, Simonon A, Hitimana D, et al. Infective and anti-infective properties of breastmilk from HIV-1-infected women. Lancet 1993;341:914-918.

Van de Perre P, Hitimana DG, Simonan A, et al. Postnatal transmission of HIV-1 associated with breast abscess. Lancet 1992;339:1490-1491

Wiktor SZ, Ekpini E, Karon JM et al. Short-course oral zidovudine for prevention of mother-to child transmission of HIV-1 in Abidjan, Cote d'Ivoire: a randomised clinical trial. Lancet 1999;353:773-80.

Ziegler JB, Johnson RO, Cooper D, Gold J. Postnatal transmission of AIDS-associated retrovirus from mother to infant. Lancet 1985;i:896-898.

19

SUBCLINICAL MASTITIS AS A RISK FACTOR FOR MOTHER-INFANT HIV TRANSMISSION

JF Willumsen,[1] SM Filteau,[1] A Coutsoudis,[2] KE Uebel,[2] M-L Newell,[3] and AM Tomkins[1]

[1]Centre for International Child Health, Institute of Child Health, London; [2]Department of Pediatrics and Child Health, University of Natal, Durban, [3]Department of Epidemiology and Population Health, Institute of Child Health, London

Key words: mastitis, breast milk, sodium, inflammation, HIV

Abstract: Subclinical mastitis, as diagnosed by an elevated sodium/potassium ratio in milk accompanied by an increased milk concentration of the inflammatory cytokine, interleukin-8 (IL8), was found to be common among breast feeding women in Bangladesh and Tanzania. Subclinical mastitis results in leakage of plasma constituents into milk, active recruitment of leukocytes into milk, and possible infant gut damage from inflammatory cytokines. Therefore, we wished to investigate whether subclinical mastitis was related to known risk factors for postnatal mother-to-child HIV transmission, that is, high milk viral load or increased infant gut permeability. HIV-infected South African women were recruited at the antenatal clinic of McCord's Hospital, Durban. Risks and benefits of different feeding strategies were explained to them and, if they chose to breast feed, they were encouraged to do so exclusively. Women and infants returned to the clinic at 1, 6 and 14 weeks postpartum for an interview about infant health and current feeding pattern, a lactulose/mannitol test of infant gut permeability, and milk sample collection from each breast separately for analysis of Na/K ratio, IL8 concentration and viral load in the cell-free aqueous phase. Only preliminary cross-sectional analyses from an incomplete database are available at this point. Moderately (0.6 - 1.0) or greatly (>1.0) raised Na/K ratio was common and was often unilateral, although as a group right and left breasts did not differ. Considering both breasts together, normal, moderately raised or greatly raised Na/K was found, respectively, in 51%, 28%, 21% of milk samples at 1 week (n=190); 69%, 20%, 11% at 6 weeks (n=167); and 72%, 16%, 12% at 14 weeks (n=122). IL8 concentration significantly correlated with both Na/K and viral load at all times. Na/K correlated with viral load at 1 and 14, but not 6 weeks. At 1 and 14 weeks, geometric mean viral loads in samples with Na/K > 1.0 were approximately 4 times those in samples with Na/K < 0.6. At 1 week but not later times, exclusive breast feeding was associated with lower milk viral load than was mixed feeding. Gut permeability was unrelated to milk Na/K ratio or IL8 concentration and was not significantly increased by inclusion of other foods than breast milk in the infant's diet. The results suggest that subclinical mastitis among HIV-infected women may increase the risk of vertical transmission through breast feeding by increasing milk viral load. The importance of various causes of subclinical mastitis, which likely differ at 1 week from at later times and may include local infection or sterile inflammation, systemic infection, micronutrient deficiencies, or poor lactation practices, needs to be further clarified so that appropriate interventions can be implemented.

1.   BACKGROUND

1.1   Breast feeding and mother to infant HIV transmission

Breast feeding is estimated to account for about a third of mother-to-infant HIV transmission among African populations.[1] This has resulted in a major public health dilemma since the advantages of breast feeding for preventing infant morbidity and mortality are well established. HIV-infected women who have reliable access to safe, clean breast milk substitutes are advised not to breast feed. However, in much of Africa, provision of clean breast milk substitutes cannot be guaranteed and women must balance the risks of HIV transmission through breast feeding against the risks of infant mortality associated with not breast feeding. A woman's choice is further complicated by the fact that the protection against diarrhea and respiratory infections which is provided by breast milk may be particularly important for infants already HIV-infected before or during delivery. Furthermore, in cultures where breast feeding is almost universal, not breast feeding may disclose HIV status which could have serious social consequences. Therefore, it is important to try to identify which women or which feeding practices are associated with breast milk transmission of HIV so that the subgroup of mother-infant pairs at risk can be supported in safe use of breast milk substitutes and the remaining pairs can be supported in optimising infant health through breast feeding.

A recent study from South Africa found that exclusive breast feeding was associated with a lower risk of mother-to-infant transmission before 3 months than was mixed feeding.[2] There are biologically plausible mechanisms whereby mixed feeding may carry the highest risk of HIV transmission. Breast milk, in addition to virus, contains antibodies and glycosaminoglycans which may inhibit virus binding to cells in the infant gut,[3, 4] various factors which can actively promote the infant's own immune function,[5] and factors which promote development of gut integrity.[6] Therefore, with exclusive breast feeding, the net result may be a low level of postnatal transmission. Feeding of other foods can damage the infant's gut and increase permeability. In breast feeding mixed with other foods, this increased permeability, together with decreased total amounts of breast milk immune factors, may tip the balance between virus and protective factors in milk and permit virus to enter infant cells more readily. An additional factor which we have recently considered is that supplementation of a breastfed infant's diet with other foods may, by decreasing milk intake, result in milk stasis and subclinical mastitis with consequent adverse effects on the infant.

1.2   Subclinical mastitis

The biology of mastitis has been extensively studied by dairy researchers. Inflammatory cytokines such as IL8, IL1 and tumour necrosis factor-α are produced within the mammary gland and mediate both recruitment of leukocytes and opening of the tight junctions between epithelial cells.[7-9] IL8 can be readily measured in milk[10, 11] but, in our experience, milk is a difficult matrix in which to quantitate many of the other key cytokines involved in mastitis.[11] However, sodium is an abundant and easily measurable plasma constituent which crosses into milk when tight junctions become permeable.[12]

Recently, while investigating the impact of maternal vitamin A supplementation on immune factors in the breast milk of Bangladeshi women, we wished to exclude women with mastitis since this inflammation was likely to greatly alter milk immunology.[10] Therefore, we measured milk sodium and controlled for the varying proportions of aqueous phase in spot milk samples by expressing sodium as a ratio to potassium. To our surprise, elevated milk sodium was too common - 25% of women at 2 weeks postpartum and 12% at 3 months - for us to simply exclude these women. Since the study was designed for other purposes, women were not asked about mastitis at the time of sampling, although any overt mastitis would have been noted in the general health check. We refer to high milk Na/K ratio accompanied by high IL8 concentration but in the absence of symptoms as subclinical mastitis. Importantly, infants of women with raised milk Na/K ratio at either 2 weeks or 3 months gained significantly less weight between these two time points than did infants of women with normal milk sodium.[10] Poor weight gain associated with high breast milk sodium has also been observed in American infants.[13] A possible mechanism is that poor lactation practice by the mother or weak suckling by the infant results in milk stasis, mammary gland involution,[14, 15] and consequently both raised milk sodium and poor growth.

Common features of clinical and subclinical mastitis

often occurs unilaterally
high milk sodium
high milk IL8
high milk pH
associated with systemic inflammation
decreased by dietary anti-oxidants

Since subclinical mastitis was common among Bangladeshi women and was associated with poor infant, and possibly also maternal, health, we extended our investigations to other populations. Of Tanzanian women participating in a trial of food-based micronutrient supplementation, 13% at 1 month postpartum and 11% at 3 months had subclinical mastitis.[11] Milk Na/K ratio correlated with maternal plasma acute phase proteins. Biologically it seems more plausible that subclinical mastitis may result from systemic infection or inflammation than that a localised and subclinical inflammation can result in a detectable systemic inflammation. Systemic illness is common in the first few months postpartum[16] and can increase permeability of other epithelia such as that of the gastrointestinal tract.[17] We also found in the Tanzanian cohort that supplementation of women during the last trimester of pregnancy and the first 3 months postpartum with vitamin E-rich sunflower oil, but not with vitamin A-rich red palm oil, could decrease milk Na/K.[11] A possible mechanism is that antioxidant micronutrients such as vitamin E can decrease both production of inflammatory cytokines and tissue damage caused by free radicals produced during inflammation.[18] Antioxidant micronutrient supplementation is well recognised in the dairy industry as a means of decreasing mastitis.[19] The box summarises the similarities between subclinical and clinical mastitis.

Our South African studies are the first for which the primary aim was to investigate subclinical mastitis in a population. We first conducted a cross-sectional study of women attending vaccination clinics in the Durban area with their infants (Willumsen *et al* submitted). We specifically inquired about symptoms of mastitis or problems with breast feeding and we collected milk from each breast separately. Problems of breast pain, cracked nipples or other breast feeding difficulties were reported by only 3% of the women and could not explain the high prevalence of raised Na/K ratio. Of 269 women with infants 20 weeks old or less, 71 (26%) had Na/K ratio > 0.6 in milk from one breast and 77 (29%) had raised Na/K ratio in both breasts. Unilateral inflammation thus seems common for both subclinical and clinical mastitis, indicating that local inflammation or infection may be an important cause. Although the different sampling methods prevent simple comparisons across studies, raised Na/K ratio appeared more common in this population than in those we studied in Bangladesh and Tanzania. One possible reason for this is the high prevalence of HIV infection in Durban although for ethical and logistic reasons we did not test for HIV in this cross-sectional, vaccination clinic-based study. We inquired about infant feeding practices within the previous 24 hours and found that exclusive breast feeding was associated with lower Na/K ratio (0.58, 95% CI 0.53 - 0.62, n = 320 breasts) than mixed breast milk and formula feeding (1.05, 95% CI 0.82 - 1.35, n = 104), although mixed feeding with breast milk and other foods resulted in the lowest Na/K ratio (0.43, 95% CI 0.38 - 0.47, n = 166 breasts; P<0.05 in each case).

There is little comparable population-based data on Na/K ratios in milk of well-nourished European or North American women since breast feeding in these populations is not universal and the women recruited to research studies have been generally of high socioeconomic status. Of 22 women we have recruited to date from a general practice clinic in a middle class suburb of London, 18 had normal Na/K ratio in both breasts, 2 had a slightly elevated Na/K in one breast and 2 had bilateral subclinical mastitis. We have also analysed Na/K ratios in repeated samples from a small group of women expressing milk regularly to feed very sick infants in hospital. Although many samples in this group have high Na/K since infants were mostly premature and/or too ill to suckle, Na/K ratios were found to be quite consistent for an individual woman across time.

2. SUBCLINICAL MASTITIS AND RISKS FACTORS FOR MOTHER TO INFANT HIV TRANSMISSION IN SOUTH AFRICA

2.1   Rationale

We next investigated subclinical mastitis among a group of women known to be HIV-infected since these women and their infants were likely to suffer the most serious consequences of subclinical mastitis. The increased mammary epithelial permeability which results in raised milk sodium[12] could permit nonspecific leakage of virus into milk and the elevations in inflammatory cytokines such as IL8 could specifically recruit leukocytes, possibly carrying cell-associated virus, into the milk. In addition, certain milk cytokines appear able to pass functionally intact through the infant's stomach[5] and we wished to investigate whether the high milk levels of inflammatory cytokines in subclinical mastitis had adverse effects on infant gut integrity.

2.2   Methods

HIV-infected pregnant women were recruited from the antenatal clinic at McCord's Hospital, Durban, South Africa in connection with a trial of the effect of vitamin A supplementation on mother-to-child HIV transmission. The study showed that vitamin A supplementation had little effect on transmission[20] but infant feeding practices were important.[2] Exclusive formula feeding was associated with 19% of infants becoming HIV-infected by 3 months of age, exclusive breast feeding for at least 3 months with 15% infection, and breast feeding mixed with other foods with 24% infant infection which was a significantly higher proportion than in the other two feeding groups.

The subclinical mastitis study recruited women who were enrolled during the later part of the main study and who elected to breast feed. Women returned to the clinic when their infants were 1, 6 and 14 weeks old for clinical examination, a questionnaire about infant feeding and breast health, a lactulose/mannitol dual sugar test of infant gut permeability,[21, 22] and donation of spot milk samples from each breast.

2.2.1   Laboratory analyses

Milk sodium and potassium were measured by flame photometry as described previously.[10] Milk IL8 was measured using a commercial ELISA kit (CLB, Eurogenetics, Middlesex, UK). Lactulose and mannitol in urine were measured enzymatically using an autoanalyser.[22] Milk viral load was measured in the aqueous cell free fraction by RNA PCR (Amplicor, Roche Diagnostics). The method had a detection limit of 200 copies/ml. Infant HIV infection was determined by positive blood antibody tests at 9 months or greater and/or by detection of RNA in samples taken at earlier time points according to a protocol described previously.[20]

2.2.2   Statistical analyses

Biochemical data were log-transformed to normalise distributions. Na/K ratios <= 0.6 were considered normal, 0.6 to 1.0 were considered moderately raised, and > 1.0 greatly raised. These cutoffs were based partly on histograms of the distribution of Na/K ratios, which were remarkably similar to those in our other studies,[10, 11] and partly on published values of milk electrolytes. Na/K ratios in milk of healthy women at one month postpartum generally averaged 0.6 or less[23] which is about twice the value expected if milk electrolyte levels reflect intracellular levels.[12] Na/K >1.0 is approximately equivalent to 18 mmol/L sodium which, after the first few days postpartum and in the absence of weaning, is indicative of mastitis.[15]

2.3   Results and Discussion

The trial is ongoing so results presented are based on preliminary cross-sectional analysis of an incomplete set. The subsample of women from the main study who were examined for subclinical mastitis did not differ in general from those in the whole study except that women who did not breastfeed at all were excluded. Of the 108 infants (only 104 mothers since there were 4 pairs of twins) 26 infants were HIV-infected by 3 months of age.

The prevalence at each time point of raised milk Na/K ratio in one or both breasts, for women from whom paired samples were available, is shown in Table 1. Results are similar to those of the cross-sectional survey. Unilateral raised milk sodium was more common than bilateral, except at 1 week where it is likely that in some women lactation was not fully established and the mammary epithelium tight junctions had not yet closed completely. Na/K ratio and milk viral load were not significantly affected by infant birth weight or gestational age or mode of delivery.

Table 2. Subclinical mastitis among South African women with HIV infection

Na/K level in both breasts*	1 week (n = 94)	6 weeks (n = 83)	3 months (n = 61)
bilateral low	35 (37%)	44 (53%)	33 (54%)
unilateral raised			
Moderate	17 (18%)	19 (23%)	10 (16%)
Severe	11 (12%)	9 (11%)	12 (20%)
bilateral raised			
both moderate	11 (12%)	5 (6%)	3 (5%)
one moderate, one severe	12 (13%)	4 (5%)	3 (5%)
both severe	8 (8%)	2 (2%)	0 (0%)

*low: Na/K $\leq$ 0.6; moderate: Na/K > 0.6 and $\leq$ 1.0; severe: Na/K > 1.0

Since left and right breasts seemed to behave independently, for some analyses we used breast, rather than woman, as the sampling unit. Milk IL8 was always highly correlated with Na/K ratio as we have shown in other populations previously (Table 2). Milk IL8 was also correlated with viral load at all times but viral load was significantly correlated with Na/K ratio only at 1 and 14 weeks. A similar relation between milk sodium and viral load has been found in HIV-infected Malawian women.[24] IL8 acts to recruit leukocytes and we actually measured cell-free virus so we do not believe the relationship between IL8 and viral load is directly causal but that both are related to the changes that occur during subclinical mastitis. It is slightly surprising that Na/K ratio, which indicates non-specific permeability, is not more closely related to cell-free virus than is IL8 concentration.

Table 3. Correlations between logarithmic values of milk Na/K ratios, HIV viral loads and IL8 concentrations in samples from both breasts

Correlations (r, n, P)	1 week	6 weeks	14 weeks
Na/K with IL8	0.56, 189, <0.001	0.50, 166, <0.001	0.56, 120, <0.001
Na/K with viral load	0.33, 128, <0.001	0.13, 137, 0.12	0.32, 110, 0.001
IL8 with viral load	0.28, 127, 0.001	0.24, 138, 0.005	0.45, 116, <0.001

At 1 and 14 weeks viral load in milk samples with Na/K $\leq$ 0.6 was significantly lower than in samples with Na/K>1 (Table 3). Interestingly, the proportion of samples with undetectable virus decreased with increasing Na/K ratio category at 6 and 14 weeks but not at 1 week. It appears that the cause of subclinical mastitis and its relation to inflammation and viral load differs at 1 week from later times.

In the overall trial, women who exclusively breastfed were less likely to transmit HIV to their infants than women who mixed breast milk and other foods. Therefore we analysed milk viral loads (Table 4) according to feeding practice.

Table 4. Subclinical mastitis and breast milk HIV viral load in South African women[1]

Na/K ratio	1 week	6 weeks	14 weeks
<= 0.6	811 (570 - 1155) 18/66 (27%)	1018 (707 - 1465) 35/98 (36%)	829 (553 - 1245) 31/77 (40%)
0.6 - 1.0	1372 (809 - 2329) 10/39 (26%)	1550 (576 - 4172) 8/26 (31%)	1772 (639 - 4910) 5/18 (28%)
> 1.0	2751 (867 - 8729)* 9/25 (36%)	1565 (699 - 3504) 1/14 (7%)	4462 (1976 - 10077)* 1/15 (7%)

[1] Geometric mean (95% CI); proportion (%) undetectable, i.e. < 200 copies/ml.
* Different from group with Na/K <= 0.6

Mixed feeding was associated with increased viral load at 1 week only. The proportions of breasts with undetectable viral load were significantly different across groups at 6 and 14 weeks but this was mainly because of the high proportion among the small numbers in the breast milk plus water group. IL8 showed the same pattern as viral load and Na/K ratio was similar but not statistically significantly different even at 1 week, unlike in our previous cross-sectional study. However, when analysed as proportions in the different Na/K categories, there were significantly fewer samples in the moderately and greatly raised Na/K groups in the exclusive breast feeding group compared to the other groups. Feeding mode likely affects Na/K, IL8 and viral load, rather than vice versa, since there was no association of initial feeding choice with measures of maternal health (eg blood CD4 count or hemoglobin during pregnancy) or infant health (birth weight, gestational age) other than the perhaps spurious associations that women who gave breast milk plus water were slightly older and had slightly heavier babies than women in other groups.

Table 5. Breast milk HIV viral load in both breasts according to infant feeding practice[1]

	1 week	6 weeks	14 weeks
Exclusive breast feeding	936 (692 - 1265)[a] 31/100 (31%)	1267 (893 - 1799)[a] 34/115 (30%)	1288 (886 - 1875) 30/98 (31%)
Breast milk + water	1707 (706 - 4128)[ab] 2/18 (11%)	334 (173 - 646)[b] 8/12 (67%)	200 (200 - 200) 4/4 (100%)
Mixed feeding	6557 (618 - 69626)[b] 4/12 (33%)	1420 (356 - 5667)[ab] 3/13 (23%)	765 (295 - 1984) 7/16 (44%)

[1] Geometric mean (95% CI); proportion (%) undetectable, i.e. <200 copies/ml. Means in a column not followed by the same superscript are significantly different by Duncan's multiple range test, P<0.05.

Finally we investigated whether subclinical mastitis was associated with increased infant gut permeability. There was no significant association between gut permeability and either milk Na/K or feeding mode. The latter observation is not surprising since, in a larger cohort from the same trial, we found significantly increased intestinal permeability in infants given formula only but not in those who were mixed fed (Rollins, Filteau *et al*, unpublished). It appears that the amount of milk consumed by the mixed fed group was sufficient to promote gut integrity and that complementary foods in this middle income (by African standards) peri-urban community with piped water supply were not grossly contaminated.

2.4   Conclusions

Mother-to-infant transmission occurs in utero, during delivery and postpartum through breast feeding. Recent progress in reducing transmission during delivery[25, 26] means that even greater attention needs to be paid to breast feeding transmission since more women are likely to consent to testing and more of their infants will be born uninfected. Thus the results from the main study from which the present results were taken are especially exciting showing decreased transmission up to 3 months of age in infants who were exclusively breastfed, compared to mixed fed, until that age. The present substudy provides some evidence of mechanisms for this association.

Subclinical mastitis was more prevalent among those who mixed fed, rather than exclusively breastfed, their infants. Subclinical mastitis was associated with increased milk viral load at 1 and 14 weeks postpartum but, interestingly, increased viral load was associated with mixed feeding only at 1 week. The mechanisms may differ at 1 week from those at later time points. Subclinical mastitis had no effect on infant gut permeability. This may be because high milk concentrations of inflammatory cytokines such as IL8 are balanced by high concentrations of anti-inflammatory cytokines such as transforming growth factor-β.[11] Therefore, although results are preliminary, it appears that subclinical mastitis may increase risk of HIV transmission during early lactation and this risk is mediated through increased milk viral load. This supports the epidemiological data suggesting that early lactation is the major period of postnatal transmission.[27]

Extrapolating from causes of clinical mastitis,[28] subclinical mastitis is likely to result from systemic infection, breast infection, mixed feeding such that milk production decreases below about 400 ml/day[15] or poor lactation practices which lead to milk stasis and mammary gland involution. Infections, usually from skin commensals such as *Staphylococcus aureus*, are unlikely to take hold without other factors inducing milk stasis.[29] Lactation counselling to optimise breast feeding may reduce the incidence of milk stasis and raised milk sodium concentration.[13]

Policies for optimal infant feeding by African women with HIV infection are continually being revised. The present study provides mechanistic data to support the observation of a protective effect of exclusive breast feeding in a non-randomised cohort. Further studies should be conducted to determine whether promotion of exclusive breast feeding, which is cheap and safe even for women and infants unaffected by HIV, can decrease HIV transmission among other populations.

ACKNOWLEDGMENTS

We are grateful to Dolly Naicker, Jean Mshentshela and Zama Mngadi for help in the clinic and with sample collection and to Richard Beesley and Subitha Dwarika for laboratory analyses. The work was supported by the Department for International Development, UK and UNICEF, South Africa.

REFERENCES

1. Van de Perre, P., 1999, Mother-to-child transmission of HIV-1: the 'all mucosal' hypothesis as a predominant mechanism of transmission. *AIDS* **13**: 1133-1138.
2. Coutsoudis, A., Pillay, K., Spooner, E., Kuhn, L., and Coovadia, H., 1999a, Influence of infant feeding patterns on early mother-to-child transmission of HIV-1 in Durban, South Africa. *Lancet* **354**: 471-476.
3. Van de Perre, P., Simonon, A., Hitimana, D.-G., Dabis, F., Msellati, P., Mukamabano, B., Butera, J.B., van Goethem, C., Karita, E., and Lepage, P., 1993, Infective and anti-infective properties of breastmilk from HIV-1-infected women. *Lancet* **341**: 914-918.
4. Newburg, D.S., Linhardt, R.J., Ampofo, S.A., and Yolken, R.H., 1995, Human milk glycosaminoglycans inhibit HIV glycoprotein gp120 binding to its host cell CD4 receptor. *J. Nutr.* **125**: 419-424.
5. Filteau, S.M., 1999, Milk components with immunomodulatory potential. In *Advances in Nutrition Research* **10** (H. Draper and B. Woodward, eds.), Plenum, New York, in press.
6. Weaver, L.T., Laker, M.F., Nelson, R., and Lucas, A., 1987, Milk feeding and changes in intestinal permeability and morphology in the newborn. *J. Pediatr. Gastroenterol. Nutr.* **6**: 351-358.
7. Shuster, D.E., Kehrli, M.E., and Baumrucker, C.R., 1995, Relationship of inflammatory cytokines, growth hormone, and insulin-like growth factor-1 to reduced performance during infectious disease. *Proc. Soc. Exp. Biol. Med.* **210**: 140-149.
8. Waller, K.P., Colditz, I.G., Flapper, P., and Seow, H.-F., 1997, Leukocyte and cytokine accumulation in the ovine teat and udder during endotoxin-induced inflammation. *Vet. Res. Commun.* **21**: 101-115.
9. Barber, M.R., and Yang, T.J., 1998, Chemotactic activities in nonmastitic mammary secretions: presence of interleukin-8 in mastitic but not nonmastitic secretions. *Clin. Diag. Lab. Immunol.* **5**: 82-86.

10. Filteau, S.M., Rice, A.L., Ball, J.J., Chakraborty, J., Stoltzfus, R., de Francisco, A., and Willumsen, J.F., 1999a, Breast milk immune factors in Bangladeshi women supplemented postpartum with retinol or β-carotene. *Am. J. Clin. Nutr.* **69**: 953-958.

11. Filteau, S.M., Lietz, G., Mulokozi, G., Bilotta, S., Henry, C.J.K., and Tomkins, A.M., 1999b, Milk cytokines and subclinical breast inflammation in Tanzanian women: effects of dietary red palm oil or sunflower oil supplementation. *Immunol.* **97**: 595-600.

12. Peaker, M., 1974, Recent advances in the study of monovalent ion movements across the mammary epithelium: relation to onset of lactation. *J. Diary Sci.* **58**: 1042-1047.

13. Morton, J.A., 1994, The clinical usefulness of breast milk sodium in the assessment of lactogenesis. *Pediatrics* **93**: 802-806.

14. Dewey, K.G., Finlay, D.A., and Lonnerdal, B., 1984, Breast milk volume and composition during late lactation (7-20 months). *J. Pediatr. Gastroenterol. Nutr.* **3**: 713-720.

15. Neville, M.C., Allen, J.C., Archer, P.C., Casey, C.E., Seacat, J., Keller, R.P., Lutes, V., Rasbach, J., and Neifert, M., 1991, Studies in human lactation: milk volume and nutrient composition during weaning and lactogenesis. Am. J. Clin. Nutr. **54**: 81-92.

16. Li, X.F., Fortney, J.A., Kotelchuck, M., and Glover, L.H., 1996, The postpartum period: the key to maternal mortality. *Int. J. Gynecol. Obstet.* **54**: 1-10.

17. Jennings, G., Lunn P.G., and Elia, M., 1995, The effect of endotoxin on gastrointestinal transit time and intestinal permeability. *Clin. Nutr.* **14**: 35-41.

18. Grimble, R.F., 1998, Nutritional modulation of cytokine biology. *Nutrition* **14**: 634-640.

19. Hogan, J.S., Weiss, W.P., and Smith, K.L., 1993, Role of vitamin E and selenium in host defence against mastitis. *J. Dairy Sci.* **76**: 2795-2803.

20. Coutsoudis, A., Pillay, K., Spooner, E., Kuhn, L., and Coovadia, H., 1999b, Randomised trial testing effect of vitamin A supplementation on pregnancy outcomes and early mother-to-child HIV-1 transmission in Durban, South Africa. *AIDS* **13**: 1517-1524.

21. Lunn, P.G., Northrop-Clewes, C.A., and Downes, R.M., 1991, Intestinal permeability, mucosal injury, and growth faltering in Gambian infants. *Lancet* **338**: 907-910.

22. Willumsen, J.F., Darling, J.C., Kitundu, J.A., Kingamkono, R.R., Msengi, A.E., Mduma, B., and Tomkins, A.M., 1997, Dietary management of acute diarrhoea in children: effect of fermented and amylase-digested weaning foods on intestinal permeability. *J. Pediatr. Gastroenterol. Nutr.* **24**: 235-241.

23. Neville, M.C., Keller, R.P., Lonnerdal, B., Atkinson, S., Wade, C.L., Butte, N., and Moser, P.B., 1985, Measurement of electrolyte and macromineral concentrations in human milk. In *Human Lactation : Milk Components and Methodologies* (R.G. Jensen and M.C. Neville, eds.), Plenum Press, New York and London, pp. 129-140.

24. Semba, R.D., Kumwenda, N., Hoover, D.R., Taha, T.E., Quinn, T.C., Mtimavalye, L., Biggar, R.J., Broadhead, R., Miotti, P.G., Sokoll, L.J., van der Hoeven, L., and Chiphangwi, J.D., 1999, Human immunodeficiency virus load in breast milk, mastitis, and mother-to-child transmission of human immunodeficiency virus type 1. *J. Infect. Dis.* **180**: 93-98.

25. Newell, M.-L., Dabis, F., Tolley, K., and Whynes, D., 1998, Cost-effectiveness and cost-benefit in the prevention of mother-to-child transmission of HIV in developing countries. *AIDS* **12**: 1571-1580.

26. Guay, L.A., Musoke, P., Fleming, T., Bagenda, D., Allen, M., Nakabiito, C., Sherman, J., Bakaki, P., Ducar, C., Deseyve, M., Emel, L., Mirochnick, M., Fowler, M.G., Mofenson, L., Miotti, P., Dransfield, K., Bray, D., Mmiro, F., and Jackson, J.B., 1999, Intrapartum and neonatal single-dose nevirapine compared with zidovudine for prevention of mother-to-child transmission of HIV-1 in Kampala, Uganda: HIVNET 012 randomised trial. *Lancet* **354**: 795-802.

27. Miotti, P.G., Taha, T.E.T., Kumwenda, N.I., Broadhead, R., Mtimavalye, L.A.R., Van der Hoeven, L., Chiphangwi, J.D., Liomba, G., and Biggar, R.J., 1999, HIV transmission through breast feeding: a study in Malawi. *J. Am. Med. Assoc.* **282**: 744-749.
28. Fetherston, C., 1998, Risk factors for lactation mastitis. *J. Hum. Lact.* **14**: 101-109.
29. Thomsen, A.C., Espersen, T., and Maigaard, S., 1984, Course and treatment of milk stasis, noninfectious inflammation of the breast, and infectious mastitis in nursing women. *Am. J. Obstet. Gynecol.* **149**: 492-495.

20

RECOMMENDATIONS ON FEEDING INFANTS OF HIV POSITIVE MOTHERS
WHO, UNICEF, UNAIDS Guidelines

DR FELICITY SAVAGE and MS LIDA LHOTSKA
Department of Child and Adolescent Health and Development, World Health Organisation, Geneva; Nutrition Section, United Nations Children's Fund, New York

1.   INTRODUCTION

Since 1992, WHO and UNICEF, and since 1995 when it was formed, UNAIDS, have been working to develop policies and guidelines concerning the safest method of feeding for infants of HIV-positive mothers. The first policy statement put forward in 1992 was made on epidemiological grounds. In countries with high infant mortality rates due to infection, often compounded by malnutrition, women were to be advised to breastfeed, as the risk of death from not breastfeeding was likely to be greater than the risk of acquiring HIV through breastmilk. In other settings, with low infant mortality rates, where the risks of artificial feeding were less, women were to be advised not to breastfeed. These recommendations were seen as reflecting a double standard – one for the rich and one for the poor – and proved unworkable as a basis for the development of globally relevant guidelines.

Throughout the 1990s, the influence of the human rights perspective on health policy steadily increased. The second policy statement on HIV and Infant Feeding put forward jointly by WHO, UNICEF and UNAIDS in 1997[1] reflected this in its rights based approach, which called for women in

Short and Long Term Effects of Breast Feeding on Child Health
Edited by Berthold Koletzko *et al.*, Kluwer Academic/Plenum Publishers, 2000

all settings to make a fully informed decision about feeding their infants. Women would not be told or advised what to do, but would be enabled to make a decision appropriate to their particular circumstances and situation, and supported in their choice of feeding method.

2.   WHO/UNICEF/UNAIDS HIV AND INFANT FEEDING GUIDELINES

On the basis of this policy, it became possible to develop "Guidelines for Decision Makers" and "A Guide for Health Care Managers and Supervisors", which had universal applicability. These were issued in 1998[1,2], and sought to clarify the direction for implementation, as well as to identify gaps in understanding, and unresolved questions that required further research. There were many serious underlying concerns. While it was recognised that breastfeeding can transmit HIV to an infant, the exact risk of transmission remained uncertain, and appeared to vary with a number of factors including the mother's health and viral load, the condition of her breasts and of the infant's oral and intestinal mucosa. Artificial feeding of infants was also recognised to have serious risks, particularly in those countries most severely affected by the HIV epidemic. The term "replacement feeding" was coined to refer to alternative feeding of an infant of an HIV-positive mother, to draw attention to the need for full nutritional support throughout at least the first two years of life, during which time an infant would normally receive a significant proportion of high quality nutrients in the form of breastmilk. Replacement feeding is defined as "the process of feeding a child who is not receiving any breastmilk from birth to two years with a diet that provides all the nutrients that the child needs". A common assumption that an infant only needed to be provided with breastmilk substitutes for the first six months of life was inappropriate. Many complementary diets are inadequate to support satisfactory growth even if breastmilk is provided. Replacement feeds could consist of commercial infant formula, or home-prepared infant formula in families where animal milk or powdered full cream milk are more readily available. Micro-nutrient supplements would be needed with home-prepared formula, and nutrient-rich complementary foods ensured as part of all replacement feeding from about 6 months of age. The guidelines also make clear that replacement feeding is not the only alternative: modified forms of breastfeeding, such as expression and heat treatment of the mother's breastmilk, wet-nursing by an HIV-negative wet-nurse, use of uncontaminated donor breastmilk, and exclusive breastfeeding for a few months and then stopping early are other ways of reducing transmission which women may choose for at least some time.

3.   CONTINUING CONCERNS

There continues to be concern about how to provide women with the information necessary to make a fully informed choice. To do so requires investment in education of both health educators and the public, for which resources would need to be identified. To support mothers in their choice, should they wish to give replacement feeds, would in many situations require alternatives to breastmilk to be made available, instruction in their safe use to be provided, and their distribution carefully regulated.

There are also concerns about women's access to adequate fuel, water, necessary utensils and time; and about the risk of misuse and spillover of infant formula among women who are uninfected or whose HIV status is unknown, with a consequent erosion of breastfeeding. Already in some settings, there appears to be a loss of confidence in breastfeeding promotion initiatives, and a tendency for some women to feed their infants on infant formula when it is not necessary. The guidelines emphasise the need to continue to promote breastfeeding through health education promotions; to strengthen the Baby-friendly Hospital Initiative to support early mother-infant contact and optimal initiation of infant feeding, as this is relevant for both HIV-positive and HIV-negative mothers; to train infant feeding counsellors in both breastfeeding support and replacement feeding; to take measures to implement the International Code of Marketing of Breast-milk Substitutes, to protect both HIV-positive and HIV-negative women from commercial influence regarding their infant feeding decision; to avoid the distribution of bottles and teats, as it is possible and safer to feed even new-born infants by cup; and to carefully monitor exclusive breastfeeding rates, so that any spillover of replacement feeding can be detected and appropriate action taken.

There is concern also about how to ensure that women receive adequate counselling to make a decision, and support for feeding their infants accordingly, when resources for all forms of health care is limited, and unavailable to many women and children even at the most basic level. To provide health workers who have the necessary skills and time to help HIV-positive women feed their infants safely would require resources that have not yet been identified, and which might deplete other part of the health care system.

4.   PREVENTION OF MTCT OF HIV PILOT PROJECTS

In 1998, following the demonstration that various short courses of anti-retroviral drugs could reduce mother-to-child transmission (MTCT) of HIV, a series of pilot projects for the prevention of MTCT were launched by WHO, UNICEF and UNAIDS. The aim is to explore the feasibility and cost-effectiveness of a package of services, including improved obstetric care, voluntary and confidential counselling and HIV testing (VCT), and short course anti-retroviral regimes. The package includes infant feeding counselling, the use of replacement feeding by mothers who choose not to breastfeed, and follow up and support for each mother's infant feeding decision. Implementation started first in Botswana, CoteD'Ivoire, Rwanda, and Zimbabwe, to be followed by Kenya, Zambia, Tanzania, and Uganda and a number of other countries.

5.   NEW CONCERNS

The early experience gained in the pilot projects has raised a series of new concerns. It has been found that even when infant formula for replacement feeding is available, many women prefer not to use it, and choose to breastfeed, in many cases because of fear of stigmatisation. There is growing interest in possible ways to make breastmilk and breastfeeding safer. New evidence has become available that anti-retroviral drugs are effective even if women breastfeed[3]. The feared rebound increase in transmission of HIV during breastfeeding after a short course of anti-retroviral drugs has been shown not to occur. There is also new evidence that exclusive breastfeeding may be less likely to transmit HIV to the infant than mixed feeding[4], though this is an observational study and not conclusive. It is postulated that mixed feeding might increase transmission, because of damage to the infant's intestinal mucosa. Mastitis and sub-clinical mastitis, which may affect up to 16% of mothers, are associated with increased viral load in breastmilk, and may increase the risk of HIV transmission[5,6]. A good breastfeeding technique is likely to prevent mastitis, and might therefore reduce the risk of transmission of HIV.

Although it has been suggested that WHO, UNICEF and UNAIDS should revise the 1998 guidelines in the light of the new study, this has not been found necessary, because by itself the study is not conclusive, and for those mothers who choose to breastfeed, it is already recommended that they do so exclusively. The range of options for feeding infants remains the same, and what is important is to make the new information clear in implementation of prevention of mother-to-child transmission. Renewed emphasis is needed on what has long been recommended for all breastfeeding women: to breastfeed exclusively, without any additional fluids, even water and tea; and to ensure that a baby is well attached to the breast during suckling and removing milk effectively, to prevent milk stasis and mastitis. There is now greater confidence that these long standing recommendations might also reduce the risk of transmission of HIV through breastmilk. To breastfeed optimally, and then to stop early, sometime between 3 and 6 months, depending on when adequate replacement feeding becomes feasible, could be the most appropriate option for many women for whom replacement feeding is difficult, and possibly the safest in many settings in terms of overall risk of infant mortality.

6.   TRAINING IN HIV AND INFANT FEEDING COUNSELLING

As a tool to aid implementation of the guidelines, WHO, UNICEF and UNAIDS are collaborating on the development of materials for a 3-day course called "HIV and Infant Feeding Counselling"[7], which aims to provide training for health workers who will counsel women about infant feeding. The course is designed to be used in conjunction with an existing course on breastfeeding counselling[8], and to train a cadre of infant feeding counsellors who can counsel all women on their choice of infant feeding method, and support them in either breastfeeding, modified breastfeeding or replacement feeding. These materials will reflect the latest understanding, and will be revised and adapted as new information becomes available.

7.   RESEARCH QUESTIONS

1. Implementation is urgently needed, and must proceed on the basis of what is known now. However, there are a number of important research questions, relating to both breastfeeding and replacement feeding, answers to which must be sought to guide implementation in future. These include:
2. What is the risk of transmission of HIV through exclusive breastfeeding compared with mixed feeding? Additional evidence is urgently needed to confirm or refute the early report.
3. What is the acceptability and feasibility of the modified breastfeeding options?
4. How effectively does help to ensure a good breastfeeding technique prevent mastitis and sub-clinical mastitis?

5. What is the feasibility of replacement feeding in resource poor settings? How can mothers measure and prepare feeds accurately and hygienically?
6. What instruction and help is necessary to ensure that women can give adequate replacement feeds?
7. How can mothers overcome practical difficulties such as management of replacement feeds at night, for example in village settings?
8. What is the infant mortality and morbidity associated with replacement feeding?

8.   CONCLUSION

Despite the evidence that HIV can be transmitted by breastfeeding, there is much that we need to know about factors that affect the rate of transmission, and about the risks and feasibility of replacement feeding, before adequate information can be provided to affected families to enable them to make the most appropriate decision about feeding their infants.

REFERENCES

1. HIV and Infant Feeding: Guidelines for Decision Makers WHO/FRH/NUT/CHD/98.1, UNAIDS/98.3, UNICEF/PD/NUT/(J)98-1.
2. HIV and Infant Feeding: A Guide for Health Care Managers and Supervisors WHO/FRH/NUT/CHD/98.2, UNAIDS/98.4, UNICEF/PD/NUT/(J)98-2.
3. Dabis F, Msellati P, Meda N, Welffens-Ekra C, You B, Manigart O, Leroy V, Simonon A, Cartoux M, Combe P, Ouangre A, Ramon R, Ky-Zerbo O, Montcho C, Salamon R, Rouzioux C, Van de Perre P, Mandelbrot L for the DITRAME Study Group, 1999. 6-month efficacy, tolerance, and acceptability of a short regime of oral zidovudine to reduce vertical transmission of HIV in breastfed children in Cote d'Ivoire and Burkino Faso: A double blind placebo-controlled multicentre trial. The Lancet; **353**: 786-92.
4. Coutsoudis A, Pillay K, Spooner E, Kuhn L, Coovadia HM, 1999. Influence of infant-feeding patterns on early mother-to-child transmission of HIV-1 in Durban, South Africa: a prospective cohort study. The Lancet; **354**: 471-76
5. Semba RD, Kumwenda N, Hoover DR, Taha TE, Quinn TC, Mtimavalye L, Biggar RJ, Broadhead R, Miotti PG, Sokoll LJ, van der Hoeven L, Chiphangwi JD, 1999. Human Immunodeficiency Virus Load in Breast Milk, Mastitis, and Mother-to-Child transmission of Human Immunodeficiency Virus Type 1. The Journal of Infectious Diseases; **180**: 93-98
6. Filteau SM – ED: please refer to the previous article in this publication, as presented in the ISRHML meeting
7. HIV and Infant Feeding Counselling: A Training Course (in preparation). WHO/UNICEF/UNAIDS.
8. Breastfeeding Counselling: A Training Course. WHO/UNICEF, 1993. WHO/CDR/93.3,4,5,6; UNICEF/NUT/93-1,2,3,4.

21

TRANSMISSION OF CYTOMEGALOVIRUS INFECTION THROUGH BREAST MILK IN TERM AND PRETERM INFANTS
The role of cell free milk whey and milk cells

[1]Klaus Hamprecht, [1]Simone Witzel, [2]Jens Maschmann, [2]Christian P. Speer and [1]Gerhard Jahn
[1]Department of Medical Virology and Epidemiology of Viral Diseases, [2]Department of Neonatology, University Hospital of Tübingen, Calwerstr. 7/6, 72076 Tübingen, Germany

Key words: Cytomegalovirus (CMV), milk whey, milk cells, breastfeeding

Abstract: We investigated the reactivation of cytomegalovirus during lactation and analysed the role of human milk whey and milk cells in mother–to–child-transmission. In contrast to term infants, preterm infants may be infected symptomatically by breastfeeding. Human milk whey is the material of choice for detection of maternal DNAlactia and virolactia, whereas milk cells not necessarily have to be infected in transmitters.

1.   INTRODUCTION

Mother-to-child transmission of CMV-infection can occur during pregnancy in the intrapartum period or postnatally. Primary CMV infection of pregnant mothers poses a 30% to 40% risk of intrauterine transmission[1]. The resulting congenital CMV infection has an incidence of about 1% of all live births in the United States [2]. 10-20% of the infants of primary infected mothers have symptomatic CMV infection at birth, whereas the presence of maternal antibody to CMV before conception provides substantial protection against severe congenital

CMV infection [3, 4]. Perinatal virus transmission has been associated with exposure of the infants to CMV containing cervical secretions at birth and occurs in approximately 40% in offspring of seropositive virus excreting women [5, 6]. However, most definitions of perinatal CMV transmission also include breast-feeding as maternal source for the acquisition of postnatal virus infections [6, 7]. The increasing popularity of breastfeeding has a major influence on the epidemiology of postnatal CMV infections [8].

More than 30 years ago cytomegalovirus was first isolated from human milk [9]. In initial studies using unseparated breast milk, the rate of isolation of infectious virus from milk in fibroblast cultures (virolactia) ranged from 9% (19/200) [10] to 32% (13/41) [11]. All of the term infants under study had normal newborn courses without long-term sequelae such as sensorineural hearing loss [11]. With the availability of PCR, a first report using milk fractionation into an aqueous layer and milk cells showed quite low rates of CMV virolactia (20% or 7/35) and also low detection rates for viral DNA from milk cells or the aqueous milk fraction [12]. Preliminary data of a longitudinal prospectively performed study on HCMV transmission by breastfeeding mothers to their preterm infants revealed a high incidence of CMV reactivation during lactation and the knowledge, that virus transmission to preterm infants in contrast to term infants may be associated with a symptomatic CMV infection. The most immature infants are at the greatest risk to acquire an early and symptomatic CMV infection [13].

This paper presents data on CMV detection in cell free milk whey and milk cells during the course of lactation and reflects the problems concerning the identification of the target vehicle for CMV transmission in human breast milk.

2.   ROLE OF MILK WHEY IN CMV DETECTION DURING LACTATION

Human cytomegalovirus can be detected in different compartments of breast milk. Viral DNA has been detected by means of PCR in supernatants of human milk [14]. A detailed protocol for preparation of milk whey and milk cells was used to describe CMV excretion of breastfeeding mothers of preterm infants during lactation [15]. The resulting whey fraction is cell free (Fig 1).

Sequences of HLA-DRBI were used to detect cellular contamination of whey preparations by PCR. The presence of CMV DNAlactia was verified by a nested PCR using primers of the CMV IE-Exon4 gene [15].

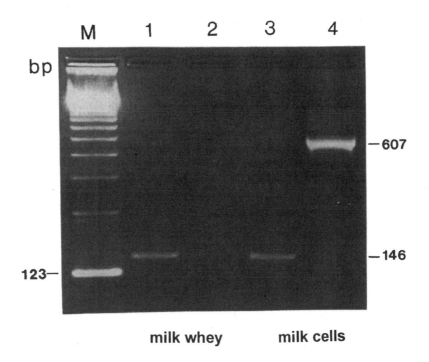

Figure 1: Detection of CMV DNA in cell free human milk whey and in milk cells (146 bp) and HLA-DRBI DNA (607 bp) in milk cells only (Agarose gel electrophoresis, ethidiumbromide staining).

Using this method, it is possible to detect 200 viral genome equivalents/ml in milk whey. To avoid cellular contamination of whey preparations, it is necessary to use milk specimens without any prior storing. Milk whey is the material of choice to detect CMV during any phase of lactation. Viral DNAlactia is most reliably detected in milk whey at the onset and the end of virus excretion into milk. During these periods, CMV DNA in milk cells is often not detectable. In cell free milk whey virolactia is more frequently detectable than in milk cells. There exists a strong correlation between the detection of DNAlactia and virolactia in milk whey.

3.   ROLE OF MILK CELLS IN CMV DETECTION DURING LACTATION

The highest concentration of leukocytes in human milk is observed in colostrum (1-3 x10^6/ml). In the milk of the first few days after birth, the different leukocyte types are distributed as follows: neutrophils, 55-60%, macrophages, 30-40%, and lymphocytes, 5-10% [16]. Phenotypic and functional differences between milk leukocytes and peripheral blood leukocytes are summarized in Table 1. In contrast to blood T-cells, the milk CD3-cells express phenotypic activation markers such as HLA-DR, IL2-receptor (CD25) and CD45RO (primed/memory cells). Phagocytes in human milk are also activated. The density of HLA-DR expression on macrophages is higher compared to peripheral blood monocytes [17].

Table 1. Phenotypic and functional characteristics of human milk leukocytes in comparison to blood leukocytes

milk cell type	phenotype	function	reference
T-cells	Tγ/δ ↑ > Tα/β	IFN γ prod. ↑	[18]
	CD45RO ↑		[19]
	CD45RA ↓		
	CD4/CD8 ↓		[20]
	CD3CD25 (Il2R) ↑		[21]
	CD3 HLA-DR ↑		
macrophages	HLA-DR ↑	Motility ↑	[17]
	Fcγ ↓	PGE2 prod	[22]
	LactoferrinR	Lysozyme	[23]
		C3, C4	
		Lactoferrin	
neutrophiles	CD11b ↑	Motility ↓	[24]
	L-selectin (Leu-8) ↓	chemotactic response ↓	[25]

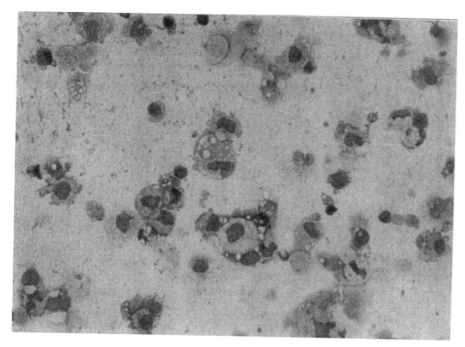

Figure 2: Cytospin preparation of milk cells at the onset of CMV DNAlactia in milk whey at day ten after delivery. May-Grünwald-Giemsa stain (400x).

Monocytes/macrophages and myeloid progenitor cells are potential target cells for CMV. Monocytes and late stage infected macrophages are discussed to be involved in the hematogenous spread of CMV as well as in the persistent virus infection during latency. Endothelial as well as epithelial cells also seem to be involved in the virus entry and dissemination, respectively (for review see: [26]). However, up to now the sites of CMV persistence and the molecular mechanisms for reactivation are quite undefined.

In Figure 2 a cytospin preparation of milk cells at the onset of CMV DNAlactia in milk whey at day ten after delivery (transient milk) is shown. At the onset of viral DNA detection in milk whey neither viral DNA nor late pp67 mRNA were detectable in milk cells. Virolactia was also not found in both milk cells and milk whey. Typical fat vacuoles and granular material in neutrophils and macrophages are visible. Most cells belong to the macrophage and lymphocyte lineage. Only few neutrophils are present.

In Figure 3 milk leukocytes of mature milk (day 30 after birth) are shown. The α-naphthyl acetate esterase staining used, allows identification of macrophages expressing diffuse red-brown granulation. The fat vacuoles remain unstained. Neutrophils are characterised by their typical polymorphonuclear shape in the methylgreen counterstain. CMV excretion into milk has begun 21 days before. On day 30 after birth CMV DNAlactia, pp67 mRNAlactia and virolactia was detected in both milk cells and milk whey suggesting an active virus replication in milk cells. Interestingly, the frequency of neutrophils seems to be enhanced compared to transient milk (Figure 2).

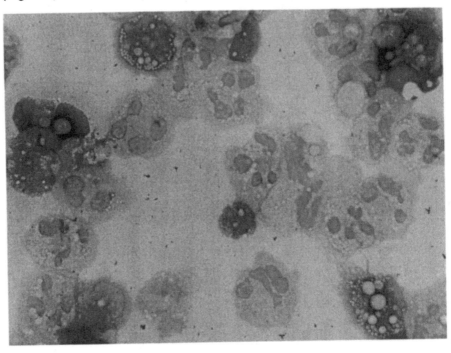

Figure 3: Cytospin preparation of milk cells on day 30 after birth. α-naphthylacetate esterase stain, methylgreen counterstain (1000x). In this milk cell preparation CMV infection was productive, since viral DNA, pp67 late mRNA and infectious virus were detectable.

The target cell for CMV in human milk has not been identified up to now. Cell separation experiments and cell sorting of distinct milk cell populations (as CD14+ macrophages) failed to proof the CMV infected vehicles in human milk. Thus, the role of milk cells in virus transmission remains to be elucidated. A main problem in this context is the fact, that milk cells are not CMV infected during all stages of lactation. Furthermore, we found evidence that the frequency of infected cells is quite low, since for successful amplification of viral DNA at least $5 \times 10^4 - 10^5$ milk cells are necessary. Additionally, some mothers excrete milk cells which remain uninfected during the whole course of lactation. The only source of CMV in the breast milk of these mothers is the cell free milk whey.

4.   CONCLUSION

Postnatal CMV transmission by breastfeeding mothers represents the main route for the acquisition of this virus, since the incidence of CMV excretion into breast milk during lactation is very high. Additionally, a high CMV seroprevalence in most countries of the world (up to 100%) and a transmission rate of about 40% as well as high feeding rates especially in non-industrialized countries promote the spread of CMV. Therefore, the epidemiology of CMV is dominated by breastfeeding. Despite the fact, that the presence of CMV in breast milk has been shown 30 years ago, the mechanisms, vehicles and the kinetics of viral reactivation remain elusive. Fractionation of human milk into milk whey and milk cells is a first step in describing risk factors for transmission. CMV is detectable in cell free milk whey during all stages of viral reactivation in the course of lactation. In milk whey CMV DNA, CMV RNA and the infectious virus can be detected. The source of this cell free virus remains unclear: milk cells are not infected at all stages of lactation and some mothers excrete only uninfected milk cells. Transmission of CMV by breastfeeding mothers to their preterm infants may be associated with symptomatic CMV infection, such as sepsis-like syndroms [27]. Therefore, efficient and gentle inactivation methods for infected milk samples are an urgent need for a risk group of preterm infants with extremely low birth weight (GA<30 weeks, BW<1000g).

ACKNOWLEDGMENTS

This study was supported by a grant from DFG (Ha 1559/2-1). We thank Mrs Andrea Baumeister for excellent technical assistance.

REFERENCES

[1] Stagno, S., Pass, R.F., Cloud, G., Britt, W.J., Henderson, R.E., Walton, P.D., Veren, D.A., Page, F., Alford, C.A., 1986, Primary cytomegalovirus infection in pregnancy. Incidence, transmission to fetus, and clinical outcome. *JAMA* **256:** 1904-1908

[2] Alford, C., Britt, W., 1990, Cytomegalovirus. In: Fields, B.N., Knipe, D.M., Chanock, R.M.

et al , *eds. Virology. 2ⁿᵈ ed.* New York.   *Raven Press.*, 1981-2010

[3] Fowler, K.B., Stagno, S., Pass, R.F., Britt, W.J., Boll, T.J., Alford, C.A., 1992, The outcome of congenital cytomegalovirus infection in relation to maternal antibody status. *N Engl J Med* **326**: 663-667

[4] Boppana, S.B., Britt, W.J., 1995, Antiviral antibody responses and intrauterine transmission after primary maternal cytomegalovirus infection. *J Infect Dis* **171**: 1115-1121

[5] Reynolds, D.W., Stagno, S., Hosty, T.H., Tiller, M., Alford, C.A., 1973, Maternal cytomegalovirus excretion and perinatal infection. *N Engl J Med* **289**: 1-5

[6] Mussi-Pinhata, M.M., Yamamoto, A.Y., Figueiredo, L.T.M., Cervi, M.C., Duarte, G., 1998, Congenital and perinatal cytomegalovirus infection in infants born to mothers infected with human immunodeficiency virus. *J Pediatr* **132**: 285-290

[7] Adler, S.P., 1996, Current prospects for immunization against cytomegaloviral disease. *Infect Agents Dis* **5**: 29-35

[8] Stagno, S., Cloud, G.A., 1994, Working parents: the impact of day care and breast-feeding on cytomegalovirus infections in offspring. *Proc Natl Acad Sci USA* **91**: 2384-2389

[9] Diosi, P., Babusceac, L., Nevinglovschi, O., Kun-Stoicu, G., 1967, Cytomegalovirus infection associated with pregnancy. *Lancet* **1**: 1063-1066

[10] Stagno, S., Reynolds, D.W., Pass, R.F., Alford, C.A., 1980, Breast milk and the risk of cytomegalovirus infection. *N Engl J Med* **302**: 1073-1076

[11] Dworsky, M., Yow, M., Stagno, S., Pass, R.F., Alford, C., 1983, Cytomegalovirus infection of breast milk and transmission in infancy. *Pediatrics* **72**: 295-299

[12] Asanuma, H., Numazaki, K., Nagata, N., Hotsubo, T., Horino, K., Chiba, S., 1996, Role of milk whey in the transmission of human cytomegalovirus infection by breast milk. *Microbiol Immunol* **40**: 201-204

[13] Vochem, M., Hamprecht, K., Jahn, G., Speer, C.P., 1998, Transmission of cytomegalovirus to preterm infants through breast milk. *Pediatr Infect Dis J* **17**: 53-58

[14] Hotsubo, T., Nagata, N., Shimada, M., Yoshida, K., Fujinaga, K., Chiba, S., 1994, Detection of human cytomegalovirus DNA in breast milk by means of polymerase chain reaction. *Microbiol Immunol* **38**: 809-811

[15] Hamprecht, K., Vochem, M., Baumeister, A., Boniek, M., Speer, C.P., Jahn, G., 1998, Detection of cytomegaloviral DNA in human milk cells and cell free milk whey by nested PCR. *J Virol Methods* **70**: 167-176

[16] Goldman, A. S., 1993, The immune system of human milk: antimicrobial, antiflammatory and immunmodulating properties. *Pediatr Infect Dis J* **12(8)**: 664-671

[17] Rivas, R.A., El-Mohandes, A.A.E., Katona, I.M., 1994, Mononuclear phagocytotic cells in human milk: HLA-DR and Fc-gammaR ligand expression. *Biol Neonate* **66**: 195-204

[18] Lindstrand, A., Smedman, L., Gunnlaugsson, G., Troye-Blomberg, M., 1997, Selective compartmentalization of gamma-delta-T lymphocytes in human breastmilk. *Acta Paediatr* **86**: 890-91

[19] Eglinton, B.A., Roberton, D.M., Cummins, A.G., 1994, Phenotype of T cells, their soluble receptor levels, and cytokine profile of human breast milk. *Immunology and Cell Biology* **72**: 306-313

[20] Richie, E.R., Bass, R., Meistrich, M.L. et al., 1984, Distribution of T lymphocyte subsets in human colostrum. J Immunol 129: 1116-1119

[21] Wirt, D.P., Adkins, L.T., Palkowetz, K.H., Schmalstieg, F.C., Goldman, A.S., 1992, Activated and Memory T Lymphocytes in Human Milk. *Cytometry* **13**: 282-290

[22] Bartal, L., Padeh, S., Passwell, J.H. ,1987, Lactoferrin inhibits prostaglandin E2 secretion by breast milk macrophages. *Pediatr Res* **21**: 54-57

[23] Pitt, J.,1979, The milk mononuclear phagocyte. *Pediatrics* **64 (suppl)**: 745

[24] Keeney, S.E., Schmalstieg, F.C., Palkowetz, K.H., Rudloff, H.E., Le, B.-M., Goldman, A.S., 1993, Activated neutrophils and neutrophil activators in human milk: increased expression of CD11b and decreased expression of L-selectin. *J of Leukocyte Biol* **54**: 97-104

[25] Thorpe, C.W., Rudloff, H.E., Powell, L.C. et al, 1986, Decreased response of human milk leukocytes to chemoattractant peptides. *Pediatr Res* **20**: 373-377

[26] Sinzger, C., and Jahn, G., 1996, Human cytomegalovirus cell tropism and pathogenesis. *Intervirology* **39**: 302-319.

[27] Ballard, R.A., Drew, W.L., Hufnagel, K.G., Reidel, P.A., 1979, Aquired cytomegalovirus infection in preterm infants. *Am J Dis Child* **133**: 482-485

22

PHYSIOLOGY OF OLIGOSACCHARIDES IN LACTATING WOMEN AND BREAST FED INFANTS

Kunz Clemens[1], Rudloff Silvia[2]
[1] Institute of Nutrition, University of Giessen, Wilhelmstr.20, 35392 Giessen; [2] Research Institute of Child Nutrition, Heinstueck 11 44225 Dortmund

1.   BACKGROUND

Human milk is composed of 50-70 g/l lactose and 5-8 g/l lactose derived oligosaccharides[1]. It seems likely that among other components milk oligosaccharides play an important role in the infant's defense against bacterial and viral adhesion in particular within the gastrointestinal tract[2, 3, 4,5]. A prerequisite for systemic effects is that milk oligosaccharides are absorbed and distributed via the blood to different organs and cells. To increase our knowledge with regard to oligosaccharide metabolism in the infant it would be of great advantage if suitable methods would be available.

Currently, a dietary influence on the biosynthesis of carbohydrates in the mammary gland is considered not to be of any importance. However, we hypothesized that lactating women have an exogenous demand for galactose (Gal) because they may produce up to several liters of milk per day with a

Short and Long Term Effects of Breast Feeding on Child Health
Edited by Berthold Koletzko *et al.*, Kluwer Academic/Plenum Publishers, 2000

high lactose and oligosaccharide content and one of the major constituent of these carbohydrates is Gal, and not glucose [6, 7].

Therefore we investigated whether an orally given ^{13}C-labeled galactose bolus to lactating mothers leads to a specific labelling of milk lactose and oligosaccharides in the human mammary gland (Fig. 1). If the ^{13}C-enrichment of milk carbohydrates would be high enough we should then be able to follow some metabolic pathways of milk oligosaccharides in the infant.

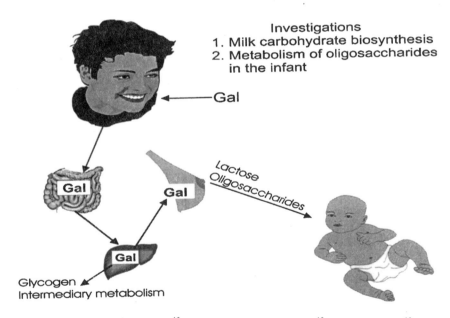

Fig. 1: Scheme of our studies with ^{13}C-labeled monosaccharides (^{13}C-Galactose and ^{13}C-Glucose) to investigate questions with regard to a) milk carbohydrate biosynthesis and b) oligosaccharide metabolism in the infant.

2.   STUDY DESIGN

The study design is shown in figure 2.

Fifteen breastfeeding women (3rd - 4th month of lactation) received directly after their breakfast an oral Gal bolus (25 g Gal + 2 g ^{13}C-Gal; D-Gal; 1-^{13}C,99 %). During the following 24 - 36 h they collected 5 - 10 ml milk at each nursing and urine (in 4 h fractions). Most of the mothers also collected breath at each nursing. The milk volume was determined by weighing the infant immediately before and after suckling. We also collected urine from 2 infants during 24 – 36 h after the gal bolus was given to their mothers.

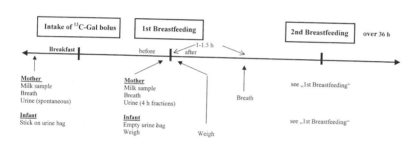

Fig. 2: Outline of the study design.

The ^{13}C-enrichment in breath, urine, whole milk and in milk fractions with fat, protein and carbohydrates was determined after total combustion by isotope ratio mass spectrometry (IR-MS) (Delta S, Finnigan, Bremen, Germany). To identify ^{13}C-labelled components protein- and fatfree milk was separated into individual fractions by Sephadex G25 gel filtration and characterized by high pH anion exchange chromatography with pulsed amperometric detection (HPAEC-PAD), high performance thin layer chromatography (Silica-HPTLC), fast atom bombardment mass spectrometry (FAB-MS) and ^{13}C-nuclear magnetic resonance spectroscopy (^{13}C-NMR) [6, 7, 8]

To exemplify the potential of applying stable isotopes in lactating mothers and to follow the metabolic fate in their infants we report the data from one mother-infant pair. More detailed information is given in references 6 and 7.

3. RESULTS

IR-MS (expressed as $\delta^{13}C_{PDB}$[‰]) of whole milk from all women revealed a maximum ^{13}C-enrichment during the first 2 h to 8 h after the oral intake of ^{13}C-Gal, followed by a continuous decrease of $\delta^{13}C_{PDB}$[‰]. An example is given in Figure 3 which shows the $\delta^{13}C_{PDB}$-values in whole milk and in the milk fat, protein and carbohydrate fraction of one woman. In milk the maximum $\delta^{13}C_{PDB}$ was reached within 8 h after the Gal-bolus was given which then rapidly declined in the following hours. The highest ^{13}C-enrichment was observed in milk carbohydrates followed by milk proteins. However, parts of the high $\delta^{13}C_{PDB}$[‰] in the protein fraction are due to residual lactose present. Only a low amount of ^{13}C-enrichment was detectable in fat. The cumulative ^{13}C-enrichment over the first peak was about 7 % of the oral ^{13}C-dose.

To identify ^{13}C-enriched components, the carbohydrate fraction was separated by Sephadex G25 gel filtration in individual fractions and investigated by HPAEC-PAD, silica-HPTLC and IRMS. As can be seen in Fig. 4, the highest $^{13}C_{PDB}$-values were found in lactose, followed by neutral and to a lesser extent by acidic oligosaccharides.

Figure 5 shows, as an example, the characterization of the Sephadex G25 fractions by HPAEC-PAD. The major components have also been identified by FAB-MS.

^{13}C-NMR of the isolated lactose from milk samples collected during 36 h after the Gal intake demonstrated that a ^{13}C was present only at the C_1-position of Gal and at the C_1-position of glucose. Moreover, in milk from some women there seemed to be a preferential labelling of Gal compared to glucose immediately after the Gal intake. As the orally given ^{13}C-Gal was only labelled at C_1-atom the data indicate that a significant part of dietary Gal is directly transported to the lactating mammary gland without being metabolised by the liver [6, 7].

To be able to answer the question whether milk oligosaccharides are absorbed in the infants' intestinal tract we collected urine from 5 infants and analysed it by the method described above.

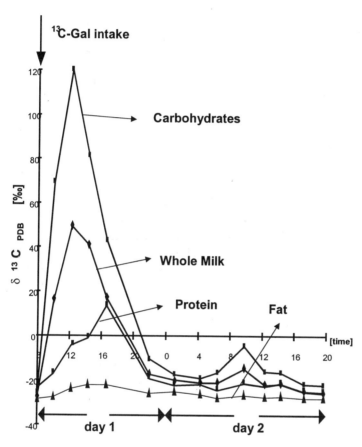

Fig. 3: ^{13}C-enrichment (expressed as $\delta^{13}C_{PDB}$[‰]) of whole milk and milk fractions from one woman during the first 36 h after a single oral galactose bolus (25 g Gal + 2 g ^{13}C-Gal; D-Gal; 1-^{13}C,99 %).

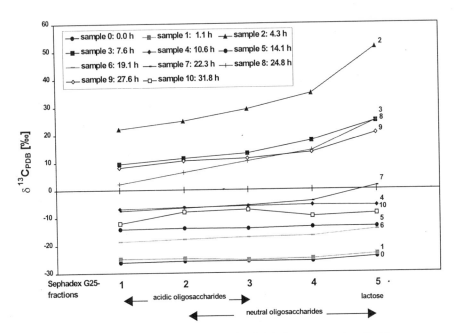

Fig. 4: ^{13}C-enrichment in fractions after Sephadex G 25-chromatography of milk carbohydrates. $\delta^{13}C_{PDB}$ values are shown from the fractions with lactose, neutral and acidic oligosaccharides from 10 milk samples collected during 32 h after the gal bolus was given.

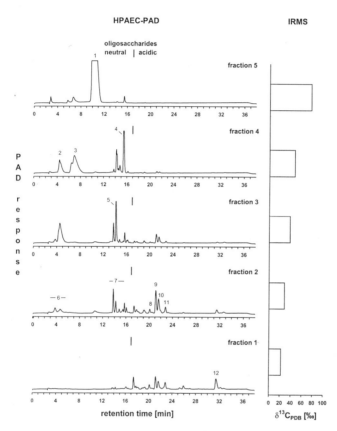

Fig. 5: HPAEC-PAD of fractions after Sephadex G 25-chromatography of milk carbohydrates.

1   Lactose
2   Fuc$_2$-Lacto-N-Tetraose
3   3-Fucosyl-Lactose
4   Lacto-N-Tetraose
5   Lacto-N-Fucopentaose I
6   multiple fucosylated Tetraoses, Hexaoses etc
7   monofucosylated Hexaoses, Octaoses, Decaoses etc
8   NeuAc-Lacto-N-Tetraose (LSTc)
9   NeuAcα2-6Lactose
10   NeuAcα2-3Lactose
11   NeuAc-Lacto-N-Tetraose (LSTa)
12   NeuAc$_2$-Lacto-N-Tetraose and multiple sialylated components
     (only the main components are given)

In figure 6, the ^{13}C-enrichment in the milk of one mother and in the urine of her infant is shown. Compared to the milk, the maximal $\delta^{13}C_{PDB}$ of infant's urine was delayed with -10.7 ‰ as the highest ^{13}C-enrichment (in mother's milk 34,3 ‰).

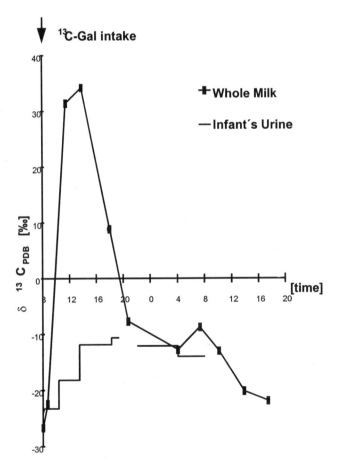

Fig 6: ^{13}C-enrichment in mothers milk and in urine of her infant.

To further investigate which urinary component contributed to the ^{13}C-enrichment, deproteinized urine was separated by gel filtration into six fractions which were then directly subjected to IRMS or after further chromatographic purifications. IRMS analysis of lactose and these oligosaccharides revealed the highest $\delta^{13}C_{PDB}$-value in lactose, followed by fucosyl-lactose (Fuc-Lac), lacto-N-tetraose (LNT), Fuc-LNT and Fuc$_2$-Lac (listed in order of decreasing amounts of ^{13}C-enrichment).

4.   CONCLUSIONS

Our data demonstrate that a part of orally applied Gal is directly incorporated into milk lactose, neutral oligosaccharides and acidic components. Moreover, there seems to be a preferential labelling of Gal compared to glucose within the lactose moieties. The metabolic fate of *in vivo* labelled lactose and oligosaccharides in the recipient infant is currently investigated. So far, determining the amount of specific oligosaccharides in milk and their excretion via urine in the infant we found that about 0.5 to 1.0 % of lacto-N-tetraose and lacto-N-fucopentaose 1 can be detected in urine. The data confirm our previous studies comparing the urinary oligosaccharide profile of breast-fed and bottle-fed infants[9]. The conclusion is that some milk oligosaccharides are absorbed without being digested in the gastrointestinal tract. Hence, a variety of physiological effects of milk oligosaccharides may be possible not only locally in the infant's gastrointestinal tract. Therefore, an influence of oligosaccharides on leukocyte endothelial interactions may be of significant importance with regard to immunological reactions (see the following chapter by Klein et al.).

ACKNOWLEDGMENTS

This work was supported by the German Research Foundation (DFG; Ku 781/8-3).

REFERENCES

1. Kunz C, Rudloff S, Schad W, and Braun D, 1999, Lactose-derived oligosaccharides in the milk of elephants: comparison with human milk. *Brit J Nutr* **82**: 391-399
2. Kunz C, Rudloff S, 1993, Biological functions of oligosaccharides in human milk. *Acta Paediatr* **82**: 903-912

3. Zopf D, Roth S, 1996, Oligosaccharide anti-infective agents. *Lancet* <u>347</u>: 1017-1021

4. Varki A, 1993, Biological roles of oligosaccharides : all theories are correct. *Glycobiology* <u>3</u>: 97-130

5. Kunz C, 1999, Microbial receptor analogs in human milk - Structural and functional aspects. In *Probiotics, other nutritional factors and intestinal microflora..* (L A Hanson, Yolken R, eds). 42nd Nestlé Nutrition Workshop in Beijing (China). Raven Press, New York, pp 157-174

6. Obermeier S, Rudloff S, Hartmann R, Pohlentz G, Brösicke H, Lentze MJ, Kunz C, (submitted) Isotope ratio mass spectrometry of *in vivo* ^{13}C-labeled carbohydrates in milk and urine of lactating women

7. Kunz C, Obermeier S, Rudloff S, Brösicke H, Hartmann R, Pohlentz G, Lentze MJ (submitted) Incorporation of oral ^{13}C-galactose into lactose and oligosaccharides of human milk

8. Kunz C, Rudloff S, Hintermann A, Pohlentz G, Egge H, 1996, High-pH anion exchange chromatography with pulsed amperometric detection and molar response facto of human milk oligosaccharides. *J Chromatogr B* <u>685</u>: 211-221

9. Rudloff S, Pohlentz G, Diekmann L, Egge H, Kunz C, 1996, Urinary excretion of lactose and oligosaccharides in preterm infants fed human milk or infant formula. *Acta Paediatr* <u>85</u>: 598-603

23

IMMUNOMODULATORY EFFECTS OF BREAST MILK OLIGOSACCHARIDES

N. Klein, A. Schwertmann, M. Peters, C. Kunz, and S. Strobel

Immunobiology Unit, Institute of Child Health, 30 Guilford Street, London WC1N 1EH. England and The Research Institute of Child Nutrition, Dortmund, Germany.

Key Words: Oligosaccharides, adhesion molecules

Abstract: Breast milk oligosaccharides are excreted in urine in amounts that suggest that they may exist in the circulation at levels compatible with a physiological function. Some oligosaccharides have structural similarity to cellular adhesion molecules and may influence adhesion of cells in breast fed infants. In this study, breast milk oligosaccharides were purified and incubated in assays of cell adhesion. They were found to inhibit neutrophil adhesion to stimulated vascular endothelial cells in a dose dependent fashion. In contrast they enhanced platelet-neutrophil complex formation. These results indicate that breast milk oligosaccharides may play a physiological role in modulating cellular adhesion in vivo.

1.   INTRODUCTION

Apart from nutritive aspects of breast milk, a number of physiological and immunomodulatory and protective properties have long been known.

Important protective factors in breast milk have been associated with secretory IgA [sIgA], lactoferrin and lysozyme which have direct antibacterial properties. The role of cellular components of breast milk during early lactation such as neutrophils, macrophages and lymphocytes in early immunological protection are unresolved but are thought to assist in local mucosal immunity.

More recently, non-immunological components of breast milk such as complex oligosaccharides with anti-inflammatory and anti-infectious properties have become the topic of continued scientific interest.

1.1   Structural aspects of oligosaccharides

The amount of oligosaccharides in breast milk changes during lactation. The oligosaccharide concentration in breast milk is around 5-8g/l which is around 5-10% of the Lactose concentration and as such a major component of breast milk. The oligosaccharide spectrum is determined through the blood group and secretor status of the mother. Around 70% of the Caucasian population belongs to the Le [a-b+] status with a1-2, 1-3 and 1-4 linked fucose molecules. About 20% of the population have an inactivation of a secretor gene and the milk lacks mainly a1-2 fucosyl components. Around 10% Le [a-b-] have a specific fucosyltransferase and do not secrete any a1-4 fucosyl structures [1].

1.2   Absorption of breast milk oligosaccharides

In order for breast milk oligosaccharides to operate systemically, they need to be absorbed to have a systemic effect at other surfaces, for example the endothelium. Intact breast milk oligosaccharides have been demonstrated in the urine only of those premature infants who have been breast fed when compared to formula fed premature infants. 13C stabile isotope studies revealed that in-vivo labelled lactose given to mothers was incorporated into oligosaccharides which were taken up by the infant as indicated by the occurrence of complex 13C labelled carbohydrates with partial identity with breast milk oligosaccharides from mothers [1].

1.3   Oligosaccharides as receptor analogues

The adhesion of pathogens to the host cell is one of the crucial first steps during infection and inflammation. This contact occurs frequently through carbohydrate sequences which are ubiquitously expressed on cell surfaces. These receptors often contain neutral, fucosyl - or sialyl-carbohydrate structures, similar to those in breast milk oligosaccharides. These oligosaccharides can fulfil the role of receptor analogues and are such in a position to prevent adhesion of pathogens [bacteria and viruses]. This concept has been demonstrated in vitro for *Streptococcus. pneumoniae*, *Haemophilus.. influenza*, and *campylobacter* binding to epithelial cells [2].

1.4   Oligosaccharides as ligands of cell adhesion molecules

Leucocyte adhesion to endothelium and extravasation at sites of inflammation is a multi - step process. Low avidity binding by sialyted and fucosylated oligosaccharides and members of the selectin (CD62) family results initially in slowing down (rolling) of passing leucocytes. This is then followed by firm adhesion and transmigration mediated by activated β1 and β2 integrins and members of the immunoglobulin supergene family particularly VCAM-1 and ICAM-1. The migration of leucocytes, such as neutrophils, lymphocytes and monocytes at sites of inflammation is therefore determined by the expression of adhesion molecules which in turn are regulated by signals mediated by surface costimulatory molecules and by cytokines [3].

There is increasing evidence that the complex multi-cellular processes of inflammation, haemostasis and thrombosis are closely linked. It has been established that inflammatory cytokines such as TNF-α and IL-1 can induce a pro-thrombotic state. This results from increased monocyte and endothelial cell Tissue Factor (TF) expression and pathway activation and reduced fibrinolytic activity secondary to raised levels of plasminogen activator inhibitor-1 [4]. Conversely, key components of the coagulation pathways, such as thrombin, have now been shown to contribute to inflammation by inducing IL-6 and IL-8 release from monocytes and endothelial cells.

Recently, it has become apparent that platelets are pivotal in regulating this haemostatic/inflammatory axis. Platelets express surface adhesion molecules responsible for primary haemostasis, and accelerate the conversion of pro-thrombin to thrombin [4]. In addition platelets can secrete pro-inflammatory mediators such as IL-1 and express surface molecules capable of modulating inflammatory processes (e.g. CD40L).

The capacity for platelets to influence the haemostatic/inflammatory axis may rely upon direct contact with inflammatory cells. Heterotypic aggregation of platelets to neutrophils (and other leukocytes) has been observed *in vitro* and in blood taken from healthy volunteers. These interactions are mediated by platelet CD62P expression, and leukocyte β2 integrins [4,5]. Indirect evidence that these complexes may themselves have a physiological function is provided by studies which have shown changes in the numbers of, or capacity to form these heterotypic cell complexes in clinical conditions in which thrombosis and inflammation are prominent features. How platelet-leukocyte complexes contribute to these conditions has yet to be elucidated.

There is now good evidence that sialyl and fucosyl lactosamines such as sLe^x, sLe^a are critical epitopes during lectin-ligand binding steps. Similar carbohydrate structures or their precursors are abundant in breast milk and may therefore influence adhesive events in vivo[6].

2.   OBJECTIVE

On the basis of the physiological properties of breast milk oligosaccharides we have investigated the following:

(1) The modulating effects of oligosaccharide fractions [defatted breast milk, neutral and acid oligosaccharides] on cellular adhesion to human umbilical vascular endothelial cells [HUVEC].

(2) The influence of breast milk oligosaccharides on platelet neutrophil complex formation in a newly developed whole blood assay.

3.   METHODS

3.1   Cell culture and adhesion assays

Human umbilical vein endothelial cells (HUVEC) were prepared as previously described [7]. Briefly, endothelial cells were removed from human umbilical cords by collagenase II digestion, resuspended in MCDB131 medium with 20% FCS and antibiotics and grown in primary cultures for 24-48 hours until they reached 90-95% confluence. For flow cytometry and leucocyte adhesion assays, HUVEC monolayers from primary cultures were dispersed with trypsin/EDTA and re-cultured onto ECAF coated tissue culture plates in MCDB131 medium with 20% FCS, ECGF and antibiotics. Cultures were grown for 24-48 hours until confluent when ECGF containing medium was removed and medium containing cytokines and/or antibodies or leucocytes was added for the times indicated.

Peripheral blood leucocytes were prepared by collection of whole blood from normal healthy donors into heparin (10 IU/ml). The suspension was diluted 2 fold in RPMI 1640 medium and centrifuged at 200g for 10 minutes. The red cell/leucocyte pellet was washed again in the same manner then resuspended in 10 volumes of red blood cell lysing medium (150mM NH_4Cl, 20mM $NaHCO_3$, 1mM EDTA). Red cells were allowed to lyse for 10 minutes at room temperature before centrifugation at 200g for 7 minutes followed by a further 2 washes in RPMI 1640 medium with 10% FCS. The leucocyte pellet was then resuspended in endothelial cell culture medium at 2×10^6 cells/ml.

To measure leucocyte adhesion to endothelial cells, 4×10^6 leucocytes in 2ml of endothelial cell culture medium were added to endothelial cells in 24 well plates. Plates were placed on a rotary shaker to create flow and incubated for 1 hour at 37°C in 5% CO_2 in air. Non adherent cells were removed by aspiration of the supernatant and a further two washes. Endothelial cells and adherent leucocytes were dispersed by incubation in modified Puck's saline A supplemented with 0.2 % EDTA and 10% FCS at pH 7.2 for 15-20 minutes at room temperature. Both adherent and non adherent cell fractions were washed and centrifuged at 200g for 7 minutes then resuspended into equal volumes of PBS with 5% FCS and 0.02% NaN_3. Both fractions were stained for T cells (CD3), B cells (CD19), monocytes (CD14) and neutrophils (CD15).

3.2   Flow cytometry

HUVEC monolayers for antibody staining and flow cytometry were incubated with modified Puck's saline A, and resuspended by gentle mechanical action. The cells were then washed immediately in PBS containing 5% FCS and 0.02 % NaN_3, and aliquoted for staining. Cells were incubated with primary mAbs, washed and, when required, incubated with either FITC or PE conjugated goat anti-mouse IgG. The fluorescence data were acquired and analysed on a Becton Dickinson FACScalibur using CellQuest software. In some experiments, the results were expressed as median fluorescence intensity (MFI). In other experiments, calibrated FITC conjugated beads (Dako) were used to calculate the molecules of equivalent soluble fluorochrome (MESF), which allows direct comparison between experiments.

3.3   Investigation of platelet-neutrophil complexes

PNCs were investigated as previously described [4]. Briefly 50 µl of blood was added to a combination of a directly conjugated monoclonal antibody directed against a platelet antigen (CD42b PE, CD42b:FITC or CD61

PerCP) and a neutrophil antigen (CD11b:FITC, Mab24:FITC, CD62L:PE) or isotype control antibodies within ten minutes of sampling. Following gentle mixing, the samples were left at room temperature for ten minutes before the addition of 200 µl of FACSlyse. Following gentle resuspension the samples were incubated for a further ten minutes before the addition of 250 µl of 0.2% formaldehyde in PBS. Samples were analysed by flow cytometry within one hour of preparation.

3.4 **Whole blood stimulation**

Blood was drawn from non-smoking healthy volunteers who had not been on any medication for at least two weeks via a 21G butterfly needle without the use of a tourniquet. The first 2ml of blood were discarded, and the required volume collected into sodium citrate to a final concentration of 0.38%. Whole blood stimulation experiments were performed immediately after sampling as previously described [4]. ADP was used at a final concentration of 10µM, and FMLP at a final concentration of 1µM. Different concentrations of BMO (Breast milk oligossacharides) were added before samples were then analysed after incubation at 37°C with gentle mechanical agitation on a rotary shaker (~10Hz).

4.   **RESULTS**

4.1   **Adhesion molecule expression**

All BMO samples were tested for their capacity to induce the endothelial adhesion molecules, ICAM-1, VCAM-1 and E-selectin. None were found to effect either resting EC's or TNF stimulated cells.

4.2   **Leukocyte adhesion to HUVEC's**

Neutral oligosaccharides did not influence neutrophil adhesion at rest. However, when added to TNFα stimulated HUVEC, there was a dose dependent inhibition of neutrophil adhesion (Figure 1). We did not detect any consistent changes in lymphocyte adhesion under these conditions. The results with acidic oligosaccharides were usually minimal although in some experiments there was enhancement of neutrophil adhesion.

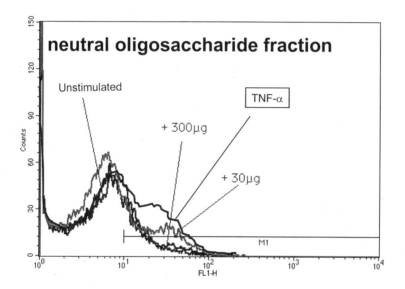

Figure 1: Effect of Neutral Breast Milk Oligosaccharides on Neutrophil adhesion to TNF stimulated Endothelial Cells

4.3   Platelet-neutrophil complex formation

Examination of the neutrophils from whole blood stained with CD42b:PE and CD11b:FITC, allowed the detection of two populations of cells: free neutrophils and platelet-neutrophil complexes (PNCs).   ADP stimulation increased the intensity of CD11b staining in both PNCs and free neutrophils. Addition of defatted breast milk led to a dose dependent increase in PNCs and an increase in neutrophil CD11b expression. This occurred in the presence or absence of ADP. Experiments with BMO also increased PNCs although in the samples used low levels of endotoxin were detected (Figure2).

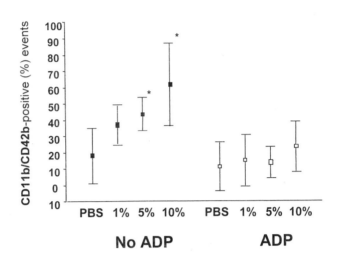

Figure 2: CD11b/CD42b expression on polymorphic neutrophiles and platelets after incubation with breast milk oligosaccharides

5.   CONCLUSIONS

(1) This study investigated the capacity for different breast milk fractions to influence the processes of adhesion involved in endothelial – leukocyte interactions and in platelet-neutrophil complex formation. Both adhesive models require selectins, integrins and members of the immunoglobulin superfamily. We found that purified neutral oligosaccharides had the capacity to inhibit binding of neutrophils to TNF stimulated endothelium. The model used examined adhesion under low flow conditions and so it is difficult to be exactly certain how these sugars were operating. It is probable that selectin mediated adhesion was most effected but further studies are required to examine this further.

(2) We also found that defatted BM and purified oligosaccharides enhanced the formation of PNCs. Again both selectins and integrins are involved in PNC formation. How the oligosaccharides are mediating this effect is unclear. They may act to bridge CD62P to its ligands on neutrophils or more probably through the crosslinking of neutrophil selectins they activate a signalling cascade which leads to increased integrin expression and activation. More work is required to understand these processes in more detail.

(3) In summary, our results indicate that breast milk oligosaccharides can influence cellular adhesion but further work is required before we can be confident that the oligosaccharides are operating in isolation and are not acting in concert with non-oligosaccharide contaminants present in the samples as a result of the purification process.

REFERENCES

1. Kunz C, Rodriguez-Palmero M, Koletzko B, Jensen R. Nutritional and biochemical properties of human milk, Part I: General aspects, proteins, and carbohydrates. *Clin Perinatol* 1999:307-33

2. Schwertmann A, Schroten H, Hacker J, Kunz C. S-fimbriae from Escherichia coli bind to soluble glycoproteins from human milk. *J Pediatr Gastroenterol Nutr* 1999:257-63

3. Hogg N, Stewart MP, Scarth SL, Newton R, Shaw JM, Law SK, Klein N A novel leukocyte adhesion deficiency caused by expressed but nonfunctional beta2 integrins Mac-1 and LFA-1. *J Clin Invest* 1999;103:97-106

4. Peters MJ, Heyderman RS, Hatch DJ, Klein NJ Investigation of platelet-neutrophil interactions in whole blood by flow cytometry. *J Immunol Methods* 1997;209:125-355

5. Peters MJ, Dixon G, Kotowicz KT, Hatch DJ, Heyderman RS, Klein NJ. Circulating platelet-neutrophil complexes represent a subpopulation of activated neutrophils primed for adhesion, phagocytosis and intracellular killing. *Br J Haematol* 1999;106:391-9

6. Schwertmann A, Rudloff S, Kunz C. Potential ligands for cell adhesion molecules in human milk. *Ann Nutr Metab* 1996;40:252-62

7. Klein NJ, Ison CA, Peakman M, Levin M, Hammerschmidt S, Frosch M, Heyderman RS The influence of capsulation and lipooligosaccharide structure on neutrophil adhesion molecule expression and endothelial injury by Neisseria meningitidis. *J Infect Dis* 1996;173:172-9

24

POLYUNSATURATED FATTY ACID SUPPLY WITH HUMAN MILK
Physiological aspects and in vivo studies of metabolism

Thorsten U. Sauerwald, Hans Demmelmair, Nataša Fidler, Berthold Koletzko
Division of Metabolic Disorders and Nutrition, Kinderklinik and Kinderpoliklinik, Ludwig-Maximilians-University of Munich, Germany

Key words: lactation, diet, fatty acid metabolism, oxidation, transfer, stable isotopes

Abstract: The origin of polyunsaturated fatty acids (PUFA) in human milk has not been studied in detail. Diet, liberation from maternal stores and endogenous synthesis from precursors may contribute to PUFA present in human milk. Other factors influencing lipid content and fatty acid composition such as gestational age, stage of lactation, nutritional status and genetical background are known. In a series of *in vivo* studies using stable isotope methodologies we investigated the metabolism of PUFA during lactation. With this techniques the transfer of single dietary fatty acids into human milk, the oxidation and the deposition in tissues were estimated. Our studies demonstrate that the major part of PUFA in human milk seems not to be derived directly from the maternal diet but from body stores. Nevertheless diet is important, because long term intakes affect composition of body stores.

1. INTRODUCTION

Human milk contains a variety of fatty acids mainly present in the form of triglycerides. The majority of these fatty acids are saturated and monounsaturated fatty acids. However, a minor but important component are the polyunsaturated fatty acids (PUFA). These PUFA are indispensable for the structure of membranes, some of them serve as precursors for eicosanoids and some of the PUFA are associated with functional outcome during infancy [1,10]. The two major families, n-6 and n-3 PUFA, are derived from the essential fatty acids linoleic and α-linolenic acid, respectively, which must be derived from the diet, because in humans they cannot be synthesized de novo. The pathways of n-6 and n-3 PUFA with the revised steps of long-chain polyunsaturated fatty acid (LC-PUFA) synthesis are shown in figure 1. The major PUFA in human milk is linoleic acid, but more than ten other PUFA are found in human milk samples. In the last years much attention has been given to the LC-PUFA arachidonic and docosahexaenoic acid, fatty acids with chain lengths of 20-22 carbons. Together, both LC-PUFA represent amounts of about 1% of total fatty acids in human milk. Their importance results from their connection to growth, neurodevelopment and visual function of the recipient infant [1,10].

After some physiological and compositional aspects of fatty acids in human milk we will summarize in this chapter some of our recent work with stable isotopes that elucidate the metabolism of PUFA during the period of lactation.

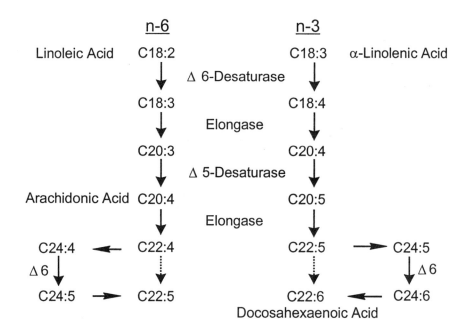

Figure 1: Simplified scheme of the revised pathways of LC-PUFA synthesis (solid lines, based on data of Sprecher et al. [21])

2. **HUMAN MILK POLYUNSATURATED FATTY ACID COMPOSITION**

2.1 Single feeding and stage of lactation

During a single feeding there is a marked increase of total fat content in human milk. At the end of a nursing cycle this milk, the so called hind milk, contains 2-3 times more total fat and thus energy than fore milk [8,17]. Hind milk has been used in nurseries with success in preterm infants to enhance weight gain [23]. The overall fatty acid composition during a single feeding is not affected by this change of fat content, but the absolute amounts of PUFA are also increased in hind milk.

With advancing lactation the fatty acid composition of human milk changes. From colostrum to mature human milk the percentages of linoleic and α-linolenic acids increase, whereas the percentages of LC-PUFA, mainly arachidonic and docosahexaenoic acid, decrease [6]. Because with advancing lactation the total fat content of milk is also increasing the total amount of LC-PUFA remains relatively stable [12]. During the first 4-6 weeks of lactation the changes in PUFA composition are more pronounced, but up to the 16th week of lactation a decrease of LC-PUFA has been observed [15]. The comparisons of breast milk from mothers of preterm and term infants have resulted in some controversies. But generally the PUFA composition of term and preterm mothers´ milk is comparable.

2.2 Human milk samples from different countries

The fatty acid composition of human milk from different countries has a similar pattern. Koletzko et al. reported data from several studies of breastfeeding mothers in Europe and Africa which resulted to have comparable median values and ranges for PUFA composition when expressed as weight percentages [13]. This finding is rather surprising if one considers the differences in ethnicity, living conditions and dietary intakes. The major PUFA in human milk is always linoleic acid with a median value of 11.0 and 12.0 wt.% in different European and African countries, respectively [13]. α-Linolenic acid, about one order of magnitude lower than linoleic acid in human milk, is most times the second major PUFA. The linoleic/α-linolenic acid ratio is used for the expression of the n-6 / n-3 balance, which seems important since both fatty acid families compete for the same enzymes in their pathways of LC-PUFA synthesis. In the above mentioned report this ratio was similar in different countries and ranged from 8.6 to 16.9 in European countries and from 8.8 to 15.7 in African countries. Likewise the median values for the percentage of total n-6 LC-PUFA of the above cited study were 1.2 and 1.5 wt.% for European and African countries, respectively, and 0.6 wt.% for the percentage of total n-3 LC-PUFA for both European and African countries. The human milk PUFA composition from seven different studies included in the report of Koletzko et al.[13] are presented in figure 2.

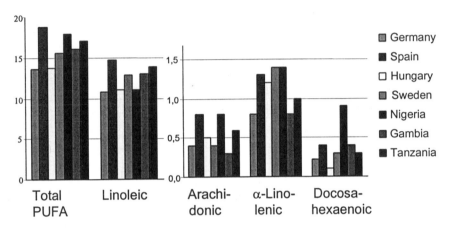

Figure 2: PUFA composition of mature human milk in different European and African countries (medians or means; wt.% of total fatty acids; from Koletzko et al.[13])

2.3   Maternal diet

Diets have an influence on the fatty acid composition of human milk. After absorption dietary fatty acids are rapidly transfered via chylomicrons, VLDL and LDL particles to the mammary gland and secreted into human milk[7]. The short term effects of a diet have recently been demonstrated after ingestion of single meals with high contents of different characteristic fatty acids, e.g. α-linolenic, linoleic or docosahexaenoic acid[5]. Within 6 hours after consumption of the test meals significant changes in marker fatty acids were observed. After 1-3 days these changes were no longer present.

The long term effects of maternal diet have been assessed by comparison of populations with vegan/vegetarian, high carbohydrate, high fish and omnivorous diets. Maternal PUFA intakes are generally reflected in the PUFA composition of human milk (see figure 3). But also the fatty acid composition of adipose tissue is influenced by long term dietary habits[18]. The high intake of linoleic and α-linolenic acid with the vegan/vegetarian diet is followed by higher values of these fatty acids in human milk of these mothers when compared to the omnivore mothers [4,19]. A high carbohydrate diet does not markedly change the PUFA composition of human milk [16], whereas a high fish diet, rich in eicosapentaenoic and docosahexaenoic acids, like that of eskimo populations, is reflected in the high levels of these n-3 LC-PUFA in their milk [9].

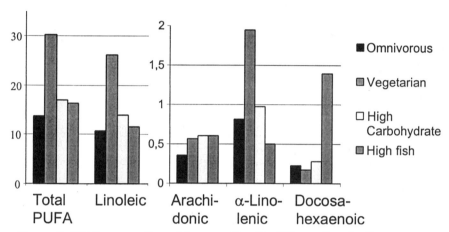

Figure 3: PUFA composition of human milk with different diets (medians or means, wt.% of total fatty acids; drawn from data of Koletzko et al. [13], Sanders and Reddy [19], Finley et al. [4], Muskiet et al. [16] and Innis and Kuhnlein [9])

3. STUDIES OF FATTY ACID METABOLISM WITH STABLE ISOTOPES DURING LACTATION

Substrates labeled with stable isotopes are ideal to trace dynamic processes *in vivo*. Their advantage in human studies is the absence of any radiation when compared with the radioactive isotopes. Stable isotopes are naturally occurring and their use has generally been considered as safe and without adverse effects. These advantages are indispensable prerequisites for studies with infants or during pregnancy and lactation. Today stable isotopes are used in a variety of applications for diagnostic and research purposes [11]. Different aspects of fatty acid metabolism such as absorption, endogenous synthesis, oxidation and transfer to several body compartments have been investigated. Even in very low birth weight infants this methodologies have recently been applied to demonstrate the *in vivo* synthesis of the LC-PUFA arachidonic and docosahexaenoic acid [20].

Already more than ten years ago Hachey et al. studied the transfer of dietary triglycerides labeled with stable isotopes in three healthy breastfeeding mothers which remained on their regular diets [7]. In their study deuterated palmitic, oleic and linoleic acids were given simultaneously with a standardized test meal to the participants. Chylomicrons and VLDL were the lipoproteins primarily involved in the transfer of the labeled triglycerides from diet to human milk. They reported a uniform secretion pattern for the three labeled fatty acids to human milk with peak enrichments between 8-10 hours after consumption of the test meal. The long-chain, diet-derived fatty acids accounted for about 29 % of the fat in human milk. In the following we report on some of our recent stable isotope studies that illustrate the metabolism of polyunsaturated fatty acids during lactation.

3.1   Linoleic acid metabolism

In a previously published study with six breastfeeding mothers we investigated repeatedly the metabolism of linoleic acid at 2, 6 and 12 weeks of lactation [2]. All women were on omnivorous diets and received an oral dose of 1 mg/kg uniformly ^{13}C-labeled linoleic acid with their breakfast. Dietary intakes were documented by 5 day home protocols during the study. Samples of breath and milk were collected over the period of 5 days at defined timepoints and measurements of ^{13}C enrichment of breath CO_2 and of fatty acids in human milk performed with isotope ratio mass spectrometry. Without any correction for a dilution of the CO_2 that might occur in the bicarbonate body pool we estimated a total of 20 % oxidation of the labeled linoleic acid within 5 days after ingestion. Peak enrichments in breath CO_2 occurred between 3-5 hours after consumption of the labeled linoleic acid and values close to the baseline were reached at 36 hours. There was no difference in the kinetics and the cumulative oxidation between the different stages of lactation.

Transfer of linoleic acid into milk peaked at about 12 hours and continously decreased until the 5th day (figure 4). The major part of dietary linoleic acid was transfered within 48 hours. Cumulative recovery of linoleic acid in milk reached about 13 % of the tracer dose over the period of 5 days. There was a considerable variation between the individual subjects but our data are in agreement with the study of Hachey et al. [7] who reported for human milk a cumulative recovery for linoleic acid of about 10 % of the dose within 3 days. We calculate that about 30 % of the linoleic acid in human milk originate from direct dietary transfer. Only a minor part of the ingested linoleic acid was used for endogenous synthesis of the longer chain metabolites dihomo-γ-linolenic and arachidonic acid which are also present in human milk. About 3-25 % of dihomo-γ-linolenic acid in human milk was derived from synthesis from dietary linoleic acid. Only about 3 % of the arachidonic acid in human milk was originating directly from dietary linoleic acid.

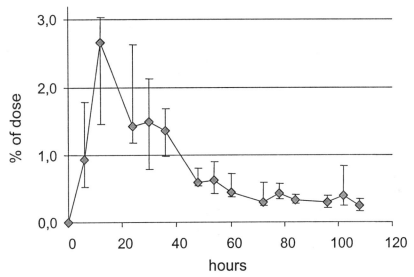

Figure 4: Time course of linoleic acid transfer from diet to milk (drawn from data of Demmelmair et al. [2])

3.2   Docosahexaenoic acid metabolism

In another study with ten mothers during the 4th and the 6th week of lactation the effects of a docosahexaenoic acid supplementation on human milk fatty acid composition and the transfer of ^{13}C labeled fatty acids from diet into human milk as well as their oxidation were assessed. Again women were on omnivorous diets and had to complete a 7 day dietary protocol during the study observation. At 4 weeks of lactation women were randomly and blindly assigned to a docosahexaenoic acid supplement (DHASCO[TM]) or a placebo. The supplement used in this study was a commercially available fatty acid mixture containing about 45 % docosahexaenoic acid. Other major components were myristic, palmitic and oleic acid (20%, 18% and 10%, respectively). The women receiving the docosahexaenoic acid supplement had signicantly higher values of DHA in human milk when compared to the control group after the two weeks of supplementation. The effects of the docosahexaenoic acid supplementation were in agreement with earlier results of Makrides et al. [14] who used the same source of supplement.

At 6 weeks of lactation all the participating mothers were given ^{13}C labeled myristic, palmitic, oleic and docosahexaenoic acid simultaneously. CO_2 and milk fatty acid enrichment were measured at defined timepoints over a period of 48 hours.

The cumulative oxidation of the fatty acid mixture in the breastfeeding women participating in this study was comparable to that of the linoleic acid oxidation in the previous study and achieved about 15% of the tracer dose within 48 hours. Results of the fatty acid oxidation have recently been reported (see figure 5, from Fidler et al. [3]).

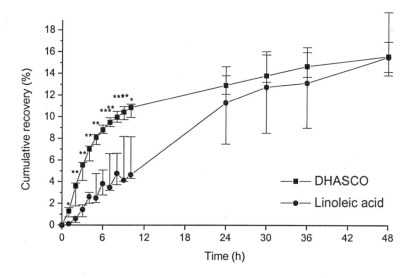

Figure 5: Cumulative recovery of ^{13}C in breath CO_2 in breastfeeding mothers after oral tracer application of ^{13}C-DHASCO™ or ^{13}C-linoleic acid (median [IQR], *p<0.05, **p<0.01, ***p<0.001, from Fidler et al. [5] and Demmelmair et al. [3])

The kinetics and the cumulative recovery of palmitic, oleic and docosahexaenoic acid in human milk were similar and not different between the supplemented and the placebo group. In contrast myristic acid recovery in human milk was always much lower, which might be explained by the observation that dietary medium chain fatty acids are oxidized readily and that medium chain fatty acids in human milk are also synthesized *de novo* from carbohydrates [22]. The transfer of fatty acids into human milk peaked between 12 and 24 hours and steadily decreased afterwards. Cumulative recovery of docosahexaenoic acid in milk reached about 8 % of the tracer dose over the period of 2 days. Values for palmitic and oleic acid cumulative recovery were comparable. Overall these values were close to those reported by Hachey et al. [7] and also to those reported by us before for linoleic acid [2].

In conclusion, milk fat contains PUFA from direct transfer of dietary fatty acids, from liberation from body stores and to a minor extent from endogenous synthesis. The major part of PUFA in human milk is derived from body stores. The latter seems to explain why PUFA content in human milk remains relatively stable after short term changes of dietary fat composition. This might be of benefit for the recipient infant. So far the few studies using stable isotope methodologies during lactation have led to a better understanding of fatty acid metabolism and further research in this area seems promising.

REFERENCES

1. Carlson, S.E. and M. Neuringer. 1999. Polyunsaturated fatty acid status and neurodevelopment: a summary and critical analysis of the literature. *Lipids* 34:171-178.
2. Demmelmair, H., M. Baumheuer, B. Koletzko, K. Dokoupil, and G. Kratl. 1998. Metabolism of $U^{13}C$-labeled linoleic acid in lactating women. *J.Lipid Res.* 39:1389-1396.
3. Fidler, N., T.U. Sauerwald, H. Demmelmair, A. Pohl, and B. Koletzko. 1999. Oxidation of an oil rich in docosahexaenoic acid compared to linoleic acid in lactating women. *Ann.Nutr.Metab.* (in press)
4. Finley, D.A., B. Lönnerdal, K.G. Dewey, and L.E. Grivetti. 1985. Breast milk composition: fat content and fatty acid composition in vegetarians and non-vegetarians. *Am.J.Clin.Nutr.* 41:787-800.
5. Francois, C.A., S.L. Connor, R.C. Wander, and W.E. Connor. 1998. Acute effects of dietary fatty acids on the fatty acids of human milk. *Am.J.Clin.Nutr* 67:301-308.
6. Genzel-Boroviczeny, O., J. Wahle, and B. Koletzko. 1997. Fatty acid composition of human milk during the first month after term and preterm delivery. *Eur.J.Pediatr.* 156:142-147.
7. Hachey, D.L., M.R. Thomas, E.A. Emken, C. Garza, L. Brown-Booth, R.O. Adlof, and P.D. Klein. 1987. Human lactation: maternal transfer of dietary triglycerides labeled with stable isotopes. *J.Lipid Res.* 28:1185-1192.
8. Harzer, G., M. Haug, I. Dietrich, and P.R. Gentner. 1983. Changing patterns of human milk lipids in the course of the lactation and during the day. *Am.J.Clin.Nutr* 37:612-621.
9. Innis, S.M. and H.V. Kuhnlein. 1988. Long-chain n-3 fatty acids in breast milk of Inuit women consuming traditional foods. *Early Hum.Dev.* 18:185-189.
10. Koletzko, B. 1992. Fats for brains. *Eur.J.Clin.Nutr.* 46:S51-S62
11. Koletzko, B., H. Demmelmair, W. Hartl, A. Kindermann, S. Koletzko, T.U. Sauerwald, and P. Szitanyi. 1998. The use of stable isotope techniques for nutritional and metabolic research in paediatrics. *Early Hum.Dev.* 53:S77-S97

12. Koletzko, B. and M. Rodriguez-Palmero. 1999. Polyunsaturated fatty acids in human milk and their role in early infant development. *J.Mammary Gland Biol.Neoplasia* 4:269-284.

13. Koletzko, B., I. Thiel, and P.O. Abiodun. 1992. The fatty acid composition of human milk in Europe and Africa. *J.Pediatr.* 120:62-70.

14. Makrides, M., M.A. Neumann, and R.A. Gibson. 1996. Effect of maternal docosahexaenoic acid (DHA) supplementation on breast milk composition. *Eur.J.Clin.Nutr.* 50:352-357.

15. Makrides, M., K. Simmer, M.A. Neumann, and R.A. Gibson. 1995. Changes in the polyunsaturated fatty acids of breast milk from mothers of full-term infants over 30 wk of lactation. *Am.J.Clin.Nutr* 61:1231-1233.

16. Muskiet, F.A.J., N.H. Hutter, I.A. Martini, J.H. Jonxis, P.J. Offringa, and E.R. Boersma. 1987. Comparison of the fatty acid composition of human milk from mothers in Tanzania, Curacao and Surinam. *Hum.Nutr.Clin.Nutr.* 41:149-159.

17. Rodriguez-Palmero, M., B. Koletzko, C. Kunz, and R. Jensen. 1999. Nutritional and biochemical properties of human milk: II. Lipids, micronutrients and bioactive factors. *Clin.Perinatol.* 26:335-359.

18. Sanders, T.A.B., F.R. Ellis, and J.W.T. Dickerson. 1978. Studies of vegans: the fatty acid composition of plasma choline phosphoglycerides, erythrocytes, adipose tissue and breast milk and some indicators of susceptibility to ischemic heart disease in vegans and omnivore controls. *Am.J.Clin.Nutr.* 31:805-813.

19. Sanders, T.A.B. and S. Reddy. 1992. The influence of a vegetarian diet on the fatty acid composition of human milk and the essential fatty acid status of the infant. *J.Pediatr.* 120:S71-S77

20. Sauerwald, T.U., D.L. Hachey, C.L. Jensen, H.M. Chen, R.E. Anderson, and W.C. Heird. 1997. Intermediates in endogenous synthesis of C22:6ω3 and C20:4ω6 by term and preterm infants. *Pediatr.Res.* 41:183-187.

21. Sprecher, H., D.L. Luthria, B.S. Mohammed, and S.P. Baykousheva. 1995. Reevaluation of the pathways for the biosynthesis of polyunsaturated fatty acids. *J.Lipid Res.* 36:2471-2477.

22. Thompson, B.J. and S. Smith. 1985. Biosynthesis of fatty acids by lactating human breast epithelial cells: an evaluation of the contribution to the overall composition of human milk fat. *Pediatr.Res.* 19:139-143.

23. Valentine, C.J., N.M. Hurst, and R.J. Schanler. 1994. Hindmilk improves weight gain in low-birth-weight infants fed human milk. *J.Pediatr.Gastroenterol.Nutr.* 18:474-477.

25

ENVIRONMENTAL EXPOSURE TO POLYCHLORINATED BIPHENYLS (PCBs) AND DIOXINS
CONSEQUENCES FOR LONGTERM NEUROLOGICAL AND COGNITIVE DEVELOPMENT OF THE CHILD LACTATION

Boersma ER and Lanting CI
Department of Pediatrics/Obstetrics and Gynecology, Perinatal Nutrition & Development Unit, University Hospital Groningen, The Netherlands

Key words: polychlorinated biphenyls, dioxins, neurodevelopment, toxicity

Abstract: Polychlorinated biphenyls (PCBs) and dioxins are environmental pollutants. Prenatally, as well as postnatally through breast feeding, large amounts are transferred from mother to the child. Formula is free of these substances. Considering their potential developmental neurotoxicity, we investigated long term effects of perinatal exposure to PCBs and dioxins on neurological and cognitive development. Given the evidence that PCBs exert oestrogenic effects, and oestrogens are known to suppress lactation, we investigated the effect of maternal PCB body load on lactation performances as well. *Methods.* A group of 418 infants were followed from birth up to 6 years of age. Half of them were fully breast fed (BF) for at least 6 weeks. Prenatal PCB exposure was measured from cord and maternal blood. Postnatal exposure was reflected by PCB and dioxin levels in breast and formula milk and plasma PCB levels at 42 months of age. Both neurological and cognitive development were taken as outcome variable at 18, 42 months and at 6 years of age. At 18 and 42 months of age neurological condition was evaluated according to Hempel and at 6 years of age according to Touwen. Condition was evaluated in terms of optimality. Separately, the fluency of movements was scored. Cognitive abilities were measured at 18 months by the Bayley Scales of Infant Development, at 42 months of age by the Kaufman Assessment Battery for Children (K-ABC) and at 6 years of age by the McCarthy Scales. Daily breast milk volume and milk fat content in relation to PCB body load was evaluated in 102 mothers. Multivariate regression models were applied to analyse associations of measured exposure variables with independant variables adjusted for confounders. *Results.* At *18 months of age* cognitive development was not affected by either pre- or postnatal exposure to the measured PCBs and dioxins. However, neurological examination showed an adverse effect of prenatal exposure to the measured pollutants on neurological optimality score. At *42 months of age* we found negative associations between prenatal PCB exposure on cognitive development. However no effect was demonstrated on postnatal exposure to the measured pollutants. Neurological development was not affected by either pre- or postnatal exposure to PCBs and dioxins. At *6 years of age* the preliminary results revealed evidence that cognitive development is affected by prenatal exposure to these pollutants in children from young mothers. An adverse effect of prenatal exposure on neurological outcome was also demonstrated in the formula fed group but not in the breast fed group. Despite a higher PCB exposures from breast milk we found at 18 months, 42 months of age, and at 6 years of age a beneficial effect of breast feeding on the quality of movements, in terms of fluency, and on the cognitive development tests. Maternal PCB body load was inversely related to 24-h breast milk volume and milk fat content. *Conclusion.* These data give evidence that prenatal exposure to PCBs do have subtle negative effects on neurological and cognitive development of the child up to school-age. Human breast milk volume and fat content is adversely affected by the presently encountered PCB levels in W. Europe. Our studies showed evidence that breast feeding counteracts the adverse developmental effects of PCBs and dioxins.

1.   INTRODUCTION

Both PCBs and dioxins are aromatic structures with different possibilities to bind a chlorine atom. There are 209 different PCB congeners and 210 different dioxin congeners The planar PCBs, because of their planar structure, resemble more closely to the dioxins. In general, 4 non planar marker congeners (PCB 118, 138, 153 and 180) are measured to characterise PCB-levels in environmental media or biological tissues. Sum of these 4 congeners makes up more than 50% of the total PCB-content. At present, these PCBs can be measured in a precise and accurate way.

PCBs are resistant to high temperatures and can conduct heat very easily. They have electrical insulating properties. Because of these favourable properties they became very attractive for the chemical industry after World War II. Consequently, PCBs were produced commercially in mixtures for use in carbonless copy paper, as plasticizer, fire retardants, heat transfer fluids, hydraulic fluids and as dielectric fluids in capacitors and transformers. Over 800 million tons of PCBs have been produced until the late 1970s, when the production was banned in most Western countries. However, worldwide, and in particular in some Eastern European countries, large scale production continued up to mid 80s.

Dioxins are unwanted by products of thermal and chemical processes (e.g. waste incineration). Both, PCBs and dioxins, are lipophilic, chemically stable, and highly resistant to biological detoxification. The half life of these compounds very between 4 and 15 years. Food is the major source (>90%) of human exposure. Other routes e.g. water and soil contribute to less than 10% of total exposure. In The Netherlands, dairy products are the major dietary source of these compounds (Huisman *et al* 1995a). Prolonged intake of small amounts of PCBs and dioxins from early life, in combination with the low metabolic degradation and rate of excretion, will eventually lead to high levels at reproductive age. This applies in particular to species at the top of the food chain, like fish, birds, wildlife, and human beings. Short term dietary regiments with a low intake of PCBs and dioxins did not reduce the levels in breast milk (Pluim *et al* 1994).

PCBs can be found in all fat compartments of the human body, including blood, adipose tissue, brain and human milk. PCBs cross the placenta easily from early gestation (Lanting *et al* 1998a). Maternal PCB-stores accumulate in foetal tissues that contain relatively high levels of storage lipids, in particular triglycerides. Consequently, on a fat basis, liver contains 80% and brain 20% of the PCB levels encountered in adipose tissue. Fetal adipose tissue PCB levels are similar with those in human milk (Lanting *et al* 1998a). This indicates that the vulnerable foetus is exposed to maternal levels of these environmental pollutants.

Postnatally PCBs and dioxins are also transferred in large quantities from the breast-feeding mother to her rapid developing child. On a body weight basis, daily intake of the breast fed child is about 80 times higher than the median intake of an adult (Huisman *et al* 1995a). In contrast, most formula milks are free of these compounds, owing to the fact that the manufacturers usually replace cow's milk fat by vegetable fats or oils free of PCBs and dioxins. Consequently, levels of the PCB congeners at 42 months of age of children, who received exclusive breast feeding are between 3.5 and 4.5 times higher than those in children who received formula milk (Lanting *et al* 1998b, Patandin *et al* 1997). At 42 months of age, PCB concentrations are lower in formula fed children than those in cord blood (median 0.20 vs. O.34 µg/L), whereas in breast feeding children remarkably higher than those at birth (median = 0.78 vs. 0.43 µg/L). Thus, human milk contributes substantially to postnatal PCB-intake.

1.1   Neurotoxicity studies in humans

Although relatively large amounts of PCBs are ingested with breast milk, most of available evidence suggests an adverse effect of prenatal exposure in producing long term postnatal neurotoxicity.

In the United States higher levels of intrauterine exposure to PCBs, as determined by PCB levels in maternal and cord plasma, have been found to result in deficits in fetal and postnatal growth (Fein *et al* 1984, Jacobson *et al* 1990, Gladen *et al* 1996), a lower score on psychomotor developmental tests up to the age of 2 years (Jacobson *et al* 1990, Rogan *et al* 1991), and a lower intelligence quotient at 11 years of age (Jacobson *et al* 1996). In Taiwan, cognitive deficit was affected in children who had been prenatally exposed to elevated PCB and dibenzofuranes concentrations through contaminated rice oil consumed by their mothers during pregnancy. These effects persisted until at least 7 years of age. (Chen *et al* 1992).

In Europe an ongoing study (the Dutch PCB/dioxin study), revealed 2 weeks after birth an adverse effect of a combination of prenatal and early postnatal exposure of PCBs, polychlorinated- *p*-dioxins (PCDDs) and polychlorinated dibenzofurans (PCDFs) on neurological condition, evaluated by the Prechtl neurological examination (Huisman *et al* 1995b). Higher levels of PCBs in breast milk were associated with a higher incidence of hypotonia. In a subgroup, visual recognition memory at 3 and 7 months of age was not affected by the measured perinatal exposures to PCBs and dioxins (Koopman-Esseboom 1995). In the same subgroup of children at 3 and at 7 months of age, there was no effect of perinatal exposure to PCBs and dioxins on the mental scale of the Bayley.

In this chapter, we will review the results of the "**Dutch PCB/ dioxin study**" during the follow up till 6 years of age. The following aspects will be discussed in more details:
- PCB-levels in maternal blood, cord blood and breast milk, and dioxin levels in breast milk.
- The effect of perinatal exposure to PCBs and dioxins on the cognitive and neurological development at 18 and 42 months of age, and briefly the preliminary results at 6 years of age.
- The effect of maternal PCB body load on lactation performances.

2.STUDY DESIGN "DUTCH PCB DIOXIN STUDY"

Detailed description of the sampling and analytical methods as well as the results of this follow up study have been published in numerous papers.

During the 10-years course of this project all clinical studies have been reviewed by Koopman_Esseboom (1995) and Huisman (1996) and more recently by Patandin (1999a) and Lanting (1999).

Some years ago these Dutch cohorts were combined with two newly recruited cohorts from Duesseldorf and the Faroe Islands to form a more comprehensive set of data. The aim of this multidisciplinary follow-up study was to look into a broad spectrum of PCB and dioxin related effects in order to determine if current W-European background concentrations are relevant to develop neurotoxicity early in life.

Apart from the effect of early exposure of PCBs and dioxins on long term development, the effect of these pollutants on lactation performances was evaluated. Given the experimental evidence that several PCBs and their metabolites exert estrogenic effects and estrogens adversely influence maternal milk output and fat metabolism we investigated the relationship between maternal PCB body burden on the one hand, and the 24-h breast milk output, and triglyceride (TG) content of mature breast milk on the other.

2.1   Sample recruitment

From June 1990 until June 1992, healthy pregnant women living in the Rotterdam and Groningen area were asked to participate.

In each area the planned sample size was 100 breast-feeding and 100 formula-feeding mother and infant pairs. Eligible women were approached by their midwives or obstetricians. Inclusion criteria were: (1) pregnancy and delivery without complications or serious illnesses; (2) first or second born infants; (3) born at term (37-42 weeks); and (4) white race. In the BF group, we only included mothers who were able to sustain full breast-feeding for at least 6 weeks. In the FF group, formula milk from a single batch was provided (Almiron M2; Nutricia N.V.; The Netherlands). In the latter group, children were exclusively fed on formula-milk during the first 6 months after birth. A wide range of perinatal factors, including maternal age, body weight and height, parity, formal education, dietary intake and smoking habits were recorded. In addition, the maternal pre-pregnancy body weight and height were measured and used to calculate the body mass index (BMI; weight [kg]/height^2 [m]). Data on the number of weeks of full and partial breast-feeding were also collected.

2.2   Exposure Variables

Prenatal exposure to PCBs was reflected by the PCB levels in maternal and cord blood. Maternal blood samples were obtained in the last month of pregnancy. The 4 non planar PCB congeners (Nos. 118, 138, 153 and 180) were determined by gas-liquid chromatography/electron capture detection with the use of two capillary columns of different polarity (Berg *et al* 1995). In W. Europe these congeners are relatively high and they can be measured accurately. The sum of these four congener concentrations was calculated for cord (ΣPCB_{cord}) and maternal plasma (ΣPCB_{mat}). ΣPCB_{cord} and ΣPCB_{mat} were used as a measure of prenatal exposure.

Postnatal exposure to PCBs and dioxins was estimated in breast milk samples and in the formula batch. Breast milk was collected as a 24-hour sample at 2 and 6 weeks after delivery. In all milk samples 17 ubiquitous 2,3,7,8-substituted dioxin congeners were determined by gas chromatography high ressolution mass spectrometry (GC-HRMS). The 26 PCB congeners were analysed by gas chromatography with electron capture detection (GC-ECD; Tuinstra *et al* 1993). Postnatal exposure was calculated in breast-fed infants as ΣPCB_{milk} times duration of lactation. To express the toxic potency of the mixture of dioxins and dioxin-like PCBs in breast-milk, the toxic equivalent factor (TEF; Safe 1994) was used to calculate the toxic equivalents (TEQ). In addition as a reflection of the body exposure to PCBs up to the age of 42 months, sum of the four plasma PCBs were measured at 42 months of age.

2.3   Outcome variables

2.3.1   Neurological Examination and Psychodevelopmental tests

At 18 months, neurological condition was assessed using the age-specific neurological exam according to Hempel (1993). This technique focuses on the observation of motor functions (grasping, sitting, crawling, standing, and walking) in a free field situation On the basis of this examination each toddler was classified as normal, mildly abnormal, or abnormal. The classification 'abnormal' implies the presence of an overt circumscript neurological syndrome, which usually leads to handicap in daily life, such as cerebral palsy. "Mildly abnormal" signifies the presence of mild signs which do not necessarily lead to a handicapping condition, e.g. slight asymmetries, or mild hypo-, and hypertonia. The neurological findings were also evaluated by means of a list of 57 precept criteria for optimality. For each child, a neurological optimality score (NOS) was established by counting the number of items considered optimal. The quality of movements in terms of fluency was evaluated separately as a fluency cluster score. Fluency of movements has been shown to be an indicator for the integrity of brain function (Prechtl *et al* 1997).

Mental (MDI) and psychomotor development (PDI) was evaluated by the Dutch standardized version of the Bayley Scales of Infant Development. All tests were performed at the infants' homes.

At 42 months of age, the age specific neurological examination was carried out by the same technique as described for the 18 months exam. In addition to the clinical diagnosis ("normal", "mildly abnormal" and "abnormal").a neurological optimality score (NOS) was established by counting the number of items considered optimal. The quality of movements in terms of fluency was evaluated separately as a fluency cluster score.

Cognitive ability was assessed by the validated Dutch version of the Kaufman Assessment Battery for Children (K-ABC; Neutel *et al 1996*). The K-ABC is constructed to assess two types of mental function: sequential and simultaneous processing. Both scores can be combined to calculate the overall cognitive score.

At 6 years of age, neurological condition was assessed by means of a standardized age-specific neurological examination *(Touwen 1979)* On the basis of this examination, each child was classified as normal, as having "minor neurological dysfunction" (MND), or as definitely abnormal. A child was diagnosed abnormal in case of a neurological disorder which resulted in a handicapping condition (e.g. cerebral palsy) A child was classified MND if it showed minor neurological signs, such as choreiform dyskinesia, mild diffuse hypotonia, or mild problems in coordination of fine manipulative ability, which did not result in a overtly handicapping condition. The neurological findings were also evaluated in terms of optimality. Separately a fluency cluster score regarding the quality of movements was developed.

The Dutch version of the "McCarthy Scales of Development (MCSD;)" was used for the cognitive and motor assessment. The MCSD is a well standardised psychometric tool yielding a "General Cognitive Index (GCI)", comparable to an IQ-measure, as well as a memory and a motor score.

2.3.2   24-hour breast milk sampling. Determination of breast milk volume and total fat content

To evaluate the effect of PCBs on lactation performances, mothers were instructed to pump their breasts before each feed. Milk was collected during a total period of 24 h. Milk volume was measured and documented immediately after each collection. From this a 10% aliquot was taken . All 10% aliquots were pooled immediately after completion of the 24-h collection and stored at -20 C until analysis. Total milk fat was calculated from the total fatty acid content of milk fat. Fatty acid concentrations were determined by capillary gas chromatography with split injection and flame ionisation detection as described in previous papers (Lanting 1999)

2.4   Statistical analysis

Multivariat analysis were applied to determine the association between the measured exposure variables with the outcome variables adjusted for confouding factors

3.   RESULTS

3.1   Characteristics of the study population

No differences were found between the study centres, Groningen and Rotterdam, for maternal age, weight, percentage of smoking during pregnancy for both women and their partners, gender, 1-minute APGAR scores and obstetrical optimality scores.

From the overall cohort of 418 children, 209 were breast-fed and 209 were formula-fed during infancy. A total of 207 subjects were living in Rotterdam, and 211 in Groningen. In Groningen, the educational level achieved by both the mothers and their partners was higher than in Rotterdam, as was the maternal alcohol consumption during pregnancy. Duration of gestation, based on reported last menstrual period, was also significantly different, but the difference was considered to be too small to have any biological significance. Mean birth weight was slightly higher in Groningen (3.56 ± 0.44 vs. 3.47 ± 0.44 kg). Baseline characteristics of the study group as a whole and that of the breast and formula feeding group at birth are given in *Tables 1 and 2.*

Table 1. Baseline characteristics of the whole study group

Variables	Outcome (n=418)
Education*	
Lower secondary school/higher secondary school/university	20% / 37% / 43%
Parity of child	
First born/second or third born	48% / 52%
Smoking during pregnancy; yes/no	26% / 74%
Alcohol consumption during pregnancy*	
No/sporadic/regular (at least 1/wk)	72% / 25% / 3%
Sex of child: male/female	54% / 46%
Neonatal jaundice: no/mild/severe	43% / 57% / 0%
Maternal age (years): mean (SD)	29 (4)
Maternal weight (kg): mean (SD)	65 (10)
Maternal height (cm) *: mean (SD)	170 (6)
Quetelet index: mean (SD)	22 (3)
Birth weight (kg) *: mean (SD)	3.52 (0.44)
Gestational age (weeks) *; mean (SD)	40.3 (1.2)
Apgar 1 min: median (range)	9 (3-10)
Obstetrical Optimality Score: median (range)	64 (50-70)

*Significant difference between Groningen and Rotterdam (p<0.05)

Table 2. Characteristics of the breast- and formula-fed group at birth.

At birth	Breast-fed n=209	Formula-fed n=209
Maternal age (years) ± SD	30 ± 4*	28 ± 4
Education		
Mother, higher education (%)	132 (63%)*	50 (24%)
Father, higher education (%)	130 (62%)*	64 (31%)
Maternal smoking during pregnancy, yes (%)	34 (16%)*	74 (35%)
Maternal alcohol use during pregnancy, yes (%)	78 (37%)*	18 (18%)
Sex: male (%)	115 (55%)	107 (51%)
Birth order, first born (%)	107 (51%)	94 (45%)
Gestational age (weeks) ± SD	40.3 ± 1.2	40.3 ± 1.2
Birth weight (g) ± SD	3544 ± 460	3487 ± 428

* P-value <0.01: significantly different from the formula-fed group

3.2   PCB LEVELS IN MATERNAL BLOOD, CORD BLOOD, AND BREAST MILK; DIOXIN LEVELS IN BREAST MILK. PCB LEVELS IN 42 MONTH-OLDS

Maternal and cord plasma concentrations of the measured PCB congeners and the ΣPCB are presented in *Table 3*. Formula-feeding mothers consumed less dairy products and beef, which are relatively rich in PCBs, compared with their breast-feeding counterparts (Huisman 1995a). The postnatal exposure levels measured in 24-hour breast milk samples (n=195) and formula milk are given in *Table 4*. In the formula milk samples, the levels of the measured PCB congeners were found to be below the limit of detection. ΣPCB concentrations in the BF children at 42 months of age (ΣPCB$_{42months}$) was 4 times higher than that in the FF group (median 0.78 vs 0.2 μg/L).

Table 3. Prenatal exposure variables: maternal and cord plasma levels of PCB 118, 138, 153, and 180 (IUPAC)

Exposure levels (μg/L) (p5,p5o,p90)	Breast-fed N=209	Formula fed N=209
ΣPCB-maternal	1.1,2.2,4.0	0.95,1.9,3.6
ΣPCB-cord	0.20,0.43,0.99	0.16,0.34,0.80

Table 4. Postnatal exposure levels, median (range), from breast milk and formula milk

Postnatal exposure levels	Breast milk		Formula milk
ΣPCBmilk (μg/kg fat) δ	n=193;	405 (158-1226)	ND
Σdioxin-TEQ (ng/kg)@	n=177;	29(11-76)	ND
ΣPCB-TEQ (ng/kg) +	n=186;	33(13-103)	ND
Total TEQ (ng/kg)*	n=168;	63(25-155)	ND

δ ΣPCBmilk, sum of Polychlorinated biphenyl (PCB) congeners IUPAC Nos 118, 138, 153 and 180 in breast milk
@ Σdioxin-TEQ, sum of toxic equivalents (TEQs) of 17 dioxins in breast milk.
+ ΣPCB-TEQ, sum of TEQs of 8 dioxin-like PCBs in breast milk.
* Total TEQ, sum of dioxin-TEQ and PCB-TEQ measured in breast milk.
ND: not detectable.

3.3   EFFECTS OF PERINATAL EXPOSURE TO PCBs AND DIOXINS ON NEUROLOGICAL AND COGNITIVE DEVELOPMENT AT THE AGE OF 18 and 42 MONTHS AND AT 6 YEARS OF AGE

At *18 months of age.* The age specific neurological examination and cognitive abilities were tested in 418 and 207 children, respectively. Prenatal exposure had a negative effect on neurological condition (Huisman *et al* 1995c). However, cognitive development appeared to be unaffected; thus, neither mental nor psychomotor score was related to prenatal or postnatal exposure to PCBs and dioxins (Koopman-Esseboom *et al* 1996). Postnatal PCB exposure through breast milk did not show any adverse effects on neurological examination and on the cognitive development. On the contrary a beneficial effect of breast feeding on the fluency of movements was found (Huisman *et al* 1995c).

At *42 months of age.* Neurological condition and cognitive abilities were evaluated   in   394   and   395   children,   respectively.   The   neurological examination revealed that neither prenatal exposure to PCBs nor postnatal exposure to PCBs and dioxins was associated with the neurological optimality score (Lanting *et al* .1998c) Despite a high lactational exposure to PCBs and dioxins, a beneficial effect of breast-feeding was found on the quality of movements in terms of fluency (Lanting *et al* 1998d).

Cognitive ability showed after adjustment for confounding factors that prenatal PCB exposure was negatively associated with the overall cognitive score as well as with both individual subscales of the Dutch K-ABC. The effect of prenatal PCB exposure was greatest in the FF group: the high exposure group had a 6-8 point reduction in score compared with the low exposure group. In contrast, hardly any effect could be detected in the breast-fed group. Moreover, children who were breast-fed performed better than formula fed children (Patandin *et al* 1999b).

At *6 years of age.* Cognitive development was assessed in 376 children (90 %) of the original cohort of 418 children. The preliminary results showed, after adjustment for confounders, a negative association between prenatal PCB exposure and general cognitive development at 6 years of age among children of young mothers only. Postnatal exposure to PCBs and dioxins was not related to cognitive development. Moreover, by univariate analysis, BF children scored significantly higher on the general cognitive index   as   well   as   on   the   memory   score   as   compared   to   FF children.(Vreugendenhil *et al* 1999).

Neurological development was evaluated in 374 children (90%) of the original cohort of 418 children. The preliminary results revealed in the formula fed group a significant adverse effect of prenatal PCB exposure on the NOS. In contrast, hardly any effect could be detected in the breast-fed group. No relationship was found between the measured postnatal exposure levels and the NOS. Similar as documented at 18 and at 42 months of age, a significant beneficial effect of breast-feeding on the fluency of movements was shown at school age

3.4   Effect of maternal PCBs on human milk output and fat content

Data on 24 h milk volumes were available for 102 women. Milk volume was inversely related to the PCB body burden (p=0.001) and it increased with height of the mother (p=0.016). Maternal smoking had a borderline negative effect (p=0.052). Milk TG level was also inversely related to maternal PCB level (p=0.015) (Lanting 1999).

4.COMMENT AND CONCLUSION

Levels of PCBs and dioxins presently encountered in The Netherlands are among the highest in the Western world. However, levels approximately twice as high are encountered in some territories belonging to the sphere of influence of the former USSR and in areas with a high consumption of fish (e.g Faroe Islands). In the present study we followed a cohort of 400 children, considered to be of low risk for brain dysfunction, from birth up to the age of 6 years.

Cognitive development at 18 months of age was neither related to prenatal exposure to PCBs nor to postnatal exposure to PCBs and dioxins. However,at the age of 3½ years and at 6 years of age, among children of young mothers, an adverse effect of prenatal PCB exposure on cognitive development , was found.

Neurological examination at 18 months and at 6 years of age, but not at 3½ years of age, revealed a negative effect of prenatal PCB exposure on neurological performance. Previous results of the same cohort examined 2 weeks after birth demonstrated an adverse effect of a combination of prenatal and early postnatal exposure to the measured PCBs and dioxins on neurological performance evaluated by the Prechtl neurologic examination. Higher levels of the planar PCBs in breast milk were associated with a greater incidence of hypotonia. (Huisman *et al* 1995b)

Our results do agree with reported cognitive deficits in the Yu cheng study and the 2 US studies, one in N.Carolina and the other around Lake Michican . In the latter cohort adverse effects of prenatal PCB exposure were found on short term memory on both verbal and numeric tests at 4 years and on the verbal IQ scores at 11 years of age.

Unfortunately, exposure data are difficult to compare and probably not justified because the analytic methods are different between the Yu-Cheng,, the US and the Dutch studies. In the Michican study, exposure was defined from total PCB levels measured in cord and maternal blood as well as in breast milk by summing 10 Webb-McCall peaks, using packed column gas chromatography. In North Carolina two Webb-Mc Call peaks were quantified. With these analytic methods the correlations between maternal blood and the corresponding milk values were for the Michican study 0.16-0.42, and for North Carolina 0.56-077. Because of the limitations in the Webb-McCall method PCBs were not detectable in 70% of the cord blood samples and in 22 % of maternal blood samples obtained in Michican (PCB detection limit 3.0 ng/L). For North Carolina 88% of the cord blood samples and 13-26% of the maternal blood and milk samples were below the detection limit. Although the Webb-McCall method was state of the art when these US studies were initiated (circa 1980), gas-chromatography with electron capture detection (GC-ECD), as used in our study to quantify the 4 PCB congeners, did improve the precision and detection limit remarkably. By this method maternal blood concentrations were closely associated with the corresponding milk sample (0.70-0.79) as were the maternal plasma levels with those in cord blood (0.52 - 0.74). Only 2.5% of the samples PCB 118 fell below the detection limit of 0.01 ng/L and in none of the other three PCB congeners. Whereas in the Dutch studies the 17 most abundant PCDD and PCDF congeners and three planar PCB congeners (77, 126 and 169) were accurately quantified in breast milk by gas chromatography–high-resolution mass spectrometry (GC-HRMS), in the US no exposure levels for the dioxins were measured.

The mechanisms behind the widely documented risks for fetal development of *prenatal* exposure to a mixture of PCB's remain unclear. Various alternatives have been proposed from evidence collected in animal studies. For example, a high binding affinity for the Aryl-hydrocarbon (Ah) receptor and subsequent consequences for brain metabolism have been described. In vitro the Ah receptor has shown to be a mediator in the production of toxic compounds after exposure to TCDD and structurally identical non-ortho planar PCBs. Second, an effect on the neuro-transmittor systems in the brain (e.g., dopamine, serotonin, and the noradrenergic systems) may play a role. Unfortunately, conversion of these findings to the human species is hampered by toxico-kinetic differences and in differences of the body distribution of these compounds between the human and most experimental animals. Moreover, from the early stages of gestation and for many years after birth, large morphological changes take place in the central nervous system involving outgrowth and retractions of dendrites and axons, myelination, and synapse reorganization. The effects of these maturational changes are reflected in the functional development of the child. Thus, results found at different ages can not be compared, as they are generated by quite different brains.

More recently, the endocrine-disrupting capacity of these compounds and their metabolites during the most vulnerable transient period of rapid cell multiplication during   fetal organ development has received special attention. The timing and duration of these periods of rapid fetal cell multiplication differ between organs, which process is most likely controlled by   a complex balance of various hormones. Maternal PCBs are easily transferred across the placenta, and they seem to equilibrate among the apolar parts of fetal and maternal lipids from the early stages of gestation (Lanting 1998a). This may imply that all fetal organs are equally at risk of the endocrine-disrupting capacity of some of the PCBs and, in particular of their more polar hydroxylated metabolites. These hydroxylated PCBs appeared to be potent modulators of both thyroidogenic and the estrogenic endocrine systems. As a result, these compounds may permanently alter the fetal programming of susceptible organs, which may have long-term consequences on hormone-related pathology in later life.

Lactational exposure to PCBs and dioxins, in contrast to foetal exposure, had no effect on neurological and cognitive development of term infants at age 18, 42 and 72 months, despite 4 times higher PCB exposure levels at 42 months in BF children as compared with FF counterparts. In contrast , a beneficial effect of breast-feeding on the fluency of movement at 18, 42 as well at 72 months of age was found after adjustments for social, obstetric, perinatal, and neonatal neurologic differences. This effect on the quality of movements can be regarded as a reflection of the differentiation of cortex and basal ganglia. In fetuses and preterm infants, fluency of movement has been found to reflect brain integrity and to be a marker of behavioral and cognitive ability at a later age (Prechtl et al 1997). In the same population a favorable effect of breast feeding on cognitive development at 18 months, 42 months and at school age was found. These findings points to a favorable effect of breast feeding on brain development and moreover, that breast feeding counteracts the adverse developmental effects of PCBs on neurological and cognitive development of the brain.

Various mechanisms might be responsible for the beneficial effect of breast feeding on early development of the term child. Firstly, the psychosocial aspects of nursing may play a role. Secondly, the specific composition of human milk, e.g. the transfer of hormones and biologically active peptides from the mother to her infant via breast milk, may affect brain development. Moreover, the fat composition of human milk differs considerably from that of most formula milks for term infants. Human milk contains, in contrast to most formula for term infants, various long-chain polyunsaturated fatty acids, which are considered to be essential nutrients for brain development during fetal life and early infancy.

The inverse relationship between background levels of PCB exposure on 24 hours output and fat content of mature human milk may also point to an oestrogenic activity of the PCB mixture to which the Dutch women are exposed. Oestrogens and and oestrogen containing contraceptives are well known to suppress lactation.(WHO 1988). The effect of PCBs on milk fat content might be explained by a decreased activity of enzyme lipoprotein lipase, which may reduce the supply of plasma lipid building blocks for subsequent milk fat synthesis In animals a low dose of dioxins have shown to exert an adverse effect on LPL activity Given the importance of this finding for public health, further studies are needed to confirm or refute the outcome of these studies, If confirmed, we need to elucidate the mechanisms responsible for such effects.

In summary, Prenatal exposure to the measured PCB's at current background levels, are associated with adverse effects on cognitive and neurological development up to 6 years of age. This adverse developmental effect was counteracted by the beneficial effect of breast-feeding for at least six weeks after birth. Our data showed evidence that presently encountered maternal PCB levels are negatively related to breast milk volume and fat content.

ACKNOWLEDGMENTS

This study is part of an international research project entitled: `Early PCB exposure and neurodevelopmental deficit: Application and validation of indicators for the early detection of deficit', which is funded by the European Community (contract no. EV5V-CT92-0207).

REFERENCES

Berg M van den, Sinnige TL, Tysklind M, Bosveld B, Huisman M, Koopman-Esseboom C, Koppe JG, 1995, Individual PCBs as predictors for concentrations of non and mono-ortho PCBs in human milk. Environmental Sciences and Pollution Research 2(2):78-82.

Boersma ER, Janoušek V, Krijt J. et al, 1994, The Czech/Dutch/German/Polish Research team. Cord blood levels of potentially neurotoxic pollutants (polychlorinated biphenyl's, lead and cadmium) in the areas of Prague (Czech Republic) and Katowice (Poland). Comparison with reference values in the Netherlands. Centr Eur Jf Public Health 2:73-6.

Chen YC, Guo YL, Hsu CC, Rogan WJ, 1992, Cognitive development of Yu-Cheng ("oil disease") children prenatally exposed to heat-degraded PCBs. Jama 268(22):3213-8.

Fein GG, Jacobson JL, Jaconson SW, Schwartz PM, Dowler JK, 1984, Prenatal exposure to polychlorinated biphenyls: Effects on birth size and gestational age. J Pediatr 105(2):315-20

Gladen BC, Rogan WJ, Ragan NB, 1996, Preliminary results on prenatal and lactational exposure to PCBs and DDE and pubertal growth and development. Organohalogen compounds 30:215-17.

Hempel MS, 1993,The neurological examination for toddler-age [Dissertation]. Groningen: University of Groningen.

Huisman M, Eerenstein SEJ, Koopman-Esseboom C, Brouwer M, Fidler V, Muskiet FAJ, Sauer PJJ, Boersma ER, 1995, Perinatal exposure to polychlorinated biphenyls and dioxins through dietary intake. Chemosphere 31(10):4273-87.

Huisman M, Koopman-Esseboom C, Fidler V, Hadders-Algra M, Paauw CG van der, Tuinstra LGMTh, Weisglas-Kuperus N, Sauer PJJ, Touwen BCL, Boersma ER, 1995, Perinatal exposure to polychlorinated biphenyls and dioxins and its effect on neonatal neurological development. Early Hum Dev 41:111-27.

Huisman M, Koopman-Esseboom C, Lanting CI, Paauw CG van der, Tuinstra LGMTh, Fidler V, Weisglas-Kuperus N, Sauer PJJ, Boersma ER, Touwen BCL, 1995, Neurological condition in 18-month-old children perinatally exposed to polychlorinated biphenyls and dioxins. Early Hum Dev 43:165-76.

Huisman M, 1996, Effects of early infant nutition and perinatal exposure to PCBs and dioxins on neurological development. A study of breast-fed and formula-fed infants [Dissertation]. Groningen. University of Groningen. ISBN 90-3670688-2.

Jacobson JL, Jacobson SW, Humphrey HEB, 1990, Effects of in utero exposure to polychlorinated biphenyls and related contaminants on cognitive functioning in young children. J Pediatr 116:38-45.

Jacobson JL, Jacobson SW, 1996, Intellectual impairment in children exposed to polychlorinated biphenyls in utero. N Engl J Med 335:783-9.

Jensen AA, 1987, Polychlorobiphenyls (PCBs), polychlorodibenzo-p-dioxins (PCDDs), and polychlorodibenzofurans (PCDFs) in human milk, blood and adipose tissue. Sci Total Environ 64:259-293.

Koopman-Esseboom C, 1995, Effects of perinatal exposure to PCBs and dioxins on early human development [Dissertation].Rotterdam. University of Rotterdam. ISBN 90-75340-03-6.

Koopman-Esseboom C, Weisglas-Kuperus N, de Ridder MA, Paauw van der CG, Tuinstra LG, Sauer PJ, 1996, Effects of polychlorinated biphenyl's/dioxins exposure and feeding type on infants ' mental and psychomotor development. Pediatrics 97:700-6

Lanting CI, Huisman, Muskiet FAJ, Paauw van der CG, Essed CE, Boersma ER, 1998, Polychlorinated biphenyls in adipose tissue, liver and brain from nine stillborns of varying gestational ages. Pediatr Res 44:1-4.

Lanting CI, Fidler V, Huisman H, Boersma ER, 1998, Determinants of polychlorinated biphenyl levels in plasma from 42 month-old children. Arch Environ ContamToxicol 35(1): 135-39.

Lanting CI, Patandin S, Fidler V, Weisglas-Kuperus N, Sauer PJJ, Boersma ER, Touwen BCL, 1998, Neurological condition in 42-month-old children in relation to pre- and postnatal exposure to polychlorinated biphenyl's and dioxins. Early Hum Dev 50:283-92.

Lanting CI, Patandin S, Weisglas-Kuperus N, Touwen BCL, Boersma ER, 1998, Breastfeeding and neurological outcome at 42 months. Acta Pediatrica 87:1224-9.

Lanting CI,1999, Effects of perinatal PCB and dioxin exposure and early feeding on child development [Dissertation]. Groningen. University of Groningen. ISBN 90-3671002-2

Neutel RJ, Meulen van der BF, Lutje Spelberg HC, 1996, Groningse Ontwikkelingsschalen. (Dutch version of the Kaufman Assessment Battery for Children [K-ABC]). 1st ed. Lisse: Swets & Zeitlinger BV.

Patandin S, Weisglas-Kuperus N, de Ridder MAJ, Koopman-Esseboom C, Staveren van WA, Paauw van der CG, Sauer PJJ, 1997, Plasma polychlorinated biphenyl levels in Dutch preschool children either breast-fed or formula-fed during infancy. Am J Public Health 87:1711-14.

Patandin S, 1999, Effects of environmental exposure to Polychlorinatedbiphenyls and dioxins on growth and development in young children. [Dissertation].Rotterdam. University of Rotterdam. ISBN 90-9012306-7.

Patandin S, Lanting CI, Mulder PG, Boersma ER, Sauer PJ, Weisglas-Kuperus N, 1999, Effects of environmental exposure to PCBs and dioxins on cognitive abilities in Dutch children at 42 months of age. J Pediatr 134:33-41.

Pluim HJ, Boersma ER, Kramer I, Olie K, van der Slikke JW, Koppe JG, 1995, Influence of short-term dietary measurements on dioxin concentrations in human milk. Environ Health Perspect 102:968-71.

Prechtl HFR, Einspieler C, Cioni G, Bos,AF, Ferrari F, Sontheimer D, 1997, An early marker for neurological defecits after perinatal brain lesions. Lancet 349(9062):1362-3.

Rogan WJ, Gladen BC, 1991, PCBs, DDE, and child development at 18 and 24 months. Ann Epidemiol 1(5):407-13.

Safe SH, 1994, Polychlorinated biphenyls (PCBs): environmental impact , biochemical and toxic responses, and implications for risk assessment. Crit Rev Toxicol 24:87-149.

Touwen BCL, 1979, The neurological examination of the child with minor neurological dysfunction. In: Clinics in Developmental Medicine. No 71, SIMP. Heineman Medical Books: London.

Tuinstra LGMTh, van Rhyn JA, Traag WA, van de Spreng P, Zuidema T, Horstman HJ, 1993, Method for the determination of dioxins, planar and other PCBs in human milk. Organohalogen Compounds 11:181-3.

Vreugdenhil H, Lanting C, Boersma R., Weisglas-Kuperus N, 1999, Dutch PCBs and Dioxin Study. Prenatal and postnatal PCB and dioxin exposure and the McCarthy Scales of children abilities. Poster presented at DIOXIN '99.

World Health Organization, 1988, Task Force on Oral Contraceptives, Special Programme of Research, Development, and Research Training in human Reproduction. Effects of hormonal contraceptives on breast milk composition and infant growth. Studies in Family Planning 16(6):361-9.

26

TRANSITION OF NITRO MUSKS AND POLYCYCLIC MUSKS INTO HUMAN MILK

B. Liebl[1], R. Mayer[1], S. Ommer[2], C. Sönnichsen[2], B. Koletzko[2]
[1] *Landesuntersuchungsamt für das Gesundheitswesen Südbayern, D-85762 Oberschleißheim;*
[2] *Dept. of Pediatrics, University of Munich, Lindwurmstr. 4, D-80337 Munich, Germany*

Key words: nitro musks, polycyclic musks, human milk

Abstract: Synthetic musks are widely used in various consumer products. The identification of nitro musks in human milk in the early 1990s in connection with evidence for cancerogenicity in animal experiments have caused public concern. However, the validity of previously reported quantitative data has been questioned. Polycylic musks have hardly been investigated so far. The present study aimed at providing accurate current data on the occurrence of nitro and polycyclic musks in human milk. Samples from 40 healthy breast feeding mothers were analysed under carefully controlled conditions avoiding secondary contamination. As in earlier studies, among the nitro compounds musk xylene and ketone were the most frequently detected substances. However, much lower concentrations (roughly by a factor of 10) were found (musk xylene: median 6.1 ng/kg fat). Among the polycyclic musks HHCB was found in most samples (median 64 ng/kg fat). Scientific knowledge on possible routes of exposure and health risk aspects is summarized and discussed.

1.   INTRODUCTION

Musk is one of the most important fragrances used in various consumer products such as cosmetics, soaps and laundery detergents[1,2]. Since consumption cannot be met by natural sources and chemical synthesis of the natural odorous compounds (macrocyclic ketones and alcohols)[3] is expensive, easier accessible substitutes were developed. The annual worldwide production rate of artificial musks is in the range of several thousand tons[4].

Despite their similar odour, the compounds mainly used are structurally very different from the natural musk compounds.

Nitro musks are highly substituted benzenes with at least two of the substituents being nitro groups. Musk xylene, the first synthetic musk still in use, is known already since 1888[5]. It was followed by several similar nitroaromatic compounds (*Figure*1). Nitro musks are highly lipophilic substances. The octanol-water partition coefficients are of similar order of magnitude as those of some well-known environmental pollutants, e.g. lower chlorinated PCB (poychlorinated biphenyls)[6]. The identification of nitro musks in environmental samples indicated that they might be just as persistent and caused first doubts concerning the safety of these chemicals. Domestic wastewaters are assumed to be the major route of environmental pollution. Musk xylene and musk ketone were detected in the aquatic environment at first in Japan in 1981[7]. In the early 1990s, these compounds were also found in German surface water, fish and other aquatic organisms[8,9,10] and for the first time in human fat and milk[11,12]. These findings in connection with evidence for cancerogenic effects of musk xylene in animal experiments[13] led to public concern and to a controversial discussion in view of regulatory consequences. The production and use of musk xylene in Germany has decreased in recent years after the toiletries and detergent industries voluntarily stopped including it in their products[14].

Polycyclic musks, i.e. highly substituted indane and tetraline derivatives (*Figure*1), represent another group of industrially important synthetic musk odorants, which were introduced in the 1950s[15]. It has been presumed that the critical discussion about nitro musks is promoting their replacement by polycyclic musks[16]. The share in the annual world production of polycyclic musks is increasing rapidly[4,17]. However, little is known about the environmental and toxicological properties of these compounds so far. HHCB and AHTN, the most frequently used representatives, have even higher octanol-water distribution coefficients than musk xylene indicating an even higher potency for bioconcentration[18]. Recently polycylic musks have also been found in surface water and fish[19,2,20], as well as in human adipose tissue and milk[21,22].

Human milk is widely used to identify and monitor body burden of lipophilic, persistent environmental pollutants in man. However, validated procedures are required to obtain reliable results[23]. In particular, the methods used for fat extraction have been a matter of discussion[24]. Sample contamination is another critical point, especially in the case of synthetic musk compounds[25].

nitro musks

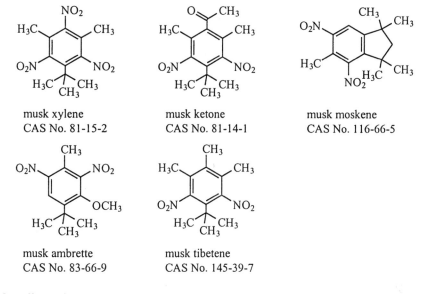

musk xylene
CAS No. 81-15-2

musk ketone
CAS No. 81-14-1

musk moskene
CAS No. 116-66-5

musk ambrette
CAS No. 83-66-9

musk tibetene
CAS No. 145-39-7

polycyclic musks

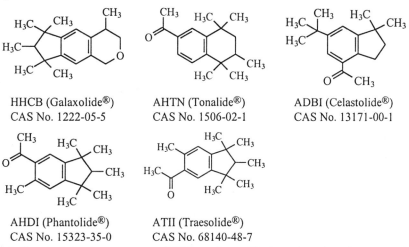

HHCB (Galaxolide®)
CAS No. 1222-05-5

AHTN (Tonalide®)
CAS No. 1506-02-1

ADBI (Celastolide®)
CAS No. 13171-00-1

AHDI (Phantolide®)
CAS No. 15323-35-0

ATII (Traesolide®)
CAS No. 68140-48-7

Figure 1. Chemical structures, names and CAS numbers of the investigated musk compounds.

The present study aimed at providing accurate current data on the occurrence of nitro musks and polycyclic musks in human milk. The state of scientific knowledge regarding possible routes of exposure and health risk aspects is summarized and discussed.

2.   EXPERIMENTAL

Sample collection and all analytical procedures were performed under controlled conditions to avoid secondary contamination. All persons involved in experimental procedures carefully avoided contact with the samples. All materials used in contact with milk were washed carefully with detergents free of musk compounds. Method blanks were proceeded with each batch of samples analysed.

2.1   Study Population, Sample Collection

Fourty healthy nursing mothers (age 24-38 years; BMI 19-34) were included into the study which had been approved by the Ethical Commitee of the Medical Faculty, University of Munich. Written informed consent was obtained before enrollment. 18 mothers had one child, 20 had two, one mother had three children and another mother had four children. Except for 4 subjects supplementing small volumes of formula, all mothers exclusively breast fed their infants. Samples were taken in 1997/1998 at the pediatric hospital. To avoid contamination from the skin the breast used was carefully cleaned with propylene glycol. Milk (ca. 50 ml per sample) was expressed using a standard electric pump (Medela, Eching, Germany) while feeding the infant from the other breast. Samples were frozen immediately and stored at -20°C until analysis.

2.2   Fat Extraction

Prior to investigation of the study population various methods for total fat extraction were compared. In all cases frozen samples were thawed, tempered to 39°C and mixed to ensure homogeneity before extraction. The method described by Bligh & Dyer (see below) was also tested with lyophilized milk (10 ml per sample using a Lyophilizator Wkf L05, Brandau, Germany) which had been reconstituted with aq. dest. (2 ml per sample). Fat contents were always determined gravimetrically using an analytical balance R-200 D from Sartorius (Göttingen, Germany).

Modified Roese-Gottlieb/Mojonnier. The AOAC protocol[26] which is regarded as the standard for comparison of methods[23] was applied according to IDF-Standard Nr.172.1995[27]. Using this procedure the extracted lipid fraction is purified by subsequent washes. In detail, 50 ml milk were mixed with 40 ml ethanol abs. and 10 ml NH_4OH. The mixture was shaken (1 min) with 50 ml diethyl ether and carefully mixed with 50 ml pentane. After removal of the aqueous fraction the lipid fraction was purified twice with 50 ml Na_2SO_4 solution (100 g/l) and then rotary evaporated to dryness.

Modified Bligh & Dyer[28]. This method is a further procedure recommended by the International Dairy Federation (IDF) for extraction of fat from milk[29,23]. Lipids are extracted in a single step using a non-polar solvent [30,31]. Briefly, 1 ml milk was mixed with 4 ml methanol:chloroform (2:1). After incubation for 15 min at 37°C, 1 ml chloroforme and aq. dest. were carefully added and the mixture was cooled in icewater (15 min). After centrifugation (2500 rpm, 20 min), the eluate (chloroforme phase) was carefully removed and evaporated to dryness in an exsiccator (>24 h, 37°C, under N_2).

Brühl [32]. Similar to the AOAC official method 605.02[33] established for extraction of fat from bovine milk for pesticides, K-oxalate is used for globule disruption by this procedure. Subsequently, the aqueous fraction is extracted once more. In detail, 50 ml milk were mixed successively with 5 ml K-oxalate solution (35 g/l), 50 ml ethanol, 50 ml *tert*-butylmethylether (TBME) and 50 ml petroleum ether. After removal of the organic fraction, the remaining aqueous fraction was extracted with 50 ml TBME and 50 ml petroleum ether. The combined organic fractions were rotary evaporated to dryness.

2.3   Cleanup

Removal of lipids and cleanup of the dried extract was performed by silica gel adsorption chromatography according to Steinwandter[34] with modifications. 0.3 g of the fat extract together with the internal standard (D3-AHTN) were dissolved in 2 ml of a mixture of petroleum ether and dichloromethane (80 + 20; v/v) and transferred to a glas column packed with 15 g silica gel (60 mesh, activated at 180°C over night) containing 10 % of water. The column was eluted with 220 ml of the solvent mixture. The eluate was rotary evaporated to dryness. The residue was dissolved in 1 ml cyclohexane and submitted to gas chromatography/mass spectrometry analysis.

2.4   Gas Chromatography/Mass Spectrometry

Analytical determination was performed using capillary gas chromatography (Carlo-Erba 8000, Milan, Italy) coupled with high resolution mass spectrometry (VG AutoSpec Ultima, Micromass, Manchester, UK). GC-separation was achieved on a 60 m DB5-MS capillary column (0.25 mm i.d., film thickness 0.25 µm; retention gap: 5 m, 0.32 mm i.d.) from J + W Scientific Products. The carrier gas was helium 5.0 from Linde (Munich, Germany) which had been purified using Oxisorb® from Messer-Griesheim (Krefeld, Germany) and an active coal filter Supelpure HC from Supleco (Bellefonte, PA, USA). The temperature program was 80°C, 1 min, 30°C/min to 180°C, 2°C/min to 220°C, 20°C/min to 280°C, 2 min. The mass

spectrometer was operated in single ion monitoring (SIM) mode at a mass
resolution of 10.000 using 2 specific mass traces per analyte and D3-AHTN
as internal standard. The fat content of the sample was used to express the
final results on a lipid adjusted basis.

2.5   Chemicals

Fat extraction. K-oxalate monohydrate was from Sigma (Deisenhofen,
Germany); chloroforme p.a., diethyl ether p.a., ethanol abs. p.a., methanol
p.a., Na_2SO_4 , petrolem ether p.a. (boiling range 40-60°C) were from Merck
(Darmstadt, Germany); NH_4OH puriss. p.a., n-pentane puriss. p.a. and *tert*-
butylmethylether puriss. (H_2O < 0.01 %) were from Fluka (Deisenhofen,
Germany); aqua ad injectabilia was from Pharmacia & Upjohn (Erlangen,
Germany).

Cleanup and analysis. Cyclohexane, dichloromethane, methanol, petroleum ether (all of purity for residue analysis) were from Promochem (Wesel,
Germany); silica gel 60 (70-230 mesh) was from Merck (Darmstadt, Germany).

Reference substances. External standard solutions were prepared in cyclohexane (50 pg/µl for each compound); musk ambrette, musk ketone,
musk xylene, ADBI, AHDI, AHTN, ATII, HHCB were from Ehrenstorfer
(Augsburg, Germany); musk moskene and musk tibetene were from Gevau-
dan-Roure (Geneve, Switzerland). D3-AHTN from Ehrenstorfer (Augsburg,
Germany) in cyclohexane (2 ng/µl) was used as internal standard.

3.   RESULTS

3.1   Fat Extraction

With untreated milk the tested methods provided similar results concerning the amounts of totally extracted fat in a number of comparatively
investigated samples (*Table 1*). However, because of technical problems the
Bligh & Dyer procedure could not be adapted to the relatively large sample
volume (ca. 50 ml milk) required for further analysis to achieve detectable
amounts of the musk compounds. This problem could not be solved by lyo-
philization of larger sample volumina (e.g. 10 ml, reconstituted with 2 ml of
water), because recovery of lipids then markedly decreased.

High yields and high inter-assay reproducibility (data not shown) were
particularly achieved using the method described by Brühl which therefore
was chosen for further analysis. Fat contents of 3.69±1.72% (mean±sd) were
determined in the 40 samples analysed for musk compounds. No loss in fat

content was observed during storage times of up to three weeks (data not shown).

Table 1. Fat contents obtained by various extraction methods.

method		Bligh & Dyer	lyophil. milk	Roese-Gottlieb	Brühl
sample volume [ml]		1	10	50	50
n		10	6	12	8
median	[% fat]	3.33	1.36	3.40	3.47
mean ± sd	[% fat]	3.38 ± 0.16	1.36 ± 0.60	3.40 ± 0.07	3.46 ± 0.02
vk		4.8 %	43.9 %	1.9 %	0.6 %

3.2   Nitro Musks

Limits of detection was 1 ng/g fat for the investigated nitro musk compounds. Procedural blanks revealed concentrations below the detection limit. *Table2* shows the concentrations measured in the study population. Relatively large interindivual differences in the degree of contamination were found. Musk xylene and musk ketone were the most frequently detected compounds. Musk moskene and ambrette were detected in only very few samples in low concentrations; musk tibetene was found in none of the samples analysed.

Table2. Detection frequency and concentrations of the investigated nitro musks.

	musk xylene	musk ketone	musk moskene	musk ambrette	musk tibetene
detection frequency	38/40	18/40	3/40	1/40	0/40
range [ng/g fat]	1.3 - 47.9	2.1 - 82.9	2.3 - 3.1	3.6	–
median [ng/g fat]	6.1	4.6	–	–	–
mean [ng/g fat]	8.6	9.6	–	–	–

3.3   Polycyclic Musks

The limits of detection were 1 ng/g fat for ADBI, AHDI and ATII. For AHTN and HHCB detection limits determined by procedural blanks (mean + 3 sd) were 15 and 20 ng/g fat, respectively. The concentrations in the investigated 40 samples of human milk are summarized in *Table 3*. In analogy to the nitro musks, the degree of contamination revealed large interindividual differences. However, the detected levels of the polycylic compounds were significantly higher than those of the analysed nitro musks. Especially HHCB was found in most samples in considerable amounts.

Table 3. Detection frequency and concentrations of the investigated *polycylic musks.*

	HHCB (galaxolide®)	AHTN (tonalide®)	ADBI (celastolide®)	AHDI (phantolide®)	ATII (traesolide®)
detection frequency	35/40	13/40	15/40	10/40	10/40
range [ng/g fat]	21 - 1316	16 - 148	1.0 - 14.1	1.0 - 19.8	1.1 - 51.3
median [ng/g fat]	64	22	1.6	3.2	1.5
mean [ng/g fat]	115	36	2.9	5.5	6.4

4.   DISCUSSION

4.1   Occurrence of Synthetic Musk in Human Milk

Carefully controlled sampling and analytical procedures are required to determine musk compounds in biological samples quantitatively[25,35,23]. Due to the widespread occurrence of musk compounds many possibilties of secondary contamination in the course of sample collection and analysis are given, e.g. from glassware, hands, nipples, soaps, solvents, aerosoles etc.. The method employed for fat extraction must be suitable to handle sufficiently large sample volumina which are required to obtain detectable absolute amounts of the analytes of interest and to reduce the influence of secondary sample contamination. On the other hand, the amount of milk available from a single nursing mother is limited. Therefore, and in order to obtain valid results on a fat adjusted basis a method ensuring complete extraction of fat is required. A number of protocols have been proposed using various mixtures of nonpolar and polar solvents to quantitatively disrupt gobule membranes and disolve the core fat[23]. Among the methods tested in the present study, the procedure published by Brühl best met the requirements mentioned above.

The present results confirm the existence of synthetic musks in human milk. In agreement with earlier studies[11,12], among the nitro musks musk xylene and musk ketone were the most frequently detected compounds. However, compared to the first reports in 1993 much lower concentrations (roughly by a factor of 10) were found (*Table4*). The former studies must be reviewed critically because investigators might not have paid enough attention to the methodological problems mentioned above, particularly to the possibility of sample contamination. In some cases the samples analysed had been collected under poorly controlled conditions, e.g. by manual expression performed by the mothers themselves, so that contamination from the skin or sampling vials certainly cannot be excluded in all cases. On the other hand, in a series of subsequent investigations in 1993 and 1994 various laboratories in Germany and Switzerland independently found similar contents of nitro musks in human milk and adipose tissue. Recently, all available data about musk xylene were summarized by Käfferlein et al.[6]. According to this comprehensive study the peak of usage and highest contents of musk xylene in human tissues obviously occurred in 1993. In the same year the German toiletries and detergent industries announced to voluntarily stop including musk xylene in their products[14], and a decrease in the level of contamination is evident since then. The considerable drop of contents documented by the present results can be explained by the comparatively short elimination half-times of nitro musks (about 100d for musk xylene in man, see 4.3.1).

In contrast to the nitro musks, higher contents of polycyclic musks, especially of HHCB and AHTN, were detected here than reported previously by Rimkus & Wolf[22] (*Table4*). It can be speculated that this supports the assumption that nitro musks are more and more being replaced by polycyclic musks in consumer products and that polycyclic musks are transferred into human tissue as well[36]. However, further investigations with larger numbers of representative samples are needed to confirm any trend in the level of contamination.

Table4. Comparison of present data (last row) with earlier studies (means given in [ng/g fat]).

year of sampling	study	n	nitro musks		polycyclic musks		
			musk xylene	musk ketone	HHCB	AHTN	ADBI
1992/1993	Rimkus & Wolf[12]	23	80	30	–	–	–
	Liebl & Ehrenstorfer[11]	391	100	40	–	–	–
1995	Rimkus & Wolf[22]	5	25	5	49	26	7
1997/1998	present data	40	8.6	9.6	115	36	3

4.2　　Route of Exposure

The relevance of various possible sources of human exposure and routes of absorption of synthetic musk compounds are still not fully clarified. In contrast to other persistent lipophilic environmental contaminants (e.g., PCB, polychlorinated dibenzodioxins and -furans PCDD/F)[37,38] which accumulate in food chains and the human body, with musk xylene no correlation was found between body burden in the general population (i.e. levels in blood plasma) and age, body mass index or nutritional habits (i.e. fish consumption)[39]. Oral uptake by consumption of fatty food (fish, meat, eggs, milk), which represents the main source (>90%) of human exposure to organochlorine compounds[40,41] does not seem to be decisive in the case of musk compounds. Among foodstuffs relevant contents have only been found in freshwater fish from polluted rivers and aquacultures but not in any other fatty foodstuffs including seafood[18] which represents the main share of the anyway limited fish consumption in Germany. Residues found in fish and other aquatic organisms do not seem to be a result of bioaccumulation (uptake with food or via food chain), but mainly of bioconcentration (uptake from polluted water)[6].

However, another route of exposure seems to be much more relevant, namely percutaneous absorption[16]. Intensive contact to the skin is obvious, due to the wide spread occurrence of musk compounds in cosmetics, soaps, detergents and washed/softened textiles. Toxicological studies in rats[42,43,44] and in-vitro tests with guinea-pig and human skin[45] demonstrated that relevant amounts may be absorbed following direct contact to the skin. The large inter-individual differences of contamination in human tissue shown in the present and in previous investigations[46] further support this hypothesis (prevalent exposure by the diet would characteristically lead to only small variation). However, no studies are available at present proving the causal relationship between levels in the human body and levels in household and body care products. Thus further studies are needed to verify the role of dermal absorption in humans[16].

4.3   Health Risk Aspects

4.3.1   Kinetics, Metabolism

Considering that the octanol-water partition coefficients and bioconcentration factors determined so far are similar to those of organochlorine compounds like PCB, it might be assumed that musk compounds just as well tend to accumulate in fatty compartments of the human body. This assumption is supported by animal studies on the tissue distribution of musk xylene[47,48]. However, at least nitro musks seem to be eliminated from the human body much faster than organochlorine compounds. While elimination half-times of PCB is in the range of several years, much shorter half-times (about 100 d) were determined in kinetic studies with ^{15}N-labeled musk xylene in volunteers[49]. Comparatively rapid elimination could also explain the missing relationship between levels of musk xylene in the human body and age or body mass index[39], as well as the observed drop in levels in human milk discussed above.

In addition, at least nitro musks seem to be eliminated mostly unchanged rather than via metabolism[6]. In contrast to other aromatic amines (e.g., di- and trinitrotoluenes) reductive degradation associated with the formation of hemoglobin- and DNA-reactive intermediates (i.e. nitroso and hydroxylamine derivatives, respectively) is inhibited, probably because contact with metabolic enzymes is hindered by the sterical relationship of the various functional groups to each other[47].

Presently no data are available on the kinetics and metabolism of polycyclic musks in mammals.

4.3.2   Toxicological data

Available data on the toxicology of artificial musk compounds is limited. Most studies published so far were performed with nitro musks, especially with musk xylene, while with polycyclic musks except for a few *in vitro* studies no data is available.

Acute toxicity of nitro musks is low. LD_{50} values in rats, mice and rabbits are in the range of several g/kg[13,50,51,52,53].

Skin tolerance. While in the first studies nitro musks showed little or no effects, clinical experiences soon revealed that musk ambrette is a photo contact allergen in man[54]. Further animal and human investigations showed that this is not true for other nitro musks[6,55]. In a study with 1323 persons using 25 fragrances most widely used in the U.S., an allergic reaction to a 0.1% solution of musk xylene in vaseline was determined in 2 persons only[56].

Subacute and chronic toxicity. In animal studies increasing paralysis of the hind paws and atrophy of the testes was observed in rats orally exposed to 25-200 mg/kg of musk ambrette over a period of 20-50 weeks[57]. Neurotoxic effects were not found with other nitro musks[42]. Feeding experiments in mice with high doses of musk xylene (>0.15%) over a period of 17 weeks[13] and dermal exposure of musk ketone to rabbits over a period of 3 weeks[51] led to slight increases of liver weights.

Carcinogenicity, Genotoxicity. In the only long-term animal study on carcinogenicity reported so far, musk xylene (75 and 150 ppm in the diet, i.e. ca. 90 and 170 mg/kg/d) significantly increased the incidence of malignant and benign liver cell tumors in mice[13]. In genotoxicity/mutagenicity experiments only musk ambrette was positive in the Salmonella/microsome assay (Ames test)[58,59,60]. Therefore and because of its photo-allergenic and neurotoxic properties (see above), musk ambrette was banned by law in cosmetics in the European Community in 1995[61]. Neither musk xylene, nor musk ketone, nor any of the polycyclic musks revealed evidence for genotoxicity in various bacterial (e.g. Ames test, SOS-chromotest)[60,62] or eucaryontic test systems (e.g. sister-chromatid exchange test, micronucleus test)[36,63,64,65,66,67]. Hence, it has been suggested that the carcinogenic effects of musk xylene observed in mice were not due to a genotoxic, tumor initiating mechanism[6]. On the other hand, epigenetic mechanisms may be invovled. Musk xylene has been shown to induce (and in some cases simultaneously inhibit) both toxifying and detoxifying liver enzymes in rats and mice, in particular cytochrome P450-dependent oxigenases (especially CYP1A2) and several phase II enzymes (DT-diaphorase, glutathione-*S*-transferase, and UDP-glucuronyltransferase)[68,69,70,71]. Moreover, musk xylene and musk ketone have been identified as cogenotoxicants by induction of toxifying liver enzyms:

the S9 liver fraction (microsomal enzymes) isolated from pretreated rats (10, 20 and 40 mg/d musk xylene or musk ketone for a period of 5d) increased the toxification rate of well-known pregenotoxicants such as 2-aminoanthracene, aflatoxine B1, and benzo[a]pyrene (only musk ketone) to DNA-reactive metabolites in the SOS chromotest[72].

Other adverse effects. Developmental studies performed with musk xylene in rats indicated significant transplacental passage and exposure of offspring via maternal milk[48]. However, even in maternal toxic doses (> 20 mg/kg/d) no adverse effects on embryo-fetal development were observed[6]. In binding studies with 17β-estradiol musk xylene showed no endocrine (i.e. estrogenic) properties[73].

4.3.3   Evaluation

There still is a considerable lack of knowledge on the toxicology of musk compounds. For instance, long term animal experiments will have to be performed in at least a second species with musk xylene in order to assess its carcinogenic properties[6]. So far no data whatever is available on long-term toxicity of polycyclic musks.

In 1995 the WHO-International Agency for Research on Cancer (IARC) evaluated musk ambrette and musk xylene as being "not classifiable as to their carcinogenicity to humans" (Group 3)[74].

Concerning cancer risk caused by exposure to nitro musks the following aspects should be considered:

a) Musk xylene and musk ketone, which are the predominant contaminants found in human tissue, do not cause DNA-damage on their own but seem to have cogenotoxic properties caused by a modulation of liver enzymes.

b) Human exposure to relevant pregenotoxicants (aminoaromtes, mycotoxins, polycyclic aromatic hydrocarbons, etc.) is evident due to their ubiquitous occurrence in air, water and food.

c) Apart from nitro musks other xenobiotics, such as PCB and PCDD/F were identified as inducers of toxifying enzymes in rodents as well. Thus synergistic (at least additive) effects must be expected[72].

d) On the other hand, it is widely accepted that liver tumors in rodents resulting from nongenotoxic chemicals shown to be mirosomal enzyme inducers are not predective of a similar risk to humans[74,75]. Carcinogenic and cogenotoxic effects were observed after animal exposure to high doses of nitro musks. Since tumor promotion (not initiation) seems to be the mechanism of tumor development, a threshold determined by induction of toxifying enzymes must be assumed. No-effect levels (NOEL) for enzyme induction in animals were ≥20 mg/kg. Contents found in human milk, however, are several orders of magnitude lower. Based on the present data an average daily uptake of 6-211 (mean 38) ng of musk xylene per kg body weight may be calculated for the breast fed infant (assumptions made: 6.6 kg body weight, 850 g daily uptake of milk containing 29 g of fat). This is lower by a factor of $>10^5$ than the NOEL. From this point of view, it is unlikely that human exposure will produce similar effects on toxifying enzymes.

5.   CONCLUSIONS

Synthetic musk compounds represent a further group of lipophilic persistent environmental pollutants now found in human milk which were not noticed there until the past few years. The presence of these chemicals in human tissue is on principal undesirable under the aspect of prospective health protection. There still is a considerable lack of knowledge, especially concerning possible long term effects in mammals. Musk ambrette is the only compound banned by law so far. It is appreciable that other nitro musks, in particular musk xylene, have voluntarily neither been produced nor used in some countries, including Germany, resulting in a marked decrease in the level of contamination of human milk. On the other hand, replacement by polycyclic musks in consumer products might lead to an increasing contamination by these. To date, except for some screening tests on genotoxicity there is a complete lack of toxicological data on polycyclic musks.

REFERENCES

[1] Sommer, C., 1993, Gaschromatographische Bestimmung von Nitromoschusverbindungen in Kosmetika und Waschmitteln. *Dtsch. Lebensm. Rundsch.* **89**: 108-111.

[2] Eschke, H.D., Traud, J., Dibowski, H.J., 1995, Untersuchungen zum Vorkommen polycyclischer Moschus-Duftstoffe in verschiedenen Umweltkompartimenten. 2. Mitteilung: Befunde in Oberflächen-, Abwässern und Fischen sowie in Waschmitteln und Kosmetika. *Z. Umweltchem. Ökotox.* **7**: 131-138.

[3] Müller, P.N., Lamparsky, M., 1991, Perfumes: art, science and technology. Elsevier Applied Science, London.

[4] Barbetta, L., Trowbridge, T., Eldib, I.A., 1988, Musk aroma chemical industry. *Perfumer & Flavorist* **13**: 60-61.

[5] Baur, A., German Patent 47'599.

[6] Käfferlein, H.U., Göen, T., Angerer,J., 1998, Musk xylene: analysis, occurrence, kinetics, and toxicology. *Crit. Rev. Toxicol.* **28**: 431-476.

[7] Yamagishi T., Miyazaki T., Horii S., Akiyama K., 1983, Synthetic musk residues in biota and water from Tama River and Tokyo Bay. *Arch. Environ. Contam. Toxicol.* **12**: 83-89.

[8] Rimkus, G., Wolf, M., 1993, Rückstände und Verunreinigungen in Fischen aus Aquakultur. *Dtsch. Lebensm. Rundsch.* **89**: 171-175.

[9] Hahn, J, 1993, Untersuchungen zum Vorkommen von Moschus-Xylol in Fischen. *Dtsch. Lebensm. Rundsch.* **89**: 175-177.

[10] Rimkus, G., Wolf, M., 1995, Nitro musk fragrances in biota from freshwater and marine environment. *Chemosphere* **30**: 641-651.

[11] Liebl, B., Ehrenstorfer, S., 1993, Nitro musks in human milk. *Chemosphere* **27**: 2253-2260.

[12] Rimkus, G., Wolf, M., 1994, Nitro musks in human adipose tissue and breast milk. *Chemosphere* **28**: 421-432.

[13] Maekawa, A., Matsushima, Y., Onodera, H., Shibutani, M., Ogasawara, H., Kodama, Y., Kurokawa, Y., Hayashi, Y., 1990, Long-term toxicity/carcinogenicity of musk xylol in B6C3F1 mice. *Food Chem. Toxicol.* **28**: 581-586.

[14] Anouncement by the German toiletries and detergent industries, 1993.

[15] Wood, T.F., 1982, Chemistry of synthetic musks. II. Benzoid musks. In *Fragrance Chemistry* (E.T. Theimer, ed.) Academic Press, New York.

[16] Rimkus, G., 1997, Synthetic musk fragrances in human fat and their potential uptake by dermal resorption. In *Fragrances, beneficial and adverse effects* (P.J. Frosch, J.D. Johansen, I.R. White, eds.), pp.136-149, Springer, Berlin.

[17] Kevekordes, S., Grahl, K., Zaulig, A., Dunkelberg, H., 1997, Genotoxicity of nitro musks in the micronucleus test with human lymphocytes *in vitro* and the human hepatoma cell line Hep G2. *Toxicol. Let.* **91**: 13-17.

[18] Rimkus, G., Brunn, H., 1996, Synthetische Moschusduftstoffe in der Umwelt – Anwendung, Anreicherung in der Umwelt und Toxikologie, Teil 1: Herstellung, Anwendung und Vorkommen in Lebensmitteln, Aufnahme durch den Menschen. *Ernähr. Umschau* **43**: 442-449

[19] Eschke, H.D., Traud, J., Dibowski, H.J., 1994, Untersuchungen zum Vorkommen polycyclischer Moschus-Duftstoffe in verschiedenen Umweltkompartimenten. 1. Mitteilung: Nachweis und Analytik in Oberflächen-, Abwässern und Fischen. *Z. Umweltchem. Ökotox.* **6**: 183-189.

[20] Winkler, M., Kopf, C., Hauptvogel, C., Neu, T., 1998, Fate of artificial musk fragrances associated with suspended particulate matter (SPM) from the River Elbe (Germany) in comparison to other organic contaminants. *Chemosphere* **37**: 1139-1158.

[21] Eschke, H.D., Dibowski, H.J., Traud, J., 1995, Nachweis und Quantifizierung von polycyclischen Moschus-Duftstoffen mittels Ion-Trap GC/MS/MS in Humanfett und Muttermilch. *Dtsch. Lebensm. Rundsch.* **91**: 375-379.

[22] Rimkus, G., Wolf, M., 1996, Polycyclic musk fragrances in human adipose tissue and human milk. *Chemosphere* **33**: 2033-2043.

[23] Jensen, R.G., Lammi-Keefe, C.J., Koletzko, B., 1997, Representative sampling of human milk and the extraction of fat for analysis of environmental lipophilic contaminants. *Toxicol. Environ. Chem.* **62**: 229-247.

[24] Jensen, R.G., 1995, Letter to the editor: Comments on the extraction of fat from human milk for analysis of contaminants, *Chemosphere* **31**: 4197-4205.

[25] Helbling, K.S., Schmid, P., Schlatter, C., 1994, The trace analysis of musk xylene in biological samples: problems associated with its ubiquitous occurrence. *Chemosphere* **29**: 477-484.

[26] AOAC (Association of Official Analytical Chemists), 1995, Official method 989.05, modified Mojonnier. In *Official methods of analysis* (P. Cunnif, ed.), AOAC Internat., Arlington, VA, 16 ed, Vol II, Ch 33, pp 18-19.

[27] IDF, 1995, International Standard 172.1995. *Milk and milk products - extraction methods for lipids and lipidsoluble compounds.* IDF-General secretary, Brussels, Belgium.

28 Bligh, E.G., Dyer, W.J., 1959, A rapid method of total lipid extraction and purification. *Can. J. Biochem.Physiol.* **37**: 911-917.

29 IDF (International Dairy Federation), 1991, International Standard 75C.1991. IDF-General secretary, Brussels, Belgium.

30 Koletzko, B., Mrotzek, M., Eng, B., Bremer, H.J., 1988, Fatty acid composition of mature human milk in Germany. *Am. J. Clin. Nutr.* **47**: 954-959.

31 Koletzko, B., Thiel, I., Abiodun P.O., 1991, Fatty acid composition of mature human milk in Nigeria. *Z. Ernährungswiss.* **30**: 289-297.

32 Brühl, L., 1994, PhD Thesis *Charakterisierung maßgeblicher Triglyceride in Muttermilch und in Rohstoffen für Säuglingsnahrung.* Wilhelms University, Münster, Germany.

33 AOAC, 1995, official method 605.02, Extraction of fat from milk for pesticides. In *Official methods of analysis* (P. Cunnif, ed.), AOAC Internat., Arlington, VA, Ref 22, Vol I, Ch 10, p 6.

34 Steinwandter, H., 1980, Beiträge zur Verwendung von Kieselgel in der Pesticidanalytik. II. Analytik und Capillar-Gas-Chromatographie von δ-HCH und anderen Chlorkohlenwasserstoff-Pesticiden. *Fresenius Z. Anal. Chem.* **304**: 137-140.

35 Rimkus, G., Butte, W., Geyer, H.J., 1997, Critical considerations on the analytical analysis and bioaccumulation of musk xylene and other synthetic nitro musks in fish. *Chemosphere* **35**: 1497-1507.

36 Kevekordes, S., Dunkelberg, H., Mersch-Sundermann, V., 1999, Evaluation of health risks caused by nitro musks. *Umweltmed. Forsch. Prax.* **4**: 107-112.

37 Beck, H., 1991, Kontamination der Frauenmilch. In *Gesundheit und Umwelt '91.Beiträge zur ärzlichen Fortbildung. Vorträge aus dem Bundesgesundheitsamt anläßlich des 40. Ärztlichen Fortbildungskongresses in Berlin* (A. Somogyi, D. Großklaus, eds), pp. 21-28, MMV Medizin Verlag, München.

38 Fürst, P., Fürst, C., Wilmers, K., 1992, PCDDs and PCDFs in human milk - statistical evaluation of a 6-years survey. *Chemosphere* **25**: 1029-1038.

39 Käfferlein, H.U., Göen, T., Angerer,J., 1997, Exposure of the general population to musk xylene. *Umweltmed. Forsch. Prax.* **2**: 169-170.

40 Beck, H., Eckart, K., Mathar, W., Wittowski, R., 1989, PCDD and PCDF body burden from food intake in the Federal Republic of Germany. *Chemosphere* **18**: 417-424.

41 Geyer, H.J., Rimkus, G., Wolf, M., Attar, A., Steinberg, C. Kettrup, A., 1994, Synthetische Nitromoschus-Duftstoffe und Bromocyclen - Neue Umweltchemikalien in Fischen und Muscheln bzw. Muttermilch und Humanfett. *Z. Umweltchem. Ökotox.* **6**: 9-17.

42 Ford, R.A., Api, A.M., Newberne, P.M., 1990, 90-day dermal toxicity study and neurotoxicity evaluation of nitromusks in the albino rat. *Food Chem. Toxicol.* **28**: 55-61.

43 Spencer, P.S., Bischoff-Fenton, M.C., Moreno, O.M., Opdyke, D.L., Ford, R.A.,1984, Neurotoxic properties of musk ambrette. *Toxicol. Appl. Pharmacol.* **75**: 571-575.

44 Spencer, P.S., Sterman, A.B., Horoupian, D.S., Fouldy, M.M., 1979, Neurotoxic fragrance produces ceroid and myelin disease. *Science* **204**: 633.

45 Hood, H.L., Wicket, R.R., Bronaugh, R.L., 1996, In vitro percutaneous absorption of the fragrance ingredient musk xylol. *Food Chem. Toxicol.* **34**: 483-488.

46 Müller, S., Schmid, P., Schlatter, C., 1996, Occurrence of nitro and non-nitro benzoid musk compounds in human adipose tissue. *Chemosphere* **33**:17-28.

47 Minegishi, K., Nambaru, S., Fukuoka, M., Tanaka, A., Nishimaki-Mogami, T., 1991, Distribution, metabolism, and excretion of musk xylene in rats. *Arch. Toxicol.* **65**: 273-282.

48 Suter-Eichenberger, R., Altorfer, H., Lichtensteiger, W., Schlumpf, M., 1998, Bioaccumulation of musk xylene (MX) in developing and adult rats of both sexes. *Chemosphere* **36**: 2747-2762.

[49] Kokot-Helbling, K., Schmid, P., Schlatter, C., 1995, Human exposure to musk xylene – absorption, pharmacokinetics and toxicology. *Mitt. Geb. Lebensmitt. Hyg.* **86**: 1-13.

[50] Opdyke, D.L., 1975, Musk ambrette. *Food Cosmet. Toxicol.* **13**: 875-876.

[51] Opdyke, D.L., 1975, Musk ketone. *Food Cosmet. Toxicol.* **13**: 877-878.

[52] Opdyke, D.L., 1975, Musk tibetene. *Food Cosmet. Toxicol.* **13**: 879.

[53] Opdyke, D.L., 1975, Musk xylene. *Food Cosmet. Toxicol.* **13**: 881.

[54] Cronin, E., 1984, Photosensitivity to musk ambrette. *Contact dermatitis* **11**: 88-92.

[55] Parker, R.D., Buehler, E.V., Newmann, E.A., 1986, Phototoxicity, photoallergy, and contact sensitization of nitro musk perfume raw materials. *Contact Dermatitis* **14**: 103-109.

[56] Frosch, P.J., Pilz, B., Andersen, K.E., Burrows, D., Camarasa, J.G., Dooms-Goossens, A., Ducombs, G., Fuchs, T., Hannuksela, M., Lachapelle, J.M., 1995, Patch testing with fragrances: results of a multicenter study of the European Environmental and Contact Dermatitis Research Group with 48 frequently used constituents of perfumes. *Contact Dermatitis* **33**: 333-342.

[57] Davis, D.A., Taylor, J.M., Jones, W.I., Brouwer, J.B., 1967, Toxicity to musk ambrette. *Toxicol. Appl. Pharmacol.* **10**: 405.

[58] Wild, D., King, M.T., Gocke, E., Eckardt, K., 1983, Study of artificial flavouring substances for mutagenicity in the Salmonella/Microsome, basc and micronucleus tests. *Food Chem. Toxicol.* **21**: 707-719.

[59] Nair, J., Ohshima, H., Malaveille, C., Friesen, M., O'Neill, I.K., Hautefeuille, A., Bartsch, H., 1986, Identification, occurrence and mutagenicity in Salmonella typhimurium of two synthetic nitroarenes, musk ambrette and musk xylene, in Indian chewing tobacco and betel quid. *Food Chem. Toxicol.* **24**: 27-31.

[60] Emig, M., Reinhardt, A., Mersch-Sundermann, V., 1996, A comparative study of five nitro musk compunds in the SOS chromotest and Salmonalla mutagenicity. *Toxicol. Let.* **85**: 151-156.

[61] Richtlinie 95/34/EG der Kommission vom 10. Juli 1995 zur Anpassung der Anhänge II, III, VI und VII der Richtlinie 76/768/EWG des Rates zur Angleichung der Rechtsvorschriften der Mitgliedsstaaten über kosmetische Mittel an den technischen Fortschritt. *ABl L* **167**: 19-21.

[62] Mersch-Sundermann, Kevekordes, S., Jenter, C., 1998, Testing of SOS induction of artificial polycyclic musk fragrances in *E. coli* PQ38 (SOS chromotest). *Toxicol. Let.* **95**: 147-154.

[63] API, A.M., Pfitzer, E.A., San, R.H.C., 1995, An evaluation of musk xylene in a battery of genotoxicity tests, *Fd. Chem. Toxicol.* **33**: 1039-1045.

[64] API, A.M., Pfitzer, E.A., San, R.H.C., 1996, An evaluation of genotoxicity tests with musk ketone, *Fd. Chem. Toxicol.* **34**: 633-638.

[65] Kevekordes, S., Grahl, K., Zaulig, A., Dunkelberg, H., 1996, Genotoxicity testing of nitro musks with the SOS-chromotest and the sister-chromatid exchange test. *Environ. Sci. Pollut. Res.* **3**: 189-192.

[66] Kevekordes, S., Mersch-Sundermann, V., Diez, M., Dunkelberg, H., 1997, In vitro genotoxicity of polycyclic musk fragrances in the micronucleus test. *Mutat. Res.* **395**: 145-150.

[67] Kevekordes, S., Mersch-Sundermann, V., Diez, M., Bolten, C., Dunkelberg, H., 1998, Genotoxicity of polycyclic musk fragrances in the sister-chromatid exchange test. *Anticanc. Res.* **18**: 449-452.

[68] Iwata, N., Minegishi, K., Suzuki, K., Ohno, Y., Kawanishi, T., Takahashi, A., 1992, Musk xylene is a novel specific inducer of cytochrome P-450IA2. *Biochem. Biophys. Res. Commun.* **184**: 149-153.

[69] Iwata, N., Minegishi, K., Suzuki, K., Ohno, Y., Igarashi, T., Satoh, T., Takahashi, A., 1993, An unusual profile of musk xylene-induced drug metabolizing enzymes in rat liver. *Biochem. Pharmacol.* **45**: 1659-1665.

[70] Lehman-McKeeman, L.D., Caudill, D., Young, J.A., Dierckman, T.A., 1995, Musk xylene induces and inhibits mouce hepatic cytochrome p-450 2B enzymes. *Biochem. Biophys. Res. Commun.* **206**: 975-980.

[71] Stuard, S.D., Caudill, D., Lehman-McKeeman, L.D., 1997, Characterization of musk ketone on mouce hepatic cytochrome p-450 2B enzymes. *Exper. Appl. Toxicol.* **40**: 264-271.

[72] Mersch-Sundermann, V., Emig, M., Reinhardt, A., 1996, Nitro musks are cogenotoxicants by inducing toxifying enzymes in the rat. *Mutat. Res.* **356**: 237-245.

[73] Jobling, S., Reynolds, T., White, R., Parker, M.G., Sumpter, J.P., 1995, A variety of environmentally persistent chemicals, including phthalate plasticizers, are weakly estrogenic. *Environ. Health* **103**: 582-587.

[74] IARC, 1995, Vol. 65, Printing processes and printing inks, carbon black and some nitro compounds, Lyon, France.

[75] Whysner, J., Ross, P.M., Williams, G.M., 1996, Phenobarbital mechanistic data and risk assessment: enzyme induction, enhanced cell proliferation, and tumor promotion. *Pharmacol. Ther.* **71**: 153-191.

27

EXPOSITION TO AND HEALTH EFFECTS OF RESIDUES IN HUMAN MILK

Hildegard Przyrembel, Barbara Heinrich-Hirsch, Baerbel Vieth
Federal Institute for Health Protection of Consumers and Veterinary Medicine, Thielallee 88-92
D-14195 Berlin, Germany

Key words: environmental pollutants; human milk; adverse effects; polyhalogenated aromatic hydrocarbons; dioxins; polychlorinated biphenyls; pesticides; exposure; prenatal; postnatal

Abstract: A great variety of drugs, cosmetics, food ingredients as well as environmental contaminants are secreted with human milk as a result of actual exposure or the accumulated body burden of the mother. Of great concern and least amenable to short-term intervention are persistent substances in the environment with long half-lives in the body due to their lipophilic properties and minimal degradation. Polyhalogenated aromatic hydrocarbons, namely organochlorine pesticides, polychlorinated biphenyls (PCB) and polychlorinated dibenzodioxins (PCDD) and dibenzofurans (PCDF) are fetotoxic, neurotoxic, immunotoxic, some are promoting carcinogens and/or interfere with hormonal receptors. They pass the placenta and equilibrate among the lipid compartments of the body including breast milk lipids. Transplacental exposure is more relevant with regard to physical development and cognitive functioning of the child than postnatal exposure via breastmilk. Restrictions for production, use and release have been successful in decreasing exposure as shown by a downward trend of their contents both in human milk and serum lipids for the last 15 to 20 years. It is difficult to evaluate the potentially late effects of the exposure via breastmilk which is 10 to 100 times higher in industrialised countries than the tolerable daily intake (TDI) of 1 to 4 toxic equivalents (WHO-TEQ) pg/kg/day established in 1998 by WHO for dioxins and dioxin-like PCBs but which lasts for 0.6% of the expected life span only. Carefully conducted long-term follow-up of cohorts with defined exposure levels, with consideration of numerous biological and psychological parameters, is expected to provide the answer.

Short and Long Term Effects of Breast Feeding on Child Health
Edited by Berthold Koletzko *et al.*, Kluwer Academic/Plenum Publishers, 2000   307

1.   Introduction

Whereas breastfeeding is considered the optimal nutrition for infants both for purely nutritional reasons and for reasons affecting health and risks for diseases in later life, the fact that a multitude of environmental and other residues have been found in human milk has raised concerns about its healthiness. The organochlorine pesticide DDT was the first to be detected in human milk [1]. Many other substances have followed because of increasingly sophisticated analytical techniques or because of being "new". The advisability of recommending breastfeeding has repeatedly been questioned.

For example the German Research Association [2] recommended in 1982 breastfeeding for four (to six) months and to analyse the levels of residues in a mother's milk after four months of lactation before continuing to breastfeed. Reference values for organochlorine pesticides and PCBs to be tolerated in the daily volume were established and cost-free analysis was offered to all mothers by the food control agencies. The negative result of that advice was a certain reluctance to start breastfeeding at all, or a tendency to stop early. The positive result was that many data on human milk residue levels exist in Germany and have been collected by the Federal Institute for Health Protection of Consumers and Veterinary Medicine (BgVV, Berlin) which allow trends to be analysed reliably over the years.

Infants' exposure to environmental pollutants via mother's milk, however, cannot be seen separately from the exposure due to transplacental transfer of residues in tissues of the mother. Several studies have shown that prenatal exposure, if at all, is more likely to produce adverse effects, probably because of greater vulnerability of the developing organs and organ functions.

Independent of the question which period of exposure is of greater concern for any short-term or long-term health effects, it must be recognised that environmental levels of various long known pollutants are continuously decreasing in industrialised countries in the last decades and consequently fall in human milk. At the same time substances not recognised before, e.g. musk compounds have been detected and identified as "new" residues in tissues of human origin.

This article deals with the different kinds of potential residues in human milk, their toxicological assessment, provides data on intake and discusses the effects as apparent from longitudinal studies.

2. Residues in human milk

Substances not naturally occurring in human milk are not only undesirably from the hygienic point of view, but are of particular importance, because of their potential health significance for nursed babies. Residues of xenobiotics in human milk normally result from the burden or contamination of the maternal organism. Hence, from the various routes of exposure the uptake of substances by the mothers may occur via skin, inhalation and by oral ingestion. Chemicals are transferred from the maternal organism into the milk according to their partitioning coefficients between maternal serum and milk and may even accumulate due to possible active secretion. *Table 1* lists the most important groups of chemicals, which can be detected in human milk. The exposure of the mothers to part of these substances is more or less avoidable. However, the intake of other groups of chemicals is practically unavoidable, because of their ubiquitous occurrence and/or entrance into the food chain.

Table 1. Possible residues in human milk

medicinal drugs	mycotoxins
cosmetics/fragrances	heavy metals
stimulants (alcohol, caffeine, nicotine)	nitrate, nitrite, nitrosamines
polycyclic aromatic hydrocarbons (PAH)	
volatile organochlorine substances (solvents)	
persistent organochlorine substances	
polybrominated biphenyls (flame retardants)	

Of greatest concern are so-called persistent chemicals. Among these are chlorinated or halogenated aromatic hydrocarbons (*Figure 1*), which, due to their high stability and low biodegradation persist in the environment and hence can be detected ubiquitously.

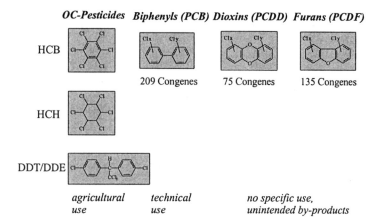

Figure 1. Persistent organochlorine substances

To these belong organochlorine pesticides (OCP), which had been used in agriculture, and polychlorinated biphenyls (PCB), which had been widely used in various industrial applications. They have been regulated in many of the industrialised countries during the past decades, which means that commercial production and use has been discontinued or banned. Further, polychlorinated dibenzodioxins and dibenzofurans (PCDD/PCDF) belong to this group of chemicals. They have never been intentionally produced, but are generated predominantly by incineration and other thermic processes and as by-products during fabrication of special chemical compounds. OCPs and PCBs – by means of certain indicator-congeners – can be determined by routine analytical methods, whereas the determination of PCDD/PCDF requires much more demanding analytical methods, which were not developed before the mid 80ties, when PCDD/PCDF were detected in human milk for the first time.

From the various sources of exposure (soil, water, air) the intake via food – predominantly from fat of animals' origin – contributes more than 95% to the human exposure and burden of such contaminants. Due to their persistence, low biodegradability and lipophilicity these substances accumulate in the food chain (*Figure 2*). Human milk can be conceived as a bioindicator, for the extent and time course of human contamination.

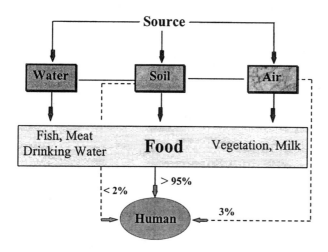

Figure 2. Pathways for human exposure and burden to PCBs and dioxins

3.   Toxicological assessment

For the evaluation of possible toxicants so-called ADI/TDI values are frequently used. For *residues*, e.g. from pesticides, but also for food additives, FAO/WHO recommended Acceptable Daily Intake values. Likewise, for *contaminants* so-called Tolerable Daily Intake values can be derived. An ADI is defined as the amount of toxicant in mg/kg body weight/day which is not anticipated to result in any adverse effects after chronic exposure to the general population of humans, including sensitive subgroups. Adverse effects are considered as functional impairment or pathological lesions which may affect the performance of the whole organism, or which reduce an organism's ability to respond to an additional challenge [3].

$$ADI/TDI = \frac{NOAEL}{Safety\ factor}$$

The **No Observed Adverse Effect Level** (NOAEL) is obtained from animal experiments. Substances under consideration are examined at various dose levels or diet concentrations in animals to determine the dosage which induces no harmful effects. To define a tolerable daily intake for humans, this value is reduced by safety factors to take into consideration the uncertainties from extrapolation of animal data to the human situation and the uncertainties because of intra-species heterogeneity. Usually a factor of 100 is applied.

4.   Applicability of the TDI concept to residues in human milk

The ADI/TDI approach implies chronic intake for the whole lifespan, which of course, does not apply to the breastfeeding period. In fact, breastfeeding for 6 months does account for less than 1% of the mean lifespan. Therefore, ADI/TDI values cannot be considered an appropriate instrument to adequately evaluate any health risk for infants' development in the context of breastfeeding. However, if daily substance intakes via breastfeeding are calculated to range below or within the ADI/TDI, it can be anticipated that any health risk is highly improbable.

This is illustrated in *Table 2*, which presents data on the current level of contamination with organochlorine pesticides in human milk samples from the Federal Republic of Germany. The milk analyses have been performed by the Federal Untersuchungsämter, which kindly provide their data to an inventory on residues in human milk at the Federal Institute for Health Protection of Consumers and Veterinary Medicine. Under quantitative aspects hexachlorobenzene (HCB), beta-hexachlorocyclohexane (β-HCH) and DDT still are relevant contaminants, whereas the other OCPs range near or at the level of determination. From the analytical data of OCP residues, the respective daily intakes can be estimated (assumptions for calculation: mean milk fat content 3.5%; mean milk fat intake 4.2 g/kg based on daily milk intake of 120 ml/kg body weight). Considering the estimates for the 95. percentile (P-95), the intake values for most of the indicated OCPs range at or below the TDI (exception HCB), some of them are even lower than the level of the NOAEL. It may be concluded therefore, that from the current levels of these OCPs no significant risk for adverse health effects can be expected and that these contaminants are of no real concern for the health of the breastfed infants.

Table 2. Estimated daily intake of pesticides and pesticide residues

	NOAEL	TDI[*]	levels in human milk[**]		estimated daily intake	
			mean	95-P	mean	95-P
	(mg/kg/d)	(µg/kg/d)	(mg/kg milk fat)		(µg/kg body weight)	
HCB	0.06	0.16-0.17	0.07	0.18	0.29	0.76
alpha-HCH	0.5	3	0.003	0.01	0.01	0.04
beta-HCH	0.1	3	0.04	0.12	0.17	0.48
gamma-HCH	1.0	3	0.006	0.02	0.03	0.08
HE	0.05	0.5	0.008	0.02	0.03	0.08
Dieldrin	0.01	0.1	0.007	0.03	0.03	0.12
DDT	0.5	20	0.31	0.90	1.32	3.86

[*] 4

[**] data from 1997 (Germany)

The situation is different, however, for PCBs and dioxins. Although continuously decreasing with time, levels of PCBs are still detectable in significant amounts in human milk from Germany (*Table 3*). For PCBs the estimated daily intakes (mean and P-95 level) amount to 2 and 4 µg/kg body weight, respectively. This is compared to a provisional TDI of 1 µg/kg body weight/day. An appropriate TDI for PCBs still remains to be established. The problem is, that the composition of PCB residues in human tissues differs in congener pattern and amount from the composition of the technical products, which have been used in animal testing so far. The testing of relevant mixtures is still an outstanding issue.

Mean levels of dioxins in human milk, given as toxic equivalents (TEq) based on international toxic equivalency factors (I-TEF), are also decreasing. However, calculations based on the current residue levels in human milk samples from Germany clearly demonstrate, that the daily intake of babies by far exceeds the TDI of 1-10 pg I-TEq/kg body weight, which had been recommended by the former German Federal Health Office [5]. At present, it is difficult to precisely figure out this excess intake during the period of breastfeeding. WHO, after reevaluation of the current data base has set the TDI at 1-4 pg WHO-TEq/kg body weight [6]. In their new concept dioxinlike PCBs are considered besides dioxins/furans and contribute to the toxic equivalents. Hence, if dioxin-like PCBs are additionally taken into consideration, the current levels of dioxinlike compounds (PCDD/F + PCB) in human milk nominally may increase two to three fold.

Table 3. Estimated daily intake of PCBs and dioxins

	levels in human milk**)		estimated daily intake	
PCBs	(mg/kg milk fat)		(µg/kg body weight)	
(1 µg/kg bw/d)	mean	P-95	mean	P-95
1997	0.50	0.94	2.1	3.9
Dioxins/Furans	(ng I-TEq/kg milk fat)		(pg I-TEq/kg body weight)	
(1-10 pg I-TEq/kg bw/d)				
(1-4 pg WHO-TEq*)/kg bw/d)	mean		mean	
1993	16.6		69.7	
			52.1 (~125 pg (WHO-TEq*))	
1997	12.4			

*) [6], including dioxin-like PCBs
**) data from Germany

WHO well recognises the particular concern evolving from their new concept of evaluating dioxinlike chemicals with respect to the occurrence of such contaminants in human milk and therefore payed special attention to the issue of breastfeeding in their Executive Summary [6]:

"Breast-fed infants are exposed to higher intakes of these compounds on a body weight basis, although for a small proportion of their lifespan. However, the consultation noted that in studies of infants, breast feeding was associated with beneficial effects, in spite of the contaminants present. The subtle effects noted in the studies were found to be associated with transplacental, rather than lactational exposure. The consultation therefore reiterated conclusions of previous WHO meetings on the health significance of contamination of breast milk with dioxin-like compounds, namely that the current evidence does not support an alteration of WHO recommendations which promote and support breast feeding."

5. Adverse effects of polyhalogenated aromatic hydrocarbons

Our knowledge on adverse effects of polyhalogenated aromatic hydrocarbons stems from animal experiments and from human data both due to acute poisoning and to chronic exposure. The effects presumably are the result of aromatic hydrocarbon receptor (AhR) mediated mechanisms but also of other mechanisms as interactions with neurotransmitter systems, signal transduction pathways, thyroid hormone metabolism and with hormone receptors both in an agonistic and antagonistic fashion.

Developmental effects in animals can grossly be divided into neurobehavioural, developmental reproductive, neurochemical and actions on the immune system (*Table 4*).

Table 4. Functional developmental effects observed in experimental animals due to perinatal exposure to polyhalogenated aromatic hydrocarbons

neurobehavioural:	cognitive function
	neuromotor behaviour
	sexual behaviour
developmental reproductive:	sperm production
	urogenital tract
	reproduction
neurochemical:	biogenic amines
	thyroid hormone levels
	markers for glial and neuronal cell
	development
immune system	

Similar effects have been seen in several studies in relation to in-utero (and postnatal?) exposure to PCBs and PCDD/Fs in human infants:

reduced birth weight and growth	7,8,9,10,11
deficits in cognitive function as infant	8,12
deficits in cognitive function as child	13,14,15
altered thyroid hormone levels	16,17,18,19
reduced psychomotor function	(8,20,21,22)

However, these findings have not been consistent in all studies performed and the studies themselves are of very different nature and quality.

6. Longitudinal studies on PCB exposed children

The references for observed effects include [8,14,16] studies which describe children born to mothers poisoned with PCB and PCDF contaminated rice oils 1968 in Japan ("Yusho") and 1978/1980 in Taiwan ("Yucheng"). The cumulative intake of on average 1 g of PCBs and 3.8 mg 2,3,4,7,8-pentachlorine and 1,2,3,4,7,8-hexachlorine dibenzofurans by pregnant women in the Yucheng incident led to the symptoms listed in *Table 5* in 118 children born during and up to five years after the poisoning period.

Table 5. Effects observed in children born during and following period of poisoning with PCB/PCDF contaminated rice oil in Taiwan 1978/79 ("Yucheng")

- infantile death
- decreased birth weight, head circumference and length
- decreased growth
- pigmentation of skin and mucous membranes
- nail deformities, natal teeth
- developmental delay
- lower IQs
- "soft" neurologic signs
- more infections upper respiratory tract
- hyperactive behaviour

Diminished growth was still apparent at 13 years, developmental delay resulted in lower intelligence quotients at seven and 12 years compared to a matched non-exposed control group, and in boys at 11 to 14 years shorter penile lengths were reported [8].

The two first studies to systematically and prospectively investigate the outcomes of background environmental contamination in infants were done almost 20 years ago. [23] studied 859 children born to 807 women volunteers between 1978 and 1982 in North Carolina. 712 of these children were followed until the age of 5 years. Both PCBs and the DDT metabolite DDE were measured in placenta, maternal and cord serum and in combined milk samples from the complete lactation period. There was no effect of contaminant levels on birth weight and head circumference. However, PCB levels >3.5 µg/g milk fat were associated with neonatal hypoactivity, hypotonia and lower reflexes. At 18 and 24 months of age children in the top fifth percentile of prenatal PCB exposure scored 4 to 9 points lower on the Bayley psychomotor scales [24]. However, breastfed children scored higher in both Bayley tests and in the McCarthy Scales of Children's Abilities from age 2 to 5 years and showed slightly higher English grades on school reports at age 10 years [25,26].

The other study conducted in Michigan with 313 children born between 1980 and 1981 was originally designed to test for fetotoxic signs in 242 infants born to mothers eating contaminated fish from Lake Michigan in comparison to 71 infants born to non-fish eating mothers. 212 of these children were followed until the age of 11 years [7,15]. Fish consumption predicted maternal serum PCB levels but not cord serum PCB levels. Higher cord serum PCB levels (> 3 ng/mL) were associated with lower birth weights (minus 160 g), smaller head circumferences (minus 0.7 cm) and shorter-duration of gestation (minus 8.8 days). However, due to then restricted analytical methods, two thirds of cord serum levels were below the detection limit of 3 ng/mL (the same problems prevailed in the North Carolina Study: 88% below the detection limit). In the follow up studies the term "exposed" is applied either to PCB levels in cord serum higher than 3 ng/mL (75 out of 241 samples) or to amount of fish consumed by the mothers. As a result an unknown number of infants from fish-eating mothers fall into the "unexposed" group.

The authors apply various calculatory measures to compensate for these analytical difficulties which tend to confuse the reader as to their real significance.

The results are listed in *Table 6* in comparison to the studies on Yucheng children and on the North Carolina cohort. Neonatal behavioural assessment (Brazelton scale) in both American studies was negatively associated with maternal serum levels and fish ingestion, respectively. There were no effects of higher cord serum PCBs on the PDI score of the Bayley test at 5 months in the Michigan study, but a negative association with the Fagan Test for Infant Intelligence was found at 7 months. At four years of age a poorer performance on the McCarthy Scales of Infant Abilities was associated with higher PCB levels in milk, especially in verbal performance and numerical memory. However, duration of breastfeeding was positively associated with performance. At 11 years of age 212 children, 167 from fish eating and 45 from non-fish eating mothers were tested with the Wechsler Intelligence Scales for Children. Children breastfed with milk containing at least 1.25 μg PCBs/g lipid, or having had at least 4.7 ng PCBs/mL in cord serum or whose mothers had had serum levels of at least 7.7 ng/mL scored lower in verbal comprehension and freedom of distractibility. Highest exposed children were three times more likely to perform poorly for full-scale IQ (mean deficit 6 points) and were two years behind in word comprehension. There was no association between performance and postnatal PCB exposure (milk content multiplied by duration of breastfeeding).

The authors compare these results to outcomes in Yucheng children. However, as *Table 7* demonstrates, exposure levels in Taiwan and Michigan are different, although due to analytical differences a direct comparison is impossible. Moreover, effects in Yucheng children were clearly more severe and persistent in follow-up.

Table 7. Exposure to PCB in "Yucheng" and children of the "Michigan" cohort

	Yucheng* 1978/1979 PCBs [ng/mL]		Michigan** 1980/1981 PCBs [ng/mL]
mother's serum	mean	49.3	5.9 ± 3.6
children's serum	1991 (at 11 y)	1.5	at 4 y 5.1 ± 3.9 (breastfed 6 m) 1.2 ± 1.6 (breastfed <6 m)
cord blood serum		–	2.5 ± 2.0
milk		–	836 ± 388 ng/g fat

* additionally exposed to PCDFs
** additionally exposed to PBB and other polyhalogenated aromatic hydrocarbons

All studies so far indicate that prenatal and not postnatal exposure correlates with the effects seen.

Table 6. Summary of findings in the three studies on exposure to PCB

	Yucheng n=118 n=118 controls	North Carolina n=859 n=712 (5y)	associated parameter	Michigan n=313 n=236 (4y) n=212 (11y)	associated parameter
Physical growth					
at birth	↓ (B.W.)			↓ (B.W.+H.C.)	C.S.
childhood	↓ (W.+H.)			↓ (5m) (W.+H.+H.C.)	C.S.
				↓ 4y (W.)	C.S.
Skin abnormalities	+	—		—	
Bronchitis	+	—		—	
Neurodevelopmental					
neonatal	Bayley MDI + PDI ↓	Brazelton ↓	M.S.	Brazelton ↓	F.I.
infancy	IQ Stanford Binet ↓	Bayley PDI ↓ (24m)	C.S.	Fagan ↓ (7m)	C.S.
preschool	WISC-R Performance IQ →	McCarthy IQ (2-5y) —	C.S.	McCarthy IQ ↓ (4y)	M.M.
childhood	←	school grades (10.5y) —		WISC-R-IQ (11y) ↓	M.M.
Behavioural disorders		—			
Activity level	↑ (10-13y)			→	

B.W. = birth weight; W. = weight; H = height; H.C. = head circumference
M.S. = maternal serum; C.S. = cord serum; F.I. = fish ingested; M.M. = mother's milk

7.   ORGANOCHLORINE BODY BURDEN

High levels in milk fat are the result of equally high levels in maternal body fat. If one accepts the toxicokinetic model of life time burden of these lipophilic persistent compounds developed by [27] with free equilibration of e.g. dioxins in all lipids of the body, breastfeeding contributes for a limited time span to the body burden. This model results in predictable concentrations of dioxins in body lipids and, at age seven years approximately, in comparable serum levels of both breastfed and non-breastfed children.

The PCB body burden of a newborn is the result of transplacental uptake and can be grossly calculated to amount to 15,4-122 µg PCB/kg body weight based on data by [28] for PCB contents in body lipids of stillborn children using the following assumptions:

> body weight 3.7 kg; 160 g lipid/kg body weight
> → total lipid mass 590 g à 97-768 ng PCB/g lipid [28]
> → 57-473 µg PCB/590 g lipid

In comparison, the total PCB intake through breastfeeding for 6 moths at 800 mL/day and assuming 3.5% fat content amounts to the values given in *Table 8* for different PCB contents in milk fat from various sources (note the different modes for content determination, which make these results not quantitatively comparable!)

Table 8. PCB-intake through breastfeeding for 6 months

800 mL/day; 3.5% fat	PCBs* (Germany 1997: 0.497 µg/g fat) =	2505 µg
	:P95: 0.90 µg/g fat) =	4536 µg
	PCBs** (NL 1990-1992: 0.54 µg/g fat) =	2700 µg
	PCBs*** (Michigan) 1980/81: 1.25 µg/g fat) =	6300 µg

*	Σ PCB (28, 52, 101, 138, 153, 180) x 1.6
**	Σ PCB 118, 138, 153, 180
***	Webb-McCall

If the cumulative intake over 6 months of breastfeeding of e.g. 2505 µg PCB is assumed to be 100% absorbed and distributed in the body fat of a 6 months old infant (fat 25% of body weight; [29]), assuming no losses, the PCB content would amount to 1.4 to 1.6 µg/g fat or a body burden of 341 to 394 µg PCB/kg body weight.

These values compare well with PCB contents measured in adipose tissue of sudden infant death probands [30]: levels are higher in infants breastfed until death than in infants dying at variable periods after weaning and they correlate with the duration of breastfeeding. Both increment in weight as well as increment in percentage of body fat result in "dilution" of the PCB content in body fat after weaning.

8.   TRENDS OF RESIDUE LEVELS IN HUMAN MILK OVER TIME

There is a downward trend in residues of polyhalogenated aromatic hydrocarbons to be observed in industrialised countries.

Figures 3 and *4* show the German observations for mean concentrations of PCB and two pesticides since 1980 and for dioxins in human milk samples since 1985.

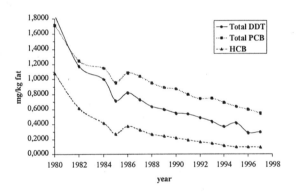

Figure 3. Trends for mean concentrations of PCB, DDT and HCB in human milk in Germany

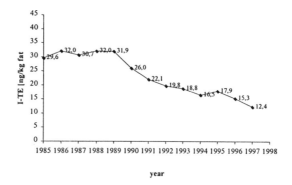

Figure 4. Trend for mean dioxin levels in human milk in Germany (n=2188)

Table 9 shows the percentage decreases from 1979/81, from 1987 and from 1993 until 1997 in human milk samples in Germany. It should be pointed out that there is a 30% decrease in mean PCB levels since 1992, when the intake of infants into the Dutch PCB/Dioxin Study (see Boersma, this volume) stopped. Conclusions that have been drawn from that study and will be drawn from future follow-up, therefore, are no longer applicable to the present levels of exposure.

Table 9. Decrease in average residue levels (in %) in human milk in Germany

from	to	β-HCH	HCB	total DDT	total PCB
1979/81	1997	87.8	93.5	82.8	71.1
1987	1997	62.1	79.1	57.8	51.3
1993	1997	19.7	48.6	28.5	31.7

(total number of samples analysed: >38 000)

German authors [31] have been able to confirm the decrease of environmental/dietary exposure to PCBs in adipose tissue biopsies from 3 year old children since 1985: median levels decreased by 86% until 1995.

Apparently strict regulation of these compounds is successful. For the future these restrictions have to be continued and, hopefully, will be combined with measures to prevent prospectively the accumulation of "new" substances with similar properties in the food chain and thereby appearing in human milk. Accumulation, once a fact is difficult to undo by individual and especially short-term measures, e.g. selective dietary choices in women planning to become pregnant. However, lifelong adherence to dietary recommendations of nutritional societies to increase the intake of plant protein to 50% of total protein intake, to prefer low-fat food from animal origin and to increase the intake of plant oils will automatically decrease the intake of polyhalogenated aromatic hydrocarbons.

9. CONCLUSION

Lipophilic persistent polyhalogenated compounds accumulate in the food chain and ultimately in human milk. In-utero exposure to these toxic compounds, however, is of greater concern than postnatal exposure via human milk. All studies looking for associated effects are hampered both by the lack of unexposed controls and by the necessity of long-term follow-up not to miss late adverse effects, which increases the number of influencing factors to be considered. Restrictive measures in production, application and release of persistent substances have to be continued and increasing awareness to control the release of "new" substances is necessary.

In view of the continuing downward trend observed with regard to contaminants in human milk in industrialised countries with the highest exposure levels, the lack of meaningful adverse effects associated with exposure through breastfeeding and the positive effects of breastfeeding on health and development there is no need to restrict breastfeeding.

10. References

[1] Lang, E.P., Kunze, F.M., and Prickett, C.S., 1951, Occurrence of DDT in human fat and milk. *Arch. Ind. Hyg. Occup. Med.* **3**: 245-246.

[2] Deutsche Forschungsgemeinschaft, 1984, Rückstände und Verunreinigungen in Frauenmilch. *Mitteilung XII der Senatskommission zur Prüfung von Rückständen in Lebensmitteln*. Verlag Chemie, Weinheim.

[3] Dourson, M.L., and Stara, J.F., 1983, Regulatory history and experimental support of uncertainty (safety) factors. *Regul. Toxicol. Pharmacol.* **3**: 224-238.

[4] WHO Food Safety Unit Programme of Food Safety and Food Aid, 1998b, *GEMS/Food International Dietary Survey* (D. Schutz, G.G. Moy and F.K. Käferstein, eds.), WHO/FSF/FOS/98.4, Geneva.

[5] Schuster, J., and Dürkop, J., (eds.), 1993, Dioxine und Furane - ihr Einfluß auf Umwelt und Gesundheit. *Bundesgesundhbl.* **36** (Sonderheft): 3-14.

[6] WHO European Centre for Environment and Health, Executive summary, 1998a, *Assessment of the health risk of dioxins: re-evaluation of the Tolerable Daily Intake (TDI)*. May 25-29, 1998, Geneva.

[7] Fein, G.G., Jacobson, J.L., Jacobson, S.W., Schwartz, P.M., and Dowler, J.K., 1984, Prenatal exposure to polychlorinated biphenyls: effects on birth size and gestational age. *J. Pediatr.* **105**: 315-320.

[8] Guo, Y.L., Lambert, G.H., and Hsu, C.-C., 1995, Growth abnormalities in the population exposed in utero and early postnatally to polychlorinated biphenyls and dibenzofurans. *Environ. Health Perspect.* **103** (Suppl. 6): 117-122.

[9] Rylander, L., Stroemberg, U., Dyremark, E., Ostman, C., Nilsson-Ehle, P., and Hagmar, L., 1998, Polychlorinated biphenyls in blood plasma among Swedish female fish consumers in relation to low birth weight. *Am. J. Epidemiol.* **147**: 493-502.

[10] Patandin, S., Koopman-Esseboom, C., de Ridder, M.A.J., Weisglas-Kuperus, N., and Sauer, P.J.J., 1998, Effects of environmental exposure to polychlorinated biphenyls and dioxins on birth size and growth in Dutch children. *Pediatr. Res.* **44**: 538-545.

[11] Vartiainen, T., Jaakkola, J.J.K., Saarikoski, S., and Tuomisto, J., 1998, Birth weight and sex of children and the correlation to the body burden of PCDDs/PCDFs and PCBs of the mother. *Environ. Health Perspect.* **106**: 61-66.

[12] Jacobson, J.L., Jacobson, S.W., and Humphrey, H.E.B., 1990, Effects of in utero exposure to polychlorinated biphenyls and related contaminants on cognitive functioning in young children. *J. Pediatr.* **116**: 38-45.

[13] Jacobson, S.W., Fein, G.G., Jacobson, J.L., Schwartz, P.M., and Dowler, J.K., 1985, The effect of intrauterine PCB exposure on visual recognition memory. *Child Dev.* **56**: 853-860.

[14] Chen, Y.-C.J., Guo, Y.-L., Hsu, C.-C., and Rogan, W.J., 1992, Cognitive development of Yu-cheng ('oil disease') children prenatally exposed to heat-degraded PCBs. *JAMA* **268**: 3213-3218.

[15] Jacobson, J.L., and Jacobson, S.W., 1996, Intellectual impairment in children exposed to polychlorinated biphenyls in utero. *N. Engl. J. Med.* **335**: 783-789.

[16] Murai, K., Okamura, K., Tsuji, H., Kajiwara, E., Watanabe, H., Akagi, K., and Fujishima, M., 1987, Thyroid function in "Yusho" patients exposed to polychlorinated biphenyls. *Environ. Res.* **44**: 179-187.

[17] Pluim, H.J., Koppe, J.G., Olie, K., van der Slikke, J.W., Kok, J.H., Vulsma, T., van Tijn, D., and de Vijlder, J.J.M., 1992, Effects of dioxins on thyroid function in newborn babies. *Lancet* **339**: 1303.

[18] Koopman-Esseboom, C., Morse, D.C., Weisglas-Kuperus, N., Lutkeschipholt, I.J., van der Paauw, C.G., Tuinstra, L.G.M.T., Brouwer, A., and Sauer, P.J.J., 1994, Effects of dioxins and polychlorinated biphenyls on thyroid hormone status of pregnant women and their infants. *Pediatr. Res.* **36**: 468-473.

[19] Winneke, G., Bucholski, A., Heinzow, B., Krämer, U., Plaßmann, S., Schmidt, E., Steingrüber, H.-J., Walkowiak, J., Weipert, S., and Wiener, A., 1997, Neurobehavioural development and TSH-levels in human infants: associations with PCBs in the neonatal period. In *Umweltbundesamt Texte 50/98: Workshop: Effects of Endocrine Disrupters in the Environment on Neuronal Development and Behavior*. Berlin, 17-18 February.

[20] Gladen, B.C., Rogan, W.J., Hardy, P., Thullen, J., Tingelstad, J., and Tully, M., 1988, Development after exposure to polychlorinated biphenyls and dichlorodiphenyl dichloroethene transplacentally and through human milk. *J. Pediatr.* **113**: 991-995.

[21] Koopman-Esseboom, C., Weisglas-Kuperus, N., de Ridder, M.A.J., Van der Paauw, C.G., Tuinstra, L.G.M.T., and Sauer, P.J.J., 1996, Effects of polychlorinated biphenyl/dioxin exposure and feeding type on infants' mental and psychomotor development. *Pediatrics* **97**: 700-706.

[22] Winneke, G., Bucholski, A., Heinzow, B., Krämer, U., Schmidt, E., Walkowiak, J., Wiener, J.-A., and Steingrüber, H.-J., 1998, Developmental neurotoxicity of

polychlorinated biphenyls (PCBS): cognitive and psychomotor functions in 7-month old children. *Toxicol. Lett.* 102-103: 423-428.

[23] Rogan, W.J., Gladen, B.C., McKinney, J.D., Carreras, N., Hardy, P., Thullen, J., Tingelstad, J., and Tully, M., 1986, Polychlorinated biphenyls (PCBs) and dichlorodiphenyl dichloroethene (DDE) in human milk: effects of maternal factors and previous lactation. *Am. J. Public Health* 76: 172-177.

[24] Rogan, W.J., and Gladen, B.C., 1991, PCBs, DDE, and child development at 18 and 24 months. *Ann. Epidemiol.* 1: 407-413.

[25] Gladen, B.C., and Rogan, W.J., 1991, Effects of perinatal polychlorinated biphenyls and dichlorodiphenyl dichloroethene on later development. *J. Pediatr.* 119: 58-63.

[26] Rogan, W.J., and Gladen, B.C., 1993, Breast-feeding and cognitive development. *Early Hum. Dev.* 31: 181-193.

[27] Kreuzer, P.E., Csanády, Gy.A., Baur, C., Kessler, W., Päpke, O., Greim, H., and Filser, J.G., 1997, 2,3,7,8-Tetrachlorodibenzo-p-dioxin (PCDD) and congeners in infants. A toxicokinetic model of human lifetime body burden by TCDD with special emphasis on its uptake by nutrition. *Arch. Toxicol.* 71: 383-400.

[28] Lanting, C.I., Huisman, M., Muskiet, F.A.J., van der Paauw, C.G., Essed, C.E., and Boersma, E.R., 1998, Polychlorinated biphenyls in adipose tissue, liver, and brain from stillborns of varying gestational ages. *Pediatr. Res.* 44: 222-225.

[29] de Bruin, N.C., van Velthoven, K.A.M., Stijnen, T., Juttmann, R.E., Degenhart, H.J., and Visser, H.K.A., 1995, Body fat and fat-free mass in infants: new and classic anthropometric indexes and prediction equations compared with total-body electrical conductivity. *Am. J. Clin. Nutr.* 61: 1195-1205.

[30] Beck, H., Mathar, W., and Palavinskas, R., 1996, Polychlorierte Dibenzodioxine, Dibenzofurane und Biphenyle in Organproben von Säuglingen und Kleinkindern. bgvv-Tätigkeitsbericht 1996, 104-110.

[31] Niessen, K.H., Helbich, H.M., Teufel, M., Witt, K., Boehm, I., Mueller, W., and Sartoris, J., 1998, Altbekannte Schadstoffe und neuentdeckte Toxaphene im Fettgewebe von Kindern. *Monatsschr. Kinderheilkd.* 146: 235-240.

28

PROMOTION OF BREASTFEEDING INTERVENTION TRIAL (PROBIT): A CLUSTER-RANDOMIZED TRIAL IN THE REPUBLIC OF BELARUS

Design, Follow-Up, and Data Validation

Kramer MS,[1,2] Chalmers B,[3] Hodnett ED,[3] Sevkovskaya Z,[4] Dzikovich I,[6] Shapiro S,[2] Collet J-P,[1,2] Vanilovich I,[6] Mezen I,[5] Ducruet T,[2] Shishko G,[6] Zubovich V,[6] Mknuik D,[4] Gluchanina E,[4] Dombrovsky V,[4] Ustinovitch A,[4] Ko T,[4] Bogdanovich N,[4] Ovchinikova L,[4] and Helsing E[7] for the PROBIT Study Group

From the Departments of Pediatrics[1] and of Epidemiology & Biostatistics,[2] McGill University Faculty of Medicine; Centre for Research in Women's Health, University of Toronto;[3] Departments of Maternal and Child Health[4] and of Foreign Relations,[5] Belarussian Ministry of Health; Belarussian Maternal and Child Health Research Institute;[6] and the Nutrition Unit, World Health Organization Regional Office for Europe[7]

Abstract: This paper summarizes the objectives, design, follow-up, and data validation of a cluster-randomized trial of a breastfeeding promotion intervention modeled on the WHO/UNICEF Baby-Friendly Hospital Initiative (BFHI). Thirty-four hospitals and their affiliated polyclinics in the Republic of Belarus were randomized to receive BFHI training of medical, midwifery, and nursing staffs (experimental group) or to continue their routine practices (control group). All breastfeeding mother-infant dyads were considered eligible for inclusion in the study if the infant was singleton, born at ≥37 weeks gestation, weighed ≥2500 grams at birth, and had a 5-minute Apgar score ≥5, and neither mother nor infant had a medical condition for which breastfeeding was contraindicated. One experimental and one control site refused to accept their randomized allocation and dropped out of the trial. A total of 17,795 mothers were recruited at the 32 remaining sites, and their infants were followed up at 1, 2, 3, 6, 9, and 12 months of age. To our knowledge, this is the largest randomized trial ever undertaken in area of human milk and lactation. Monitoring visits of all experimental and control maternity hospitals and

Short and Long Term Effects of Breast Feeding on Child Health
Edited by Berthold Koletzko *et al.*, Kluwer Academic/Plenum Publishers, 2000

327

polyclinics were undertaken prior to recruitment and twice more during recruitment and follow-up to ensure compliance with the randomized allocation. Major study outcomes include the occurrence of ≥1 episode of gastrointestinal infection, ≥2 respiratory infections, and the duration of breastfeeding, and are analyzed according to randomized allocation ("intention to treat"). One of the 32 remaining study sites was dropped from the trial because of apparently falsified follow-up data, as suggested by an unrealistically low incidence of infection and unrealistically long duration of breastfeeding, and as confirmed by subsequent data audit of polyclinic charts and interviews with mothers of 64 randomly-selected study infants at the site. Smaller random audits at each of the remaining sites showed extremely high concordance between the PROBIT data forms and both the polyclinic charts and maternal interviews, with no evident difference in under- or over-reporting in experimental vs control sites. Of the 17,046 infants recruited from the 31 participating study sites, 16,491 (96.7%) completed the study and only 555 (3.3%) were lost to follow-up. PROBIT's results should help inform decision-making for clinicians, hospitals, industry, and governments concerning the support, protection, and promotion of breastfeeding.

1.   INTRODUCTION

The potentially beneficial infant and child health effects of breastfeeding have been studied primarily in relation to two common and important sources of morbidity: infection and atopic disease. Considerable research over the past few decades has suggested a protective effect of breastfeeding against a variety of infections during infancy and early childhood.[1-8] Artificial feedings may be contaminated by enteric pathogens, particularly in developing country settings; moreover, breast milk contains potentially protective serum IgA, lactoferrin, oligosaccharides, immunocompetent mononuclear cells, and cytokines. In an extensive overview of infant feeding studies, Feacham and Koblinsky noted median relative risks of 2 to 3 for diarrheal morbidity in nonbreast-fed infants; relative risks for diarrheal mortality were even higher.[3] Although the evidence is weaker, several reviews also suggest significant protection against respiratory infection.[1,2,5-8] The protective effect of breastfeeding appears to be more striking, and thus easier to demonstrate, in settings where poverty, malnutrition, and poor hygiene are prevalent.[1-4,6] Nonetheless, partial breastfeeding for at least 3 months may confer protection even in developed country settings; a Scottish study found that nonbreastfeeding or weaning before 3 months was associated with a doubling of the incidence of gastrointestinal infection and a 50% increase in the incidence of respiratory infection during infancy.[5]

The evidence that breastfeeding protects against atopic eczema, asthma, and other atopic diseases is far less convincing than that concerning infection, especially for infants not at elevated risk due to a positive atopic history in first-degree family members.[9]   The few well-controlled epidemiologic studies[10-14] of infants at average atopic risk have reported mixed results; the largest of these[14] (based on the 1970 British Births Survey) even suggests that breastfeeding may be associated with an *increased* risk of atopic eczema.

All of the scientific evidence regarding breastfeeding and morbidity in healthy, full-term infants is based on observational studies, because it is infeasible to randomly assign such infants to be breast-fed vs formula-fed. Such studies are plagued by a number of potential sources of analytic bias, including information bias, selection bias, confounding bias, and reverse causality bias.[15-18] The multiple sources of potential bias have created doubt about the importance, and even the existence, of a protective effect of breastfeeding against infection in developed country settings.[17] Several studies have attempted to overcome these biases,[5,19-21] but the results from developed countries have been inconsistent.[5,21]

The best solution for these multiple potential sources of bias is a randomized clinical trial design in which infectious morbidity is compared in infants randomly allocated to a breastfeeding promotion intervention. Because the analysis of a randomized trial is based on the randomly allocated treatment group ("intention to treat"), information bias stemming from misclassification of feeding-type will not affect group assignment. Nor can pre-randomization selection factors influence the treatment received. Random treatment allocation ensures that potential confounding factors are also distributed randomly, and reverse causality bias is avoided by ensuring that the intervention precedes the measured outcome.

Increasing breastfeeding initiation is an important public health objective, but women's decisions concerning the initial feeding of their infants are determined prenatally and often prior to becoming pregnant.[22-24] Moreover, although one randomized trial has demonstrated that prenatal counselling can increase breastfeeding initiation rates,[25] prenatal interventions are logistically difficult and expensive to implement on a community-wide scale.

Because of these considerations, it may be preferable to focus public health interventions on improving the duration and exclusivity of breastfeeding among women who decide to initiate breastfeeding. Most of these interventions are uncomplicated and inexpensive to implement, and WHO and UNICEF have joined together in promoting a Baby-Friendly Hospital Initiative (BFHI)[26] that recommends the following 10 steps: (1) all hospitals should have a written breastfeeding policy; (2) all staff should be trained in the skills necessary to implement the policy; (3) all pregnant women should be informed about the benefits and management of breastfeeding; (4) mothers should be helped to begin breastfeeding within half an hour after a normal birth; (5) health workers should know how to assist in starting breastfeeding and how to maintain lactation during temporary separations; (6) unless medically indicated, newborn babies should have breast milk only; (7) babies should remain with their mothers 24 hours a day ("rooming-in"); (8) breastfeeding on demand should be encouraged; (9) pacifiers should not be given; and (10) the establishment of breastfeeding support groups should be fostered, and mothers should be referred to them on discharge.

Several of these recommendations have been tested in formal controlled clinical trials, systematic reviews of which are available in the Cochrane Database of Systematic Reviews (CDSR). Based on overviews contained in the CDSR, a restricted feeding schedule (i.e., at most one feeding every 4 hours) (Step 8) is associated with a summary relative risk (RR) of 1.53 (95% confidence interval = 1.08-2.15) for weaning by 4-6 weeks and 1.23 (0.08-1.87) by 12 weeks.[27] Trials of postnatal support (with or without a prenatal component) (Step 10) include a variety of in-hospital and post-discharge intervention "packages" comprising education, positioning, counselling, and help with problems; the summary RR for the effect of these interventions is 0.74 (0.65-0.86) for weaning by 2 months and 0.92 (0.83-1.01) for weaning by 3 months.[28] Early initiation of breastfeeding (Step 4) is not as well supported by the evidence from controlled trials, however, with a single small trial reporting a RR of 0.84 (0.55-1.27) for weaning by 12 weeks.[29] Interventions for improving breastfeeding techniques (Step 5) appear effective [RR for weaning by 3 months = 0.43 (0.21-0.90)] based on a single small trial.[30] The only controlled clinical trial of which we are aware concerning in-hospital formula supplementation (Step 6) is our own, which failed to show any benefit of restricting supplementation [RR = 1.13 (0.92-1.38) for weaning by 9 weeks].[31,32] A recent trial of post-discharge formula supplementation also reported a null result.[33] To our knowledge, rooming-in (Step 7) has not been formally evaluated in controlled clinical trials. Considerable evidence from observational studies supports its efficacy, however[34-40]; moreover, demand feeding is much more difficult to achieve when babies do not room in with their mothers. Several recent observational studies,[41-44] but no clinical trials, suggest that the early use of pacifiers (Step 9) may increase the risk of early weaning.

PROBIT builds on the scientific evidence concerning the components of the BFHI. Not only does PROBIT provide the first rigorous evaluation of the BFHI as a "package," but the large number of infants and mothers studied provides the first opportunity to assess the direct relationship between ***any*** breastfeeding promotion intervention and infant health. Because it is infeasible to randomize women to different forms of infant feeding, no previous study has provided an experimental link between infant feeding and infant morbidity.

2. METHODS

2.1 Research Design

The design is a multicenter randomized clinical trial using cluster randomization. (Cluster randomization · was chosen over individual randomization in order to minimize the possibility of contamination, which would inevitably occur if individual women and infants with postpartum stays at the same maternity hospital and attending the same polyclinic were exposed to different interventions.) Maternity hospitals and their corresponding polyclinics (the outpatient clinics where children are followed up for routine child care and illnesses by pediatricians) were originally paired according to geographic region (Minsk city, Minsk region, Brest, Mogilev, Gomel, Vitebsk, and Grodno), urban vs rural status, number of deliveries per year (±500 if <2500, or ≥2500), and breastfeeding initiation rates at hospital discharge ($\pm5\%$). One member of each pair was selected at random to receive the WHO/UNICEF Baby-Friendly Hospital 18-hour training course, using a double-randomization procedure. First, a random number table was used to assign a 2-digit random number to each of the study hospitals. Within each pair, the hospital/polyclinic corresponding to the higher and lower numbers were assigned to interventions A and B, respectively. Then, at a public gathering of Canadian and Belarussian investigators, a coin flip determined that B would correspond to the experimental (BFHI) intervention, whereas A sites would correspond to the control intervention. Those sites randomized to the control intervention were asked to continue their then current hospital and polyclinic practices until completion of the trial.

2.2 Selection and Enrollment of Study Sites, Mothers, and Infants

Except for a few maternity hospitals that had already begun to implement changes called for in the BFHI and a few others located near the geographic areas contaminated by radionuclides from Chernobyl (many mothers from the latter areas were advised by pediatricians not to breast-feed their infants following the disaster), all remaining maternity hospitals and their corresponding polyclinics were considered eligible for inclusion. Most of the maternity hospitals located in large cities (Minsk, Vitebsk, Brest, and Mogilev) are affiliated with several polyclinics. To maximize efficiency, we limited enrollment to mothers whose infants were to be followed at single selected polyclinic affiliated with each of these large maternity hospitals.

Within the selected hospitals, mothers were considered eligible for participation if they expressed an intention to breastfeed on admission to the postpartum ward and had no illnesses that would contraindicate breastfeeding or severely compromise its success, such as HIV positivity, active hepatitis B, or tuberculosis, coma, respiratory disease requiring mechanical ventilation, life-threatening infection, psychosis, or treatment with radionuclides or cancer chemotherapeutic agents. Infants were considered eligible for participation if they were singletons born at ≥ 37 weeks gestation, weighed at least 2500 grams, had Apgar scores ≥ 5 at 5 minutes, and had no conditions or illnesses during their postpartum hospital stay that were likely to interfere with normal breastfeeding (severe congenital anomaly, galactosemia, phenylketonuria, need for exchange transfusion or mechanical ventilation, or neurological condition interfering with their ability to suck or swallow).

Each eligible breastfeeding mother was given an information sheet informing her that the hospital was participating in a study of the effects of alternative hospital practices on infant feeding and health and that if she consented to participate, she would be asked questions on her infant's feeding and infectious illness episodes during the infant's routine health visits during the first year of life. Signed consent was obtained from all participating mothers.

2.3   Intervention

Participants from each of the experimental maternity hospitals and polyclinics (usually the head obstetrician and head pediatrician, respectively) received the 18-hour BFHI lactation management training course, which was organized by the European Regional Office of the World Health Organization. The objectives of this course were to assist hospitals in transforming their maternity facilities into baby-friendly institutions that implement the "Ten Steps to Successful Breastfeeding" and to help equip them with the knowledge to make lasting policy changes.

The 18 course hours are designed to provide a sufficient period to cover the key concepts and teach the essential skills. The course consisted of 14 lessons of 75 minutes each, with an additional 1-hour introductory lesson. Six of the lessons included a 30-minute clinical practice session. Textbooks, articles, videos, and teaching aids supplemented the course material provided. Each lesson had specified learning objectives, a lesson summary, and a self-test. Alternative learning activities were provided, including role playing, case studies, discussions, pair practice, form completion, and the viewing of illustrations and slides.

Step 10, the establishment of breastfeeding support groups to help mothers and infants following discharge from the maternity hospitals, depends on local circumstances, such as the existence of woman-to-woman support groups (e.g., La Leche League), trained community health nurses or lactation consultants, or specialized lactation clinics. Since none of these sources of breastfeeding support were available in Belarus, Step 10 focused on the experimental polyclinics, where the chief pediatricians were trained in methods of maintaining lactation, promoting exclusive and prolonged breastfeeding, and resolving common problems.

Full implementation of the intervention required at least 12 months to train all midwives, nurses, and physicians caring for study mothers and infants. After the 18-hour training course, the trial participant (usually the chief obstetrician) from the maternity hospital organized and implemented training programs for the midwives, nurses, and physicians working on the postpartum ward at his or her experimental hospital. The corresponding polyclinic participant (usually the chief pediatrician) organized and implemented a similar training program for all pediatricians, felchers (nurse-practitioners), and nurses working at the polyclinics. Monitoring visits by members of the Canadian and Belarussian Executive Committees prior to beginning recruitment at each site ensured that the hospital and polyclinic procedures and policies were consistent with the BFHI at the experimental sites, and that the control sites understood their role as controls and did not institute any changes that would render their maternity hospitals or polyclinics more baby-friendly. No control maternity hospital or polyclinic, however, was asked to "retrench," i.e., to undo changes they had already implemented prior to randomization. Monitoring visits were also undertaken once during the recruitment period and again (for the polyclinics only) during infant follow-up.

2.4   Data Collection

Data collection included information obtained both during the postpartum stay and following discharge, until each study infant reached 12 months of age. Study investigators at each maternity hospital completed an enrollment form indicating name, sociodemographic information (age, marital status, number of children <5 years living in the household, maternal and paternal education and occupation, and maternal cigarette smoking during pregnancy), general medical and obstetric history, details on feeding received during hospitalization, and telephone and other contact information. Then, at scheduled visits at 1, 2, 3, 6, 9, and 12 months, polyclinic pediatricians completed a data sheet containing information relative to infant feeding (in particular, whether the infant was still breast-fed; if so, whether exclusively or partially; and details on receipt of other liquids and solid foods in the child's diet); measurement of infant weight, length, and head circumference; and the occurrence of symptoms of gastrointestinal or respiratory infection, rash, other illness, and hospitalization since birth or the most frequent clinic visit.

Each month, the polyclinic-based study investigators sent copies of the follow-up data forms to the Data Center in Minsk, where the data were coded and entered into a dBase program with built-in checks for missing data and logical inconsistencies, which was designed by the Randomized Clinical Trial Unit (RCTU) at the Jewish General Hospital in Montreal. Missing or inconsistent data were promptly signaled by the supervisor of the Data Center in Minsk to the polyclinic-based investigator to ensure that the correct data were obtained and entered in the database. Updated copies of the database were sent electronically to the RCTU every 1-2 months.

2.5   Study Outcomes (End-Points)

The hypothesis tested was whether the BFHI-based intervention is effective in creating sufficient support for breastfeeding mothers and infants (relative to those sites not receiving the intervention) to prolong the duration of breastfeeding and, as a consequence, reduce infectious morbidity during the first 12 months of life. The primary study outcome was the risk of one or more episodes of gastrointestinal infection. Secondary outcomes included the risk of 2 or more episodes of any respiratory infection, 2 or more upper respiratory infections, atopic eczema, and recurrent (≥ 2 episodes) of wheezing; the prevalence of any breastfeeding at 3,6,9, and 12 months of age; and the prevalence of exclusive and predominant breastfeeding at 3 and 6 months. Classification of breastfeeding as "exclusive" or "predominant" was based on WHO definitions[45] applied to the cross-sectional infant feeding information at 1, 2, 3, and 6 months. The criteria for gastrointestinal and upper respiratory infection were based on the algorithms of Rubin et al,[21] modified to ensure a minimum duration of 48 hours. Rashes were considered to represent atopic eczema if they lasted at least 2 weeks or recurred after clearing for at least 1 week, were itchy, and occurred on the face and/or the extensor surfaces of the arms and/or the extensor surfaces of the legs.

2.6   Sample Size

Sample size was calculated based on estimates of the proportion of babies breast-fed (partially or exclusively) at 3 months, the effect of the intervention on increasing that proportion, and the effect of breastfeeding duration on reducing infectious morbidity.   From a prior Belarussian Ministry of Health survey, we estimated that 50% of women who initially breastfed at the control (non-intervention hospitals) would still be breastfeeding (to *any* degree) at 3 months. Based on the available evidence concerning the effectiveness of the individual components of the BFHI, we anticipated that the intervention would reduce breastfeeding discontinuation by 3 months from 50% to 35%, i.e., that 65% of mothers exposed to the intervention vs 65% of mothers not exposed to the intervention would still be breastfeeding their infants (to some degree) at 3 months. Three months of any breastfeeding was chosen as the primary basis for calculating breastfeeding prevalence based on the data of Howie et al[5]; in initially breast-fed infants who were weaned at 13 weeks vs those breast-fed any degree and for at least 13 weeks, the relative risk of gastrointestinal infection (the primary outcome) associated with early weaning was approximately 2.

Based on evidence available at the time we planned the trial, we estimated that approximately 60% of Belarussian infants would experience at least one gastrointestinal infection in the first year of life. Given a relative risk of 2 and the (control) 50:50 split of breastfeeders to nonbreastfeeders at 3 months, this overall 60% figure translated into proportions of infants experienceing one or more episodes of gastrointestinal infection of approximately 40% and 80%, respectively [(.50)(.40)+(.50)(.80)=.60]. If the experimental intervention was successful in changing the split of breastfeeders to nonbreastfeeders from 50:50 to 65:35, then the corresponding overall proportion of infants in the experimental group with one or more episodes of gastrointestinal infection was expected to be (.65)(.40)+(.35)(.80)=.54.

Because the design is based on randomizing clusters rather than individuals, we anticipated the unit of statistical analysis would be the hospital/polyclinic study site. We therefore used sample size techniques for paired cluster randomization,[46] following an approach similar to that employed in a large community-based study of smoking cessation.[47]   In addition to the elements involved in usual sample size estimates, factors to be considered in this context are the variation in outcome between unpaired clusters (study sites), the effect of matching in reducing this variation, and the size of the clusters (number of subjects per site), which was expected to vary considerably by site.

Under the null hypothesis, the average proportion of infants with one or more episodes of gastrointestinal infection was expected to be .60. We assumed three different degrees of variability between (unpaired) study sites for this proportion: 95% would be expected to have values between .50 and .70 (high variability), .52 and .68 (moderate variability), or .54 and .66 (low variability). These 95% ranges correspond to approximate standard deviations (σ) of .05, .04, and .03, respectively, assuming an approximately normal underlying distribution. In addition, we considered three different degrees of "success" in pairing, as reflected by the within-pair correlation coefficient, ρ: ineffective pairing ($\rho=0$), moderately effective pairing ($\rho=.4$), and highly effective pairing ($\rho=.7$). Even if matching was ineffective, the relative efficiency of a paired analysis to an unpaired analysis would still be .90.[48]

Assuming 500 infants enrolled at each maternity hospital, a design using 15 pairs of study sites would provide a power of greater than 80% to detect a significant difference between the two groups at a 2-sided α-level of 0.05, even assuming a "worst-case scenario" of high variability ($\sigma=.05$) between (unpaired) sites and totally ineffective pairing ($\rho=0$), provided that the risk of one or more episodes of gastrointestinal infection was in fact reduced to half by prolonged (≥3 months) breastfeeding. The design also provided power of over 80% to detect a halving of the prevalence of 2 or more respiratory infections from an assumed level of 60%, for $\sigma \leq.04$, and only marginally effective matching ($\rho \geq0.25$). The design ensured well over 90% power to detect an increase in prevalence of any breastfeeding from 50 to 65% at 3 months and from 25 to 30% at 6 months, and an increase in predominant breastfeeding from 35 to 50% at 3 months. Owing to the infrequency of hospital admission and (especially) death for infectious illnesses, we anticipated that even this large sample size (500 infants per site x 30 sites = 15,000) would be insufficient to detect differences in hospitalization rates or death from infection.

In order to ensure that 15 hospital pairs would be included in the final study sample, we randomized 17 pairs to provide a margin of security against withdrawals or unforeseen logistical problems at a few hospitals. As it turned out, two of the maternity hospitals (one experimental and one control) refused to carry out their allocated intervention following randomization. Moledechno Maternity Hospital (Minsk region) was allocated to the control intervention and refused to stop its efforts to become more baby-friendly. Luninets Maternity Hospital (Brest region) claimed to be unable to physically arrange its maternity wards to accommodate rooming-in and was therefore unwilling to accept its assignment to the experimental intervention. We then re-paired the remaining hospitals from these two original pairs, Soligorsk (experimental, Minsk region) and Stolin (control, Brest region).

3.   RESULTS

3.1   Cohort Recruitment and Retention

Recruitment began in June 1996, with gradual phase-in over the ensuing months, so that by October at all 32 remaining randomized sites (including the two re-paired sites) were recruiting mothers and infants. To ensure an adequate sample size at each of the study sites, recruitment continued until the end of December 1997. A total of 17,795 mothers were recruited at the 32 sites, making this (to our knowledge) the largest randomized trial ever undertaken in the area of human milk and lactation.

By early 1998, it became obvious to the Data Center in Minsk that one of the study sites, Novopolotsk, was reporting durations of breastfeeding that were far longer, and incidences of all infectious illnesses that were far lower, than any of the other study sites, be they experimental or control. Because of the strong suspicion that the Novopolotsk follow-up data had been falsified, we conducted an audit of 64 randomly-selected polyclinic charts and maternal interviews (by telephone or in person) in an effort to substantiate this suspicion. The audit compared the occurrence of one or more gastrointestinal infections and two or more respiratory infections according to the audit source (polyclinic chart or maternal interview) and the PROBIT study data forms. For breastfeeding at 3 months, agreement was considered present if the date of weaning in the polyclinic chart or by maternal interview was within ± 15 days of the date recorded on the PROBIT polyclinic visit forms. The results of the Novopolotsk audit are shown in Table 1 and confirm that the data recorded on the PROBIT follow-up forms substantially underestimated the incidence of both gastrointestinal and respiratory infections and grossly overestimated the duration of breastfeeding in the audited infants. Novopolotsk was therefore dropped from the trial.

Of the 17,046 subjects recruited from the 31 remaining study sites, 16,491 (96.7%) completed the study and only 555 (3.3%) were lost to follow-up. Table 2 lists the 31 sites, along with the number of subjects recruited and lost to follow-up at each. As shown in Table 3, the ages at which study infants actually attended their scheduled polyclinic visits at 1, 2, 3, 6, 9, and 12 months were extremely close to the target ages in both the experimental and control groups.

3.2   Routine Data Validation

Although no suspicion arose with respect to data validity from the remaining 31 sites, a routine audit of data validity had been planned at each. The procedure was similar to the audit carried out in Novopolotsk, although on a more modest scale. At each polyclinic, 20 polyclinic charts were selected at random, and the data contained therein bearing on gastrointestinal infections, respiratory infections, and breastfeeding at 3 months data were compared with the data on these outcomes recorded on the PROBIT polyclinic visit forms. Of the 20 audited polyclinic charts, maternal interviews were also carried out in 10. As shown in Table 4, chance-corrected agreement was high for all three outcomes, as shown by the high levels of kappa, and there was no difference in degree of over- or under-estimation according to experimental vs control status.

4.   DISCUSSION

In order for the BFHI-based training program to have an impact on reducing infectious morbidity, it must first be successful in altering maternity and polyclinic hospital practices; those practices must then effect an increase in the duration and/or degree of breastfeeding; finally, the increased duration or degree of breastfeeding must then protect the infant against infection, in general, and gastrointestinal infection, in particular. Each of these links must operate in order for our intervention to be successful in reducing infectious morbidity. Only by building in these multiple links, however, can one use a randomized experimental design to assess the "real-world" effectiveness of an intervention to promote breastfeeding in improving infant health.

After all, the potential protective effects of prolonged breastfeeding will remain largely unrealized unless we are successful in promoting it. PROBIT therefore provides an essential scientific underpinning not only for the WHO/UNICEF Baby-Friendly Hospital Initiative, but for all future breastfeeding promotion interventions in both developed and developing country settings. PROBIT was carried out in Belarus for several important reasons. Maternity hospital practices in Belarus, like those in many other former Soviet republics, resembled those in much of North America and

Western Europe several decades ago. Although the effectiveness of the intervention is therefore likely to be more effective in Belarus than it would be in western industrialized countries, such a setting provides an opportunity to examine the direct experimental link between the duration of breastfeeding and infectious morbidity. That experimental link should be generalizable to western countries, since basic health services, sanitary conditions, and other features in Belarus that may modify the effect of breastfeeding are quite similar to those in the West. PROBIT's results should therefore help inform decision-making for clinicians, hospitals, industry, and governments throughout the world concerning the support, protection, and promotion of breastfeeding.

Table 1. Results of Audit at Novopolotsk

	Polyclinic Chart	Maternal Interview
≥ Gastrointestinal Infection		
Kappa (95% CI)	.25 (.02 to .48)	.21 (.00 to .43)
Under-reporting	23%	27%
Over-reporting	3%	3%
≥2 Respiratory Infections		
Kappa (95% CI)	.39 (.19 to .58)	.42 (.19 to .65)
Under-reporting	27%	20%
Over-reporting	0%	2%
Breastfeeding at 3 Months		
Kappa (95% CI)	-.04 (-.11 to +.04)	-.04 (-.11 to +.04)
Under-reporting	2%	2%
Over-reporting	50%	44%

Table 2. Enrollment and Losses to Follow-Up at 31 Study Sites

Pair	Control	Enrolled	Lost to Follow-Up	%
1	Minsk No. 1	326	40	12.3
2	Stolin	666	18	2.7
3	Kobrin	930	5	0.5
4	Baranovitchi	747	23	3.1
5	Novopolotsk	(dropped from study)		
6	Lepel	250	8	3.2
7	Glubokoe	340	7	2.1
8	Zhlobin	799	28	3.5
9	Svetlogorsk	940	13	1.4
10	Mosty	373	3	0.8
11	Berestovitsa	232	6	2.6
12	Ostrovets	364	10	2.7
13	Volkovysk	921	2	0.2
14	Minsk regional	522	63	12.1
15	Mstislavl	310	3	1.0
16	Bobruisk	461	29	6.3
	Total	8181	258	3.2
Pair	Experimental	Enrolled	Lost to Follow-Up	%
1	Minsk No. 6	263	28	10.6
2	Soligorsk	1180	11	0.9
3	Bereuza	249	7	2.8
4	Brest	1002	74	7.4
5	Vitebsk	268	8	3.0
6	Novolukoml	250	3	1.2
7	Dokshitsy	330	7	2.1
8	Rogatchev	583	14	2.4
9	Retchitsa	1108	20	1.8
10	Shchuchin	688	19	2.8
11	Svislotch	308	11	3.6
12	Oshmiany	533	25	4.7
13	Slonim	530	13	2.5
14	Borisov	731	20	2.7
15	Klimovitchi	371	13	3.5
16	Mogilev	471	24	5.1
	Total	8865	297	3.4

Table 3. Age (in Days) at Polyclinic Visits

SCHEDULED VISIT				
Experimental Sites	Target	Median	5%ile	95%ile
1 month	30	32	28	41
2 months	61	62	57	71
3 months	91	93	89	112
6 months	183	185	176	210
9 months	274	275	266	305
12 months	365	367	360	383
Control Sites				
1 month	30	31	28	38
2 months	61	62	57	70
3 months	91	93	89	103
6 months	183	184	177	202
9 months	274	275	267	294
12 months	365	367	361	382

Table 4. Audit Results

	Polyclinic Chart		Maternal Interview	
≥1 Gastrointestinal Infection	Experimental	Control	Experimental	Control
Kappa (95% CI)	.91 (.83-.99)	.85 (.76-.94)	.76 (.61-.92)	.74 (.57-.90)
Under-reporting	1%	2%	3%	2%
Over-reporting	1%	1%	1%	4%
≥2 Respiratory Infections				
Kappa (95% CI)	.77 (.70-.85)	.86 (.80-.92)	.65 (.54-.77)	.63 (.51-.75)
Under-reporting	8%	5%	6%	4%
Over-reporting	3%	2%	11%	15%
Breastfeeding at 3 Months				
Kappa (95% CI)	.93 (.88-.98)	.91 (.87-.96)	.89 (.81-.97)	.94 (.89-.99)
Under-reporting	2%	2%	3%	1%
Over-reporting	1%	2%	1%	2%

ACKNOWLEDGMENTS

The authors gratefully acknowedge the contribution of the numerous obstetricians, pediatricians, nurses, midwives, and felchers who helped in implementing the PROBIT intervention and/or in data collection, and that of the nearly 18,000 mothers and infants who participated as subjects. Dr. Kramer is a Distinguished Scientist of the Medical Research Council of Canada.

OTHER PARTICIPATING MEMBERS OF THE PROBIT STUDY GROUP

Baranovitchi: S. Pleskatch
Berestovitsa: D. Iodkovskaya
Bereuza: S. Prihodovskaya, V. Verzhbitskaya
Bobruisk: T. Tichontchouk
Borisov: G. Khotko, Z. Liamkina
Brest: T. Avdeitchouk, A. Tcherenkevich
Dokshitsy: T. Kiva, Z. Solovjeva
Glubokoe: L. Smolskaya
Klimovitchi: A. Lazarenko, E. Pogodkina
Kobrin: L. Cheveleva
Lepel: G. Kovalevskaya
Minsk: N. Charangovitch, L. Degtiareva, L. Kebikova, L. Lazouta
Mogilev: R. Iaroutskaya, G. Ivanova
Mosty: L. Dorochevitch
Mstislavl: I. Rogatch
Novolukoml: T. Nabedo, V. Savitskaya
Oshmiany: G. Boudilovitch, I. Boulko
Ostrovets: A. Lavrentjeva
Retchitsa: V. Minkova, N. Sentchouk
Rogatchev: M. Kravtsova, L. Tcherkachina
Shchutchin: L. Bout-Gousaim, E. Koutchoun
Slonim: R. Orotchko, A. Tourly
Soligorsk: M. Kotlarova, L. Perepetchko
Stolin: R. Misioura
Svetlogorsk: N. Kotoukhova
Svislotch: P. Mosko, V. Shota
Vitebsk: E. Avsiouk, N. Belousova
Volkovysk: Y. Makovetskaya
Zhlobin: Z. Bisoukova

REFERENCES

1. Kovar MG, Serdula MG, Marks JS, et al. Review of the epidemiologic evidence for an association between infant feeding and infant health. Pediatrics 1984;74:615-638.

2. Jason JM, Nieburg P, Marks JS. Mortality and infectious disease associated with infant-feeding practices in developing countries. Pediatrics 1984;74:702-727.

3. Feachem RG, Koblinsky MA. Interventions for the control of diarrhoeal diseases among young children: promotion of breast feeding. Bull WHO 1984;62:271-291.

4. Kramer MS. Infant feeding, infection, and public health. Pediatrics 1988;81:164-166.

5. Howie PW, Forsyth JS, Ogston SA, Clark A, du V Florey C. Protective effect of breast feeding against infection. Br Med J 1990;300:11-16.

6. Cunningham AS, Jelliffe DB, Jelliffe EFP. Breast-feeding and health in the 1980's: a global epidemiologic review. J Pediatr 1991;118:659-666.

7. Beaudry M, Dufour R, Marcoux S. Relation between infant feeding and infections during the first six months of life. J Pediatr 1995;126:191-7.

8. Dewey KG, Heinig MJ, Nommsen-Rivers LA. Differences in morbidity between breast-fed and formula-fed infants. J Pediatr 1995;126:696-702.

9. Kramer MS. Does breast feeding help protect against atopic disease? Biology, methodology, and a golden jubilee of controversy. J Pediatr 1988;112:181-190.

10. Saarinen UM, Backman A, Kajosaari M, Simes MA. Prolonged breast-feeding as prophylaxis for atopic disease. Lancet 1979;ii:163-166.

11. Fergusson DM, Horwood LJ, Beautrais AL, Shannon FT, Taylor B. Eczema and infant diet. Clin Allergy 1981;11:325-331.

12. Hide DW, Guyer BM. Clinical manifestations of allergy related to breast and cows' milk feeding. Arch Dis Child 1981;56:172-175.

13. Kramer MS, Moroz B. Do breast feeding and delayed introduction of solid foods protect against subsequent atopic eczema? J Pediatr 1981;98:546-550.

14. Taylor B, Wadsworth J, Golding J, Butler N. Breast feeding, eczema, asthma, and hayfever. J Epidemiol Comm Health 1983;37:95-99.

15. Hill AB: A Short Textbook of Medical Statistics. London, Hodder & Stoughton, 1977, p 27.

16. Sauls HS. Potential effect of demographic and other variables in studies comparing morbidity of breast-fed and bottle-fed infants. Pediatrics 1979;64:523-527.

17. Bauchner H, Leventhal JM, Shapiro ED. Studies of breast-feeding and infections: how good is the evidence? JAMA 1986;256:887-892.

18. Kramer MS. Breast feeding and child health: methodologic issues in epidemiologic research. In: Goldman A, Hanson L, Atkinson S, eds. The Effects of Human Milk Upon the Recipient Infant. New York: Plenum Press, 1987:339-360.

19. Habicht J-P, DaVanzo J, Butz WP. Does breastfeeding really save lives, or are apparent benefits due to biases? Am J Epidemiol 1986;123:279-290.

20. Victora CG, Vaughan JP, Lambardi C, Fuchs SMC, Gigante LP, Smith PG, Nobre LC, Teixeira AMB, Moreira LB, Barros FC. Evidence for protection by breast-feeding against infant deaths from infectious diseases in Brazil. Lancet 1987;2:319-322.

21. Rubin DH, Leventhal JM, Krasilnikoff PA, Kuo HS, Jekel JF, Weile B, Levee A, Kurzon M, Berget A. Relationship between infant feeding and infectious illness: a prospective study of infants during the first year of life. Pediatrics 1990;85:464-471.

22. American Academy of Pediatrics. The promotion of breast-feeding. Pediatrics 1982;69:654-661.

23. Kramer MS, Gray-Donald K. Breast feeding promotion: methodologic issues in health services research. Geneva: World Health Organization, Document MCH/86.13,1988:21-38.

24. Birenbaum E, Fuchs C, Reichman B. Demographic factors influencing the initiation of breast-feeding in an Israeli urban population. Pediatrics 1989;83:519-523.

25. Kistin N, Benton D, Rao S, Sullivan M. Breast-feeding rates among black low-income women: effect of prenatal education. Pediatrics 1990;86:741-746.

26. WHO/UNICEF. Protecting, promoting and supporting breastfeeding: the special role of maternity services. Geneva: WHO, 1989.

27. Renfrew MJ, Lang S. Feeding schedules in hospitals for newborn infants. (Cochrane Review). In: The Cochrane Library, Issue 2, 1999. Oxford: Update Software.

28. Sikorski J, Renfrew MJ. Support for breastfeeding mothers. (Cochrane Review). In: The Cochrane Library, Issue 2, 1999. Oxford: Update Software.

29. Renfrew MJ, Lang S. Early vs delayed initiation of breastfeeding. (Cochrane Review). In: The Cochrane Library, Issue 2, 1999. Oxford: Update Software.

30. Renfrew MJ, Lang S. Interventions for improving breastfeeding technique. (Cochrane Review). In: The Cochrane Library, Issue 2, 1999. Oxford: Update Software.

31. Gray-Donald K, Kramer MS, Munday S, Leduc DG. Effect of formula supplementation in the hospital on the duration of breast feeding: a controlled clinical trial. Pediatrics 1985;75:514-518.

32. Gray-Donald K, Kramer MS. Causality inference in observational vs experimental studies: an empirical comparison. Am J Epidemiol 1988;27:885-892.

33. Cronenwett L, Stukel T, Kearney M, Barrett J, Covington C, Del Monte K, Reindhardt R, Rippe L. Single daily bottle use in the early weeks postpartum and breastfeeding outcomes. Pediatrics 1992;90:760-766.

34. McBryde A, Durham NC. Compulsory rooming-in the ward and private newborn service at Duke Hospital. JAMA 1951;145:625-627.

35. Jackson EB, Wilkin LC, Auerbach H. Statistical report on incidence and duration of breastfeeding in relation to personal social and hospital maternity factors. Pediatrics 36.1956;17:700-713.

36. Cole JP. Breast-feeding in the Boston suburbs in relation to personal-social factors. Clin Pediatr 1977;37:89-94.

37. Starling J, Fergusson DM, Horwood LJ, Taylor B. Breast-feeding success and failure. Aust Paediatr J 1979;15:271-274.

38. Verronen P, Visakorpi JK, Lammi A, Saarikoski S, Tamminen T. Promotion of breast feeding: effect on neonates of change of feeding routine at a maternity unit. Acta Paediatr Scand 1980;69:279-282.

39. World Health Organization. Contemporary Patterns of Breast-feeding: Report of the WHO Collaborative Study on Breast-feeding. Geneva: World Health Organization (WHO), 1981.

40. Bloom K, Goldbloom RB, Robinson SC, Stevens FE. II. Factors affecting the continuance of breast-feeding. Acta Paediatr Scand 1982;300 (Suppl):9-14.

41. Richard L, Alade MO. Sucking technique and its effect on success of breastfeeding. Birth 1992;19:185-189.

42. Victora CG, Tomasi E, Olinto MTA, Barros FC. Use of pacifiers and breastfeeding duration. Lancet 1993;341:404-406.

43. Barros FC, Victora CG, Semer TC, Filho ST, Tomasi E, Weiderpass E. Use of pacifiers is associated with decreased breastfeeding duration. Pediatrics 1995;95:497-499.

44. Gale CR, Martyn CN. Dummies and the health of Hertfordshire infants, 1911-1930. Soc Social Hist Med 1995;8:231-255.

45. World Health Organization. Indicators for assessing breast-feeding practices. WHO Document WHO/CDD/SER/91.14. Geneva: World Health Organization, 1991.

46. Shipley MJ, Smith PG, Dramaix M. Calculation of power for matched pair studies when randomization is by group. Int J Epidemiol 1989;18:457-461.

47. Gail MH, Byar DP, Pechacek TF, Corle DK. Aspects of statistical design for the community intervention trial for smoking cessation (COMMIT). Cont Clin Trials 1992;13:6-21.

48. Snedecor GW, Cochran WG. Statistical Methods, 6th ed. Ames: Iowa State University Press, 1967, p 311.

29

PROVISION OF SUPPLEMENTARY FLUIDS TO BREAST FED INFANTS AND LATER BREAST FEEDING SUCCESS

[1]Christian Kind, [2]Gregor Schubiger, [2]Uwe Schwarz, and [2]Otmar Tönz
[1] Ostschweizer Kinderspital, CH-9006 St. Gallen, Switzerland: [2] Kinderspital, CH-6000 Luzern 16, Switzerland

Key words: Breast feeding, supplementary feeding, pacifier use, randomized controlled trial

Abstract: It has been shown that altering hospital policies in a way to avoid interference of routine prescriptions with initiation of breast feeding and to provide active encouragement to mothers and personnel can result in significant benefit for later breast feeding success. It is less clear, however, which of the elements of a promotional programme such as UNICEF/WHO's "ten steps to successful breast feeding" are absolutely essential and which can be adapted to local cultural   habits.
We performed an open randomized multicenter study in Switzerland to evaluate, whether restriction of supplementary fluids for breast fed infants in the first week of life and strict avoidance of artificial teats and pacifiers affects later breast feeding success. Follow up to 6 months was ensured by mailed questionnaires.
602 mother infant pairs were enrolled. Of 294 infants in the intervention group 39% were excluded from the final analysis because of protocol violations, mainly maternal request for the use of pacifiers or bottles. Though the number of dextrin maltose supplements during the first two days (1.7 vs. 2.2 on day 1, 2.2 vs. 2.6 on day 2) and the percentage of infants receiving any supplement (85% vs. 96.6%) was significantly smaller in the intervention group, the difference was disappointingly small. The prevalence of breast feeding was 100% vs. 99% at day 5, 88% vs. 88% at 2 months, 75% vs. 71% at 4 months and 57% vs. 55% at 6 months, none of the differences being significant. We conclude that rigorous adherence to all of the ten steps may encounter obstinate resistance from cultural habits even in a population highly favourable to breast feeding. An improvement in adherence does not necessarily lead to better breast feeding success. The results of the few comparable studies in the literature show also that cultural practices during the first months of life may

Short and Long Term Effects of Breast Feeding on Child Health
Edited by Berthold Koletzko *et al.*, Kluwer Academic/Plenum Publishers, 2000

influence profoundly the long term effects of interventions during the first days of life

1.   INTRODUCTION

The relationship between maternity ward practices and later breast feeding success has been the subject of a growing number of observational and, to a lesser degree, also interventional studies. It has become increasingly clear that hospital policies avoiding interference of routine prescriptions with initiation of breast feeding and providing active encouragement to mothers and personnel, e.g. according to the World Health Organization (WHO) and United Nations Children's Fund (UNICEF)'s "ten steps to successful breast feeding"[1], can result in significant benefit for later breast feeding success. However, scientific evidence for the effectiveness of the different elements of this promotional programme varies considerably[2]. In the Swiss context the introduction of step 6 "Give newborn infants no food or drink other than breast milk, unless medically indicated" and step 9 "Give no artificial teats or pacifiers (also called dummies or soothers) to breast feeding infants" has met considerable resistance. For this reason, a summary of the available evidence for the effectiveness of these two interventions and some reflections on the usefulness of their enforcement will be presented in the following text.

There is ample evidence that the early provision of supplementary fluids to breast fed infants and the introduction of pacifiers is associated with lower rates of long term breast feeding[1]. These findings from many observational studies may easily lead to the assumption that interventions suppressing the availability of supplements in maternity wards and prohibiting the use of pacifiers will predictably increase breast feeding success. However, this conclusion is erroneous, and overzealous attempts in this direction may remind of the German proverb referring to people who are "beating the sack while meaning the donkey". There are two main reasons why interventions reducing the availability of supplements may fail. Firstly, early use of supplements may be a marker rather than a cause of breast feeding difficulties. Causation can only be demonstrated by controlled, preferably randomized, interventional trials. Secondly, mothers may be unwilling to accept an intervention running against the beliefs and practices of their cultural background. Thus even an intervention with proven efficacy will probably fail, if it is not adapted to the cultural habits of the target population.

2.   SWISS MULTICENTER RANDOMIZED TRIAL

Study design

1994 a randomized controlled study was started in 10 Swiss maternities to study the following question[3]:

Does the restriction of fluid supplementation and the elimination of any use of artificial nipples and pacifiers during the first 5 days of life in healthy breast fed term infants increase the duration of complete and partial breast feeding?

The following centers and individuals participated in the study: Bern (D. Durrer), Fribourg (F. Besson), Luzern Kantonsspital (G. Schubiger), Luzern St. Anna (F. Auf der Maur), Morges (J.-M. Choffat), Olten (I. Hämmerli), St. Gallen (C. Kind), Winterthur (R. Hürlimann), Zürich Pflegerinnenschule (P. Baeckert), Zürich Universitätsspital (D. Mieth). Participating centers all had established breast feeding promotion programmes with early initiation, unrestricted rooming-in, restricted use of formula supplements and attending lactation consultants.

Healthy full term infants (37 weeks gestation or more, birth weight 2750 - 4200g) born to mothers intending to stay a minimum of 5 days postpartum in the hospital and planning to breast feed for at least 3 months were eligible. After obtaining maternal informed consent mother-child pairs were randomized by picking the next sealed envelope to one of two groups:

– *Experimental group*: no supplemental fluids, unless medically indicated, given by cup or spoon, no bottles, artificial teats or pacifiers. Fluid supplementation with 10% dextrin-maltose solution was considered to be medically indicated in the presence of one of the following: baby agitated or screaming after breast feeding, signs of dehydration or hypoglycemia.

– *Control group*: supplemental fluids offered on a regular basis by bottle, pacifier use was unrestricted.

The experimental regimen was kept for 5 days, after which feeding methods were left to maternal choice. During the hospital stay frequency of breast feeding and supplementation, sucking behaviour and weight were recorded daily. Follow-up information was collected at 2, 4 and 6 months of age by mailed questionnaires on breast feeding, introduction of supplements and use of a pacifier. Missing informations were completed by telefone interviews.

Assuming an average breast feeding rate of 90% at age 2 months it was estimated that a sample size of 235 infants in each group would give the study a power $(1-\beta)$ of 95% to detect a 10% difference in breast feeding rate with a two-tailed α of 0.05. About the same sample size would give a power of 90% to detect a 15% difference in breast feeding rate at 6 months assuming an average of 50% for this age group. In anticipation of frequent protocol violations it was planned to enrol a total of 600 infants.

Results

A total of 602 mother-child pairs were enrolled into the study. Randomization resulted in equal distribution of gender, birth weight, gestational age, maternal age, parity and percentage of cesarean section (10.1% vs. 10.2%) among the two study groups. However, a much higher number of mother-child pairs had to be excluded from the analysis for protocol violations, mainly maternal request for a pacifier or more rarely a bottle for supplementary feedings (Table 1). Rate of follow up for assessment of breast feeding status was not significantly different between the two groups.

Table 1. Study population and results from days 1 to 5

	Experimental group	Control group
Number randomized	294	308
Lost to follow up	23	13
Protocol violations	114	17
Never received supplements	8.3%	3.4%*
Number of DM supplements:		
Day 1 (mean/child)	1.7	2.2*
Day 2 (mean/child)	2.2	2.6*

* p < 0.05

While a significant reduction in the amount of dextrin-maltose-supplementation was achieved, its extent was relatively modest, and only a minority of children in the experimental group did not receive any supplements. No differences were observed in perceived sucking behaviour, neonatal weight loss, and incidence of fever or phototherapy.

Results for breast feeding rates during follow up are shown in Fig. 1.

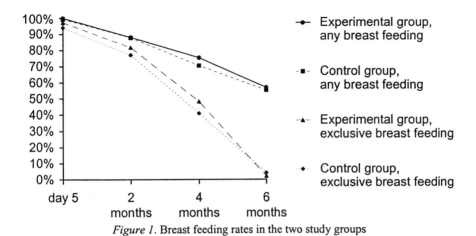

Figure 1. Breast feeding rates in the two study groups

There was no significant difference between the experimental group and the study group at any time during follow up neither for any breast feeding nor for exclusive breast feeding. An analysis extended to all mother-child pairs originally randomized (intention to treat analysis) yielded essentially unchanged results. Pacifier use at 2 and 4 months was not significantly different between groups and ranged between 69% and 76%.

3.   OTHER STUDIES ON SUPPLEMENTATION

An extensive medline search for reports on interventional studies examining the effect of restricting supplementary fluids during the first week of life on duration of breast feeding yielded two articles.

Gray-Donald et al performed a controlled prospective study of formula restriction on 781 infants in two maternity wards in Montreal, Canada[4]. In one ward a night bottle of formula was routinely offered, whereas in the other mothers were awakened for breast feeding. Breast feeding rates at 4 weeks (71% vs. 68%) and 9 weeks (55% vs. 54%) were not significantly different, but weight loss was slightly but significantly greater in the formula-restricted group (6.0% vs. 5.1%).

Martin-Calama et al have recently published their randomized controlled trial of glucose water supplementation conducted in the maternity hospital of Teruel, Spain[5]. 180 healthy full term infants were randomized by a procedure not specified in the article to an unsupplemented group and a glucose water group, being offered glucose water if hungry after breast feeding. The actual amount of supplementation in the two groups was not ascertained by the study, but weight, temperature and blood glucose were assessed at regular intervals. Follow-up was by a single telephone call at age 5 months, when duration of exclusive and partial breast feeding was asked. Loss to follow-up was apparently small, 3% in the unsupplemented and 8% in the supplemented group. Breast feeding duration was significantly longer in the unsupplemented group, with 57% vs. 41% of infants still partially or exclusively breast fed at age 20 weeks. Weight loss at 48 hours was significantly higher (5.9% vs. 4.9%) and blood glucose at 12 hours significantly lower (3.26 mil/l vs. 3.73 mil/l) in the unsupplemented group, and episodes of hypoglycaemia (17 vs. 6) and temperature >37.5 (18 vs. 7) were more frequent.

4.   STUDIES ON PACIFIER USE

The medline search found no additional study where prohibition of pacifier use was part of a controlled intervention. Observational studies on pacifier use[6,7] show consistently an association of early introduction of a pacifier with early discontinuation of breast feeding. Among women still breast feeding, intervals between feeds are greater, when their infants are regular pacifier users[6], thus suggesting that pacifier use might decrease milk production by this mechanism. Pacifier use is very widespread however, with 75% at 2 months in Switzerland[3], 68% at 6 weeks in Rochester NY, USA[6], and 85% at 1 month in Pelota, Brazil[7], even in populations with relatively high breast feeding rates. In a very interesting ethnographic study Victora et al examined psychological and behavioural variables associated with pacifier use[7]. Women who introduced pacifiers to their infants tended to be less comfortable with breast feeding, to show a more rigid breast feeding style, an increased maternal-infant distance, to express more concerns about objective aspects of infant growth, and appeared to be more willing to compare themselves to other mothers and to experience less self-confidence. Thus it appeared that mothers not completely satisfied with their breast feeding experience introduced a pacifier to their infant using it consciously or unconsciously as a weaning tool.

5.   CONCLUSIONS

On the basis of three interventional studies the evidence that restriction of supplements for breast fed infants during the first week of life prolongs the total duration of breast feeding is still equivocal. The only positive study[5] apparently achieved the greatest success in elimination of supplementary feeds. Nevertheless the positive effect was modest, a 16% increase in breast feeding rate at 20 weeks of age, and there were significant side effects with 20% of infants showing elevated temperature and a threefold increase in the frequency of hypoglycemia. The Swiss study, with a modest reduction in supplementation, showed no difference between groups but a higher overall rate of prolonged breast feeding than in the Spanish paper. There is no evidence from interventional studies that the prohibition of the use of a pacifier or artificial teat is effective in promoting breast feeding success.

In summary, a maternity policy modifying the UNICEF steps 6 and 9 in a way that mothers are allowed to offer their newborns dextrin-maltose when thirsty after breast feeding and a pacifier, if they believe this to be good for their baby, is compatible with good breast feeding success, and there is no scientific evidence that enforcement of these two rules would lead to an improvement. It could even be speculated that mothers with delayed lactogenesis who are denied the possibility to soothe their hungry babies with a supplement or pacifier during the first days might feel unsatisfied and discouraged by their early breast feeding experience and thus induced to wean prematurely.

In populations where more than 80% to 90% of newborns leave the maternity hospital fully breast fed, as in Switzerland, interventions with the goal to promote prolonged breast feeding should probably target on one hand maternal psychological factors associated with early weaning, and on the other social circumstances disturbing prolonged breast feeding.

REFERENCES

1. Saadeh, R., Akré J., 1996, Ten steps to successful breastfeeding: A summary of the rationale and scientific evidence. *BIRTH* **23**: 154-160.
2. Pérez-Escamilla R., Pollitt E., Lönnerdal B., Dewey K.G., 1994, Infant feeding policies in maternity wards and their effect on breast-feeding success: An analytical overview. *Am J Public Health* **84**: 89-97.
3. Schubiger G., Schwarz U., Tönz O., for the Neonatal Study Group, 1997, UNICEF/WHO baby-friendly hospital initiative: Does the use of bottles and pacifiers in the neonatal nursery prevent successful breastfeeding? *Eur J Pediatr* **156**: 874-877.
4. Gray-Donald K., Kramer M.S., Munday S., Leduc D.G., 1985, Effect of formula supplementation in the hospital on the duration of breast-feeding: A controlled clinical trial. *Pediatrics* **75**: 514-518.
5. Martin-Calama J., Bunuel J., Valero T., Labay M., Lasarte J.J., Valle F., de Miguel C., 1997, The effect of feeding glucose water to breastfeeding newborns on weight, body temperature, blood glucose, and breast feeding duration. *J Hum Lact* **13**: 209-213.
6. Howard C.R., Howard F.M., Lanphear B., deBlieck E.A., Eberly S., Lawrence R.A., 1999, The effects of early pacifier use on breastfeeding duration. *Pediatrics* **103**: E33

7. Victora C.G., Behague D.P., Barros F.C., Olinto M.T., Weiderpass E., 1997, Pacifier use and short breastfeeding duration: Cause consequence or coincidence? *Pediatrics* **99**: 445-453.

30

BREASTFEEDING PROMOTION—*Is Its Effectiveness Supported by Scientific Evidence and Global Changes in Breastfeeding Behaviors?*

CHESSA K. LUTTER
Food and Nutrition Program, Division of Health Promotion and Protection, Pan American Health Organization, Washington DC 20037

Key words: breastfeeding, exclusive breastfeeding, evaluation, Latin America

1. INTRODUCTION

The full impact of the scientific investment in human milk and breastfeeding research, as measured by population level reductions in infant mortality, morbidity, and improved health and development, will never be realized unless women breastfeed.   Successful breastfeeding results from the interplay of a complex series of physiological and behavioral interactions between a mother and her infant. However, whether or not an infant is put to the breast and breastfed in a manner considered optimal depends on the interaction between two factors, a woman's choice to breastfeed and her ability to act upon this choice (Figure 1). These proximal determinants must both be present for breastfeeding to occur, and are in turn, influenced most immediately by the infant feeding information a woman receives as well as by the physical and social support provided to her during pregnancy, childbirth, and post-partum. These factors are in turn, influenced by familial, medical, and cultural attitudes and norms, demographic and economic conditions (including maternal employment), commercial pressures, and national and international policies and norms. Thus, to promote optimal breastfeeding behaviors, interventions need to be targeted not only to individual women but also to changing the context in which infant feeding choices are made and implemented.

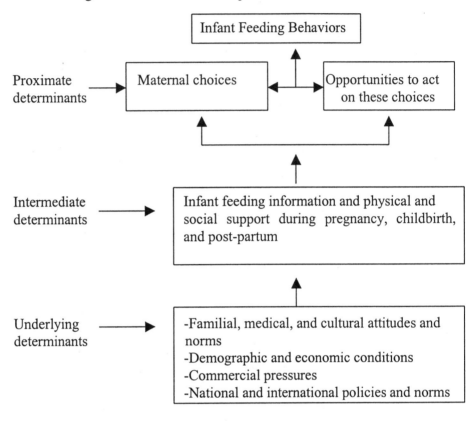

Figure 1. Model of infant feeding behaviors

Optimal infant feeding behavior is a continuum and changes as an infant and young child ages[1]. Although the term breastfeeding is used to describe the process by which an infant suckles breastmilk from his or her mother, breastfeeding actually includes a number of specific recommended behaviors. These include early initiation, the giving of colostrum, exclusive breastfeeding (defined as breast milk as the sole source of infant food and liquid), continued breastfeeding with the addition of complementary foods at about six months of age, and continued breastfeeding into the second year of life and beyond. However, because the optimal behavior varies with infant age, the timing of interventions to promote the desired breastfeeding behavior is critical as it is likely to affect a mother's decision-making process, her motivation to overcome problems should they arise, and her persistence in maintaining a recommended behavior despite negative pressures. Therefore, interventions need to be delivered as close as possible to the time of the desired behavior.

Over the past 20 years, several international policy initiatives in support of breastfeeding have been implemented and many governments have undertaken large breastfeeding campaigns addressing national policy, medical norms, and maternal behavior. Few of these initiatives have been evaluated. The best evidence of a causal or a plausibly causal relationship between breastfeeding promotion and improved behaviors comes from efficacy and effectiveness studies. However, these studies, almost exclusively directed at changing medical norms and maternal behavior, have been implemented in a broader context of national and international initiatives supporting breastfeeding. Compared to national and international campaigns, they have also reached very few women and hence, have had little opportunity to influence global indicators of breastfeeding behavior and, therefore, infant health.

In this paper, evidence from trend data, national evaluations, and efficacy and effectiveness studies are used to critically analyze the plausible causal relationship between international and national initiatives to promote breastfeeding and changes in breastfeeding behavior in Latin America. To guide future interventions, an analysis is provided of the age-specific effect of breastfeeding on infant health in relation to age-specific maternal breastfeeding behaviors and response to specific interventions. This analysis is intended to answer the following questions: 1) at what time will the effects of breastfeeding promotion on infant health be the greatest; 2) what specific behavior should be the main focus; and, 3) what interventions are likely to be most effective?

2.   INTERNATIONAL AND NATIONAL INITIATIVES

In response to concerns about changing breastfeeding behaviors with negative consequences for infant health, a number of national and international initiatives were implemented to promote breastfeeding. Three of these have been particularly important; The International Code of Marketing of Breast-milk Substitutes, the Innocenti Declaration, and the Baby Friendly Hospital Initiative. The International Code of Marketing of Breast-milk Substitutes adopted by the World Health Assembly in 1981 and subsequent relevant World Health Assembly Resolutions, collectively known as The Code, provide guidelines for the marketing of breast-milk substitutes, bottles, and teats[2]. To ensure infant feeding decisions free from the influence of marketing pressures, the Code aims to restrict such practices, including direct promotion to the public. Furthermore, World Health Assembly Resolutions 39.28, passed in 1986, and 47.5, passed in 1994, urge that there be no donations of free or subsidized supplies of breast-milk substitutes and other products covered by the Code in any part of the health care system. The Code has been adopted by almost all governments either on a voluntary basis or through legislation. Despite continued violations by infant formula manufacturers, it has had a major impact on the way formula is advertised and marketed[3]. The Code has been particularly effective in the virtual elimination of the direct marketing to women who receive services through the public sector and in the restriction of marketing to health providers.

The Innocenti Declaration, which focuses on the need to protect, promote, and support breastfeeding, was signed by over 30 countries in 1989.   This Declaration, which includes the Ten Steps to Successful Breastfeeding, forms the basis for the WHO/UNICEF Baby Friendly Hospital Initiative and was endorsed by the Forty-fifth World Health Assembly in 1992[4]. This initiative has influenced the routines and norms of hospitals throughout the world through the "Baby Friendly" certification process. To date, over 14,500 hospitals have been certified and numerous others are in the process of trying to become certified.

During the 1980s, governments throughout the world initiated national campaigns to promote breastfeeding. These campaigns generally included the adoption of the Code either as national legislation or as a norm, establishment of a national breastfeeding committee, training of health workers and changes in medical practices and norms, use of mass media, the development of written material, posters, etc., and community activities.

International and national initiatives have taken place during a period of other social and demographic changes, which are also known to affect breastfeeding. These include increased urbanization and maternal education and employment, all of which are negatively associated with breastfeeding duration, despite their overall importance to women's lives. Hypothesized to be positively associated with breastfeeding duration[5], though not established empirically, are longer birth intervals resulting from increased use of modern contraception. In the absence of such contraceptives, breastfeeding could have been truncated because of a new pregnancy. Also hypothesized to be positively associated with breastfeeding, is the economic downturn of the 1980s and lower family incomes coupled with the increased cost of commercial infant formula.

3. TRENDS IN BREASTFEEDING AND EVALUATIONS OF NATIONAL CAMPAIGNS

The most comprehensive data on breastfeeding trends come from 3 nationally representative sets of surveys. The World Fertility Surveys (WFS), conducted throughout the 1970s in many developing countries, measured the duration of breastfeeding. More detailed measures of specific breastfeeding behaviors are available from the Demographic and Health Surveys (DHS), which replaced the WFS in the 1980s and continue today. Since the 1980s, the Centers for Disease Control and Prevention (CDC) has also conducted surveys. All 3 surveys use a 24-hour infant feeding recall to assess infant feeding behaviors. WFS only collected data on breastfeeding duration and, therefore, can only be used to compare trends in this specific behavior. DHS and CDC collect data on other breastfeeding behaviors and can be used to compare changes in the duration of exclusive breastfeeding as well as other specific behaviors.

Using only those countries for which trend data are available, median durations of breastfeeding were compared for Latin America (Table 1). The results show that the median duration of breastfeeding has increased in all but 1 country and even that country, the Dominican Republic, has shown an increase during the last 2 surveys. The greatest increases are seen in Honduras (4.1 months) and Peru (5.8 months).

Table 1. Trends in breastfeeding duration

Country	Year	Median duration (months)	Reference
Bolivia	1989	16.9	18
	1993/94	17.5	19
	1998	17.5	20
Colombia	1976	9.7	5
	1986	11.6	5
	1990	12.7	21
	1995	10.3	22
Dom Rep	1975	8.9	5
	1986	9.7	5
	1991	5.9	23
	1996	7.6	24
Ecuador	1979	13.0	5
	1987	14.6	5
	1994	15.5	25
El Salvador	1993	15.5	26
	1998	17.7	27
Guatemala	1987	19.9	28
	1995	20.2	29
Honduras	1981	13.2	6
	1984	15.8	6
	1987	17.3	30
	1991/92	17.2	31
	1996	17.3	7
Mexico	1976	9.9	5
	1987	11.2	5
Peru	1997	14.4	5
	1986	17.9	5
	1991/92	17.3	32
	1996	20.2	33

Changes in the duration of breastfeeding can result from changes in behavior within population subgroups, changes in the proportion of the population in these subgroups, or both. For example, women living in urban areas have a shorter duration of breastfeeding than women living in rural areas. If over time, the population becomes increasingly urban, the duration of breastfeeding will decline even if both urban and rural women continue to breastfeed for the same length of time. The decline is thus due to the increasing proportion of the population in a subgroup that tends to breastfeed less rather than changes in behavior within the particular subgroup. The extent to which the increasing duration of breastfeeding between the 1970s and 1980s was the result of changes in behavior within population subgroups versus changes in the size of these subgroups was studied by Strawn[6]. His analysis shows that overall there was an increase in the duration of breastfeeding in all the Latin American countries ranging from 0.8 to 3.5 months, a decrease in Asian and the Pacific countries, and both increases and decreases in African countries (Table 2).

Table 2. Trends in breastfeeding duration in the World Fertility Survey and Demographic Health Survey

	Duration in months		Predicted trends		
	WFS	DHS	Overall change	Characteristic change	Behavioral change
Latin América					
Colombia	9.7.	11.6	1.9	-1.5	3.5
Dominican Republic	8.9	9.7	0.8	-2.3	3.1
Ecuador	13.0	14.6	1.6	-0.8	2.4
Mexico	9.9	11.2	1.3	-2.0	3.2
Peru	14.4	17.9	3.5	-1.2	4.6
Trinidad & Tobago	6.4	10.6	4.2	0.6	3.6
Asia and Pacific					
Indonesia	26.7	26.7	0.0	-1.5	1.5
Sri Lanka	23.4	23.2	-0.2	-0.5	0.3
Thailand	20.2	17.6	-2.6	-2.4	-0.1
Africa					
Egypt	18.2	18.2	0.0	-0.5	0.5
Ghana	19.6	22.5	2.9	-0.0	2.9
Kenya	17.9	10.9	3.0	-1.0	4.0
Morocco	16.2	15.1	-1.1	-0.8	-0.3
Senegal	19.9	20.2	0.3	-0.4	0.7
Tunisia	16.8	15.7	-1.1	-2.0	0.9

Source: Grummer-Strawn, 1996[5].

Disentangling the effects of changes in population characteristics versus changes in behavior, he showed that in the absence of changes in behavior within subgroups, the duration of breastfeeding would have declined in 13 out of the 15 countries studied. Thus, changes in behavior within population subgroups resulted in longer durations of breastfeeding than actually observed. When the net effects of changes in population characteristics associated with declines in breastfeeding duration were included (such as increased urbanization and women's education and employment), the overall effects were attenuated though still positive. Grummer-Strawn suggested three possible explanations for these positive behavioral trends: 1) increased birth intervals so that breastfeeding was not truncated by a new pregnancy; 2) the economic crisis of the 1980s and increased cost of infant formula; and, 3) national and international efforts to promote breastfeeding. Another explanation is also possible. Since data are not available from the 1960's, it is possible that despite concerns to the contrary and numerous reports out of Africa about deaths due to "bottle-babies" that breastfeeding was already increasing and this positive trend merely coincided with national and international promotion efforts.

Evaluations of national breastfeeding campaigns lend support to the interpretation that national and international efforts may be responsible for these positive trends. In Honduras, a national campaign implemented over a 5-year period between 1982 and 1988 promoted breastfeeding through changes in hospital norms, training of health providers, pre- and post-natal maternal counseling, the development of lactation clinics, educational talks in the community, and print materials. These efforts were complemented by a mass media communications campaign[7]. Because of the particularly low durations of breastfeeding in urban areas, the campaign was primarily targeted at urban populations. Nationally representative surveys conducted prior to the campaign in 1981, during the campaign in 1984, and towards the end of the campaign in 1987 demonstrate a significant increase in the duration of breastfeeding, with proportionally greater gains among urban women and early, as opposed to later, in the campaign. Among rural women, the duration of breastfeeding increased from 16.7 to 18.4 to 18.8 months while among urban women the increase was from 4.1 to 8.9 to 9.9 in 1981, 1984, and 1987, respectively.

The most recent national survey shows that these gains have been maintained among rural women (18.7 months) and significantly increased among urban women (15.1 months)[8].The Brazilian national campaign, conducted between 1981 and 1986, also focused on educating heath providers, implementing rooming-in, restricting the distribution of infant formula, and on the counseling of mothers[9, 10]. As in Honduras, these efforts were also complemented by an extensive mass media campaign. Unlike the situation in Honduras, however, the availability of nationally representative data did not coincide with the campaign. Data from 1974/75 and 1987/85 available for Sao Paulo, show a significant increase in the duration of breastfeeding among all income groups, with proportionally greater increase among women of higher socio-economic status. More recent data from Brazil show a median duration of breastfeeding of 6 months in Sao Paulo, again illustrating increases in the duration of breastfeeding[11].

4.   BREASTFEEDING PROMOTION: WHEN, WHERE, AND HOW?

In the developing world, a culture of breastfeeding exists that does not include the behavior of exclusive breastfeeding. Although the vast majority of women initiate breastfeeding and continue breastfeeding, the duration of exclusive breastfeeding tends to be very short (Table 3).

Table 3. Breastfeeding Patterns in Six Latin American Countries: DHS Surveys 1994 – 1996

	Bolivia	Colom-bia	Dom Rep	Guate-mala	Parag-uay	Peru
	(1994)	(1995)	(1996)	(1995)	(1990)	(1996)
Initiation %	96.3	94.5	93.2	95.6	92.8	96.8
Exclusive Breastfeeding						
0-1 months (%)	61.4	26.7	39.1	54.8	10.1	71.2
2-3 months (%)	47.8	9.1	17.4	45.3	5.7	54.2
4-5 months (%)	27.3	4.8	8.3	40.3	0.9	38.6
Median duration						
Exclusive (months)	1.6	0.5	0.6	1.7	0.4	2.7
Partial (months)	17.5	11.3	7.6	19.8	10.5	19.5

Breastfeeding confers a different health advantage depending on the specific behavior and age of the infant. Exclusive breastfeeding is more protective of health than partial breastfeeding. Within the period of exclusive breastfeeding, benefits are larger the younger the infant, reflecting the declining risk of death across infancy. In a case-control study on breastfeeding and mortality, Victora et al., showed that compared to exclusively breastfed infants, infants who were partially breastfed had a relative risk of death of 4.2 and those who were not breastfed had a relative risk of death of 14.2[12]. When this analysis was limited to deaths within the first 2 months of life, the risk of death of not breastfeeding compared to that of exclusive breastfeeding increased to 23.3. With respect to morbidity both Brown et al., and Popkin et al., show that the protective effect of exclusive breastfeeding is greatest for infants less than 2 months of age[13, 14].

Unfortunately, the protective effect of exclusive breastfeeding on infant health is greatest during the period when women are most likely to abandon this behavior (Table 3). The greatest declines in the proportion of women exclusively breastfeeding occurs during the first month of life. Therefore, it is important to promote exclusive breastfeeding during this critical period.

To test the efficacy of breastfeeding counseling delivered by peer counselors through home visits, women in a peri-urban community in Mexico were randomized into 3 groups[15]. One group received 6 visits (2 prenatal, and in weeks 1, 2, 4, and 8), the second group received 3 visits (1 prenatal, and in weeks 1 and 2), and the third group served as a control. Peer counselors, selected from the community, were between 25 and 30 years of age, had a high-school education, and received 1 week of in-class training, followed by 2 months of training in lactation clinics and in mother-to-mother support groups. Special training materials and visual aids were developed for the study to assist with counseling efforts. The prenatal visits focused on the benefits of exclusive breastfeeding, basic lactation anatomy and physiology, positioning of the infant and "latching-on", common myths, typical problems, and birth preparation. Post-partum visits focused on establishing a healthy breastfeeding pattern, addressing maternal concerns, providing information, and social support. Key family members were also included in these visits. The duration of exclusive breastfeeding was significantly longer in the women in the intervention group; at 2 weeks the prevalence was 80, 62 and 24 percent in the 6-visit, 3-visit, and control groups, respectively. At 3 months the prevalence was 62, 50, and 12 percent in the 6-visit, 3-visit, and control groups, respectively. A significant effect on diarrheal morbidity was also found in the intervention group. Because most women gave birth in Baby Friendly hospitals, these figures were compared to data available from historical controls. Compared to these historical controls, the current controls were 6 times more likely to exclusively breastfeed at 2 weeks (24 versus 4 percent); at 3 months there was no difference in the exclusive breastfeeding (12 percent for both groups). Thus, it appears that giving birth in a Baby Friendly hospital influences exclusive breastfeeding early in life, however, in the absence of any follow-up support there is no impact on this behavior at 3 months. Although the women with the most visits breastfed the longest, the cost of the intervention relative to the impact must also be evaluated. From a public health perspective, in which resources for breastfeeding promotion are limited, it may be more cost-effective to cover more women with 3 visits than a smaller group for 6 visits.

The efficacy of home-based counseling has also been demonstrated in Bangladesh by Haider et al. (this volume). In this study, 40 clusters with a total of 726 women, were randomized into intervention and control groups. In contrast to the extensive training in the study in Mexico (more than 2 months), training of counselors in this study lasted 2 weeks and was based on the WHO/UNICEF course "Breastfeeding Counseling: A Training Course"[16]. This course focuses not only on the clinical aspects of lactation management, but also on the equally important act of listening and communicating skillfully to achieve good rapport with a breastfeeding woman. Also in contrast to the study in Mexico, a larger number of visits (15) were made to each woman starting in the third trimester of pregnancy and continuing at least twice monthly until the infant was 5 months of age. It was believed that this large number of visits were needed because almost all women delivered at home and, hence, were not exposed to positive breastfeeding messages through health services. Also, although almost all women initiated breastfeeding and breastfed for a long period of time, initiation was delayed because the feeding of colostrum was not the norm and exclusive breastfeeding was rarely practiced. Home visits resulted in dramatic increases in these two behaviors: the feeding of colostrum was 69 percent in the intervention group versus 11 percent in the control group. At 5 months of age, 70 percent of infants in the intervention group were exclusively breastfed compared to only 6 percent in the control group. There was also a significant and positive effect of exclusive breastfeeding on weight gain at 5 months.

The 2 efficacy trials summarized above show that home visits are highly effective in extending the duration of exclusive breastfeeding. However, the feasibility of such visits outside of a research context have not been tested in an effectiveness intervention and are likely to be setting-specific and dependent on available resources. Therefore, the extent to which exclusive breastfeeding can be promoted through traditional health services is highly relevant. The largest and most comprehensive study to date of breastfeeding promotion through health services is by Kramer et al., (this volume). They report on a randomized trial of the Baby Friendly Hospital Initiative in Belarus involving 30 hospitals and 18,000 mother-infant pairs. Hospital and polyclinic staff, which provide all follow-up infant care, were trained in the 18-hour Baby Friendly course for hospital administrators. This training and the adoption of the Ten Steps in the Baby Friendly Hospital Initiative resulted in significant improvements in the duration of both exclusive and partial breastfeeding and resulted in a decline in diarrhea of 40 percent.

In a less well controlled trial[17], showed a 53 day increase in the median duration of exclusive breastfeeding at 3 months when mother-infant pairs who delivered at a hospital with a comprehensive breastfeeding promotion program were compared to mother-infant pairs that delivered in a hospital that only had rooming-in and did not give away free formula. The plausibility that the increase in exclusive breastfeeding may have been due to the maternity-ward-based breastfeeding promotion program was enhanced by rejecting alternative explanations. A key finding was the fact that women who wished to deliver at the program hospital but were unable to do so because the hospital was full and hence were sent to the control hospital had exclusive breastfeeding patterns similar to other women delivering at the control hospital. An important contribution of this study was the costing of the intervention and a cost-effectiveness analysis, which showed that breastfeeding promotion was highly cost-effective, comparable to immunization programs [18].

The efficacy and effectiveness studies summarized above provide scientific evidence that exclusive breastfeeding can be increased through carefully targeted interventions. In countries where the promotion of exclusive breastfeeding has been a key component of breastfeeding campaigns, DHS data show that exclusive breastfeeding rates can also be improved. In Peru the proportion of infants less than 4 months of age exclusively breastfed increased from 32 percent to 61 percent between 1986 and 1996. In the Dominican Republic the increase was from 10 percent to 25 percent between 1991 and 1996.

5.   CONCLUSIONS

The effectiveness of breastfeeding promotion is supported by scientific research and is a likely explanation for global changes in behavior. Because in the developing world the vast majority of women initiate breastfeeding and continue to breastfeed, future efforts to promote breastfeeding should focus on the behavior of exclusive breastfeeding for maximum health impact. To extend the duration of exclusive breastfeeding, the timing of the intervention is critical. Women must be reached early during the prenatal period, supported at birth, and within the first month post-partum when breastfeeding problems and the shift from exclusive to partial breastfeeding are most likely to occur.

The challenge ahead is to implement infant feeding counseling and support in health services and community-based programs. Research is needed to answer questions such as what is the most cost-effective methods of training and the number and timing of visits? What are the most important messages for a mother to have and how are they best delivered to her? It is also necessary to start thinking and acting on the concept of infant feeding promotion and include complementary feeding as well as breastfeeding in promotion activities. Research must emphasize not only the efficacy and effectiveness of the promotion of optimal infant feeding behaviors on infant health, but also its cost-effectiveness. It is necessary to involve health economists in future research.

Lastly, to ensure that the numerous benefits of human milk and breastfeeding on infant survival, health, and development are achieved, the potential synergies between research and the implementation and evaluation of interventions based on this research must be realized. To do this not only requires sound scientific research, but also the linking of this research to the science of public health intervention and the development of creative methodologies to evaluate multi-faceted interventions. This requires that the same level of scientific rigor, creativity, and investment that has been brought to the science of human milk and breastfeeding also be brought to the science and art of promoting optimal infant feeding behaviors.

REFERENCES

[1]Brown K, Dewey K, Allen L. Complementary feeding of young children in developing countries: a review of current scientific knowledge. WHO/NUT/98.1, 1998, Geneva.

[2]WHO, The International Code of Marketing of Breast-milk Substitutes. 1981, Geneva, Switzerland.

[3]Taylor A. Violations of the international code of marketing of breast milk substitutes: prevalence in four countries. *Br Med J* 1998;**316**:1117-1122.

[4]WHO, Baby Friendly Hospital Initiative. 1992. Geneva, Switzerland.

[5]Grummer-Strawn LM. The effect of changes in population characteristics on breastfeeding trends in fifteen developing countries. *Inter J Epidem* 1996;**25**:94-102.

[6]Popkin BM, Canahuati J, Bailey PE, O'Gara C. An evaluation of a national breast-feeding promotion programme in Honduras. *J. Bio Sci* 1991;**23**:5-21.

[7]Centers for Disease Control and Prevention, Encuesta Nacional de Epidemiologia y Salud Familiar, Honduras 1996. Atlanta, GA.

[8]Monteiro CA, Zuniga HPP, Benicio MHD'A, Rea MF, Tudisco ES, Sigulem DM. The recent revival of breast-feeding in the city of Sao Paulo, Brazil. *Amer J Public Health* 1987;**77**:964-966.

[9]Rea MF and Berquo ES. Impact of the Brazilian national breast-feeding programme on mothers in greater Sao Paulo. *Bull WHO* 1990;**68**: 365-371.

[10]Demographic and Health Surveys. Pesquisa Nacional Sobre Demografia y Saúde, Brasil, Macro International 1996;Calverton, MD.

[11]Victora CG, Smith PG, Vaughan JP, et al. Evidence for protection by breastfeeding against infant deaths from infectious diseases in Brazil. *Lancet* **iii**: 1987;319-322.

[12]Brown KH, Black RE, de Romana GL, de Kanashiro HC. Infant feeding practices and their relationship with diarrheal and other diseases in Huascar (Lima), Peru. *Pediatr* 1989;**83**:31-40.

[13]Popkin BM, Adair L, Akin JS, Black R, Briscoe J, Flieger W. Breastfeeding and diarrheal morbidity *Pediatr* 1990;**86**: 874-882.

[14]Morrow AL, Guerrero ML, Shults J, Calva JJ, Lutter C, Brazo J, Ruiz-Palacios G, Morrow RC, and Butterfoss FD. Efficacy of home-based peer counselling to promote exclusive breastfeeding: a randomised controlled trail. Lancet 1999;**353**:1226-1231.

[15]WHO, Breastfeeding counseling: a training course. WHO/CDR/93.4. 1993. Geneva, Switzerland.

[16]Lutter CK, Perez-Escamilla R, Segall A, Sanghvi, T, Teruya K, Wickham C. The effectiveness of a hospital-based program to promote exclusive breast-feeding among low-income women in Brazil. *Amer J Public Health* 1997;**87**:659-663.

[17]Horton S, Sanghvi T, Phillips M, et al. Breastfeeding promotion and priority setting in health. *Health Policy Plan* 1996;**11**:156-168.

[18]Demographic and Health Surveys, Encuesta Nacional de Demografia y Salud, Bolivia, Macro International 1990;Calverton, MD.

[19]Demographic and Health Surveys, Encuesta Nacional de Demografia y Salud, Bolivia, Macro International 1993/94;Calverton, MD.

[20]Demographic and Health Surveys, Bolivia, Encuesta Nacional de Demografia y Salud, Macro International 1996;Calverton, MD.

[21]Demographic and Health Surveys, Colombia, Encuesta Nacional de Demografia y Salud, Macro International 1990;Calverton, MD.

[22]Demographic and Health Surveys, Encuesta Nacional de Demografia y Salud, Colombia, Macro International 1995;Calverton, MD.

[23]Demographic and Health Surveys, Encuesta Nacional de Demografia y Salud, Dominican Republic, Macro International 1991;Calverton, MD.

[24]Demographic and Health Surveys, Encuesta Nacional de Demografia y Salud, Dominican Republic, Macro International 1996;Calverton, MD.

[25]Centers for Disease Control and Prevention, Encuesta Nacional de Epidemiología y Salud Familiar, Ecuador 1994;Atlanta, GA.

[26]Centers for Disease Control and Prevention, Encuesta Nacional de Epidemiologia y Salud Familiar, El Salvador 1993;Atlanta, GA.

[27]Ceters for Disease Control and Prevention, Encuesta Nacional de Epidemiologia y Salud Familiar, El Salvador 1998;Atlanta, GA.

[28]Demographic and Health Surveys, Encuesta Nacional de Demografia y Salud, Guatemala, Macro International 1987;Calverton, MD.

[29]Demographic and Health Surveys, Encuesta Nacional de Demografia y Salud, Guatemala, Macro International 1995;Calverton, MD.

[30]Centers for Disease Control and Prevention, Encuesta Nacional de Epidemiologia y Salud Familiar, Honduras 1987;Atlanta, GA.

[31]Centers for Disease Control and Prevention, Encuesta Nacional de Epidemiologia y Salud Familiar, Honduras 1991/92;Atlanta, GA.

[32]Demographic and Health Surveys, Encuesta Nacional de Demografia y Salud, Peru, Macro International 1991/92;Calverton, MD.

[33]Demographic and Health Surveys, Encuesta Nacional de Demografia y Salud, Peru, Macro International 1996;Calverton, MD.

31

APOPTOSIS IN LACTATING RAT MAMMARY TISSUE USING TUNEL METHOD

Tadashi Iizuka[1], Mitsuyo Sasaki[1], Michio Koike[2]
1Kihoku Hospital, Wakayama Medical College, Japan. 2Department of Pediatrics, Wakayama Medical College

Key words: lactation, apoptosis, rat, TUNEL-method

1.   INTRODUCTION

In previous studies, we have found that niric oxide (NO) plays a role in the secretion of human breast milk[1-2]. NO is recognized as a pluripotential molecule, with a wide spectrum of effects on diverse organs. It acts as a growth inhibitor and a trigger of apoptosis for diverse cellular types. Although apoptosis during lactation is considered a normal function of the mammary tissue, the mechanism and roles are still unknown. Our objective was to evaluate apoptotic cells in immature mammary tissues during lactation for showing the mechanism and roles of apoptosis in lactation.

2.   MATERIALS AND METHODS

Samples of breast tissue were obtained from female Wistar rats during lactation (12 rats) or after weaning (3 rats): The animals were killed with ether and the breasts removed immediately, fixed in 10% buffered formaldehyde and embeded in paraffin. The TUNEL staining was administered according to the method reported previously [4].

3.   RESULTS

1. Morphologic studies

1) Classification of epithelial cells in breast tissues

The epithelial cells in lactating rats consisted of several different types. These were divided into 3 cell types according to maturation: Type I (most immature), Type II (immature)9, Type III (mature). In the maturing process, solid epithelial buds in immature mammary tissues were transformed into tubes of sequamous epithelium of the alveoli.

2) Morphological features of the TUNEL-positive cells

The TUNEL-positive cells exhibited the characteristics of the apoptosic cell.

2. Apoptotic cells in each cell types of maturation

The incidences of apoptotic cells in total epithelial cells were 0,26±0,20 (M±SD) %in type I, 0,71±0,29 % in type II and 0,37±0,31 % in type III. The incidence of apoptotic cells in type II was statistically higher than that in type I and III.

4.   DISCUSSION

There have been a number of studies on apoptosis in involuting mammary tissue but there have only been a few in lactating tissue. Apoptosis in involuting tissue has been recognized as a mechanism by which shrinkage of a tissue is carried out without disruption of its basic form . In the present study, the TUNEL-positive cells were morphologically compatible with the apoptotic cells. Many more apoptotic cells were identified in·the cuboidal secretory epithelium (cell type II) of immature alveoli than in the sequamous actively secretory cell (III) of mature alveoli and in the columnar pre-secretory cell (I) in the most immature alveoli. Accordingly, apoptosis in lactating tissue may play a role at the beginning of secretion. We postulate that apoptosis plays a role in preparation for lactation.

REFERENCES

1. Iizuka T, Sasaki M, Oishi K, et al. Nitric oxide may trigger lactation in humans. J Pediatr 1997; 131: 839-843

2. Iizuka T, Sasaki M, Oishi K, et al. The presence of nitric oxide synthase in the mammary glands of lactating rats. Pediatr Res 1998; 44: 197-200

32

ENERGY INTAKE AND GROWTH OF BREAST-FED INFANTS IN TWO REGIONS OF MEXICO

[a]Bolaños AV, [a]Caire G, [a]Valencia ME, [b]Casanueva E, [a]Román Pérez R and [a]Calderón de la Barca AM.
[a]CIAD, P.O. Box 1735. Hermosillo 83000, Sonora, Mexico. [b]INPer, Mexico, D.F.

1.   INTRODUCTION

The Baby-Friendly Hospital Initiative (BFHI) was introduced in North-west Mexico in 1995, increasing breastfeeding from 9 to 49% [1]. In spite of this, mothers lacked confidence in their ability to breastfeed their infants, and they bought baby formulas as soon as they had some cash availability. Therefore it is necessary to reinforce the BFHI with reliable data to encourage mothers to breastfeed. Low breastfeeding is not a problem in Central Mexico, where breastfeeding is still a traditional practice. Our objective was to evaluate the quality and quantity of milk of breast-fed infants for the first 3 mo of life in Northwest and Central regions of Mexico.

2.   METHODS

After dosing the mother, D_2O concentration was determined in saliva by infrared spectroscopy and mother's body composition and infants milk intake were determined [2] . Milk protein, fat and lactose were analysed to calculate energy intake. The infants' weight and length were compared with reference data [3] and Z scores were calculated. Energy intake, growth and body composition were compared between matched cohorts (Northwest and

Central Mexico, N and C) at 1 (n=47) and 3 (n=22) mo of age. Data were analysed by Spearman coefficient, regression analysis and student's *t* test.

3.   RESULTS AND DISCUSSION

Milk's nutrients and energy intakes at 1 and 3 mo were not significantly different (p>0.05) respect to area and age (Table 1). Fat breast-milk from mothers in N region was higher (p<0.05) than in C region with 46 and 50 mg/mL vs 29 and 31 mg/mL, at 1 and 3 mo, respectively. At 3 mo, energy intake from fat and body fat were higher (p<0.05) in the infants of the N region and the higher fat content of milk was correlated to a higher mother's body fat (r= 0.48, p< 0.001). There were no differences in Z score values for weight/length (p>0.05) for infants in the two regions at 3 mo. Weight/length Z score for infants in N region, at 2 and 3 mo were above +1 compared to ranging between 0 and +0.5 for infant in C region. Mothers in N region are able to breastfeed their infants longer than mothers in C region due to their higher body fat content (31% vs 25%, respectively) at 3 mo postpartum.

Table 1. Human milk and nutrient intakes of predominantly breast-fed infants during first 3 months of life*

	Northwest Mexico		Central Mexico	
	1 mo (n=27)	3 mo (n=11)	1 mo (n=20)	3 mo (n=11)
Milk				
g/d	573 ± 220	865 ± 250	680 ± 239	857 ± 298
g/kg/d	133 ± 44[a]	130 ± 36[a]	178 ± 63[b]	137 ± 47[*]
Protein				
g/kg/d	1.7 ± 0.7[a]	1.6 ± 0.5[a]	2.2 ± 0.8[b]	1.3 ± 0.4[*]
Lactose				
g/kg/d	7.5 ± 2.7[*]	7.4 ± 2.3[a]	10.1 ± 3.4[b]	8.4 ± 2.9[*]
Lipid				
g/kg/d	5.7 ± 2.9[a]	6.3 ± 2.8[a]	5.2 ± 3.1[ac]	4.2 ± 2.1[bc]
Energy				
kcal/kg/d	89 ± 32[a]	92 ± 32[a]	96 ± 41[a]	77 ± 30[*]

* Mean±SD; different superscripts across columns are significantly different p<0.05

REFERENCES

1. Román Pérez R, Calderón de la Barca AM and Caire Juvera G. Breastfeeding and public health policies: an analysis of the last 10 years in Northwest Mexico. Conference Papers, International Conference Breastfeeding- the Natural Advantage. Sydney, Australia. 1997.
2. Calderón de la Barca AM, Bolaños AV, Caire Juvera G et al. Evaluación del consumo de leche humana por dilución con deuterio. Perinatol. Reprod. Hum. 1998; 12 (13): 142-150.
3. NCHS growth curves for children: birth-18 years. Washington, DC. DHEW, 1977.
This project was partially sponsored by the International Atomic Energy Agency (9381).

33

EFFECT OF HUMAN MILK AND RECOMBINANT EGF, TGFα, AND IGF-1 ON SMALL INTESTINAL CELL PROLIFERATION

Carol L. Wagner, M.D. and Donna W. Forsythe, B.S.

Dept. of Pediatrics, Children's Hospital, Medical University of South Carolina, Charleston, SC

Key words: human milk, growth factors, gut epithelial cells

1.   OBJECTIVE

The objective of this study was to determine the trophic and interactive effect of these growth factors compared with human milk on *in vitro* FHs-74 cell proliferation.   In the first set of experiments, the individual effects of recombinant EGF, TGFα, IGF-1, or human milk on FHs-74 cell proliferation were measured. H_o: EGF, TGFα, IGF-1, or human milk would have a dose-dependent, trophic effect on cultured human small intestinal cells. The second set of experiments was designed to ascertain whether these growth factors in combination could additively stimulate *in vitro* cell growth. H_o: The growth factors in combination would have an additive effect on cell proliferation.

2.   METHODS

Cell Preparation and Experimental Conditions

Human fetal small intestinal cells (FHs-74) in flasks were grown in Hybri-Care medium (10% FBS) to confluence, treated with trypsin-EDTA to achieve detachment, then reattached to 96-well plates.   The cells were suspended in Hybri-Care with 10% FBS then incubated. At 48 hrs, medium without serum or other factors was added to 96-well plates at a concentration of 5 X10³ cells/well. At 72 hrs, the aqueous fraction of human milk (AHM; 1:20 v/v) or recombinant EGF, TGFα or IGF-1 was added to separate wells in the range from 0.001-1000 ng/mL medium in logarithmic increments. In addition, the growth factors in combination (0.5 or 500 ng/mL medium) also were added to the cells. After 24 hr of growth factor exposure, cell proliferation (expressed as percentage above control) was measured (CellTiter AQ, Promega, Madison, WI).

3.   RESULTS

The aqueous fraction of human milk resulted in the greatest increase in FHs-74 cell proliferation: 191 ± 48% (mean ± S.D.) above basal conditions. Cell proliferation steadily increased for the 3 growth factors in the 0.001-0.5 ng/mL medium range (F=10.22; p<0.001). Whereas EGF's maximal effect (152 ± 17 % control) on cell proliferation was at the 0.5-ng/mL concentration, TGFα (150 ± 28% control) and IGF-1's (148 ± 37% control) maximal effect did not occur until 100 ng/mL (F=4.08; p<0.003). Cell proliferation following stimulation with TGFα plateaued upon reaching maximal effect at 100 ng/mL. In contrast, cell proliferation appeared to decline at concentrations above 5-ng/mL for EGF and above 100-ng/mL for IGF-1. When EGF and TGFα, IGF-1 and TGFα, or all 3 growth factors were added concomitantly, the cell proliferation profiles resembled that of TGFα. However, when EGF and IGF-1 were added in combination, cell proliferation increased above each growth factor alone.

4.   CONCLUSIONS

While FHs-74 cell proliferation was greatest in the presence of AHM, individual growth factors did increase cell proliferation above control. Cell proliferation varied as a function of growth factor type and combination. Such variation in growth factor effect supports the premise of a narrow physiologic range and combination at which each growth factor in human milk may maximally stimulate gut epithelial cells.

34

LOW BREAST MILK VITAMIN A CONCENTRATION REFLECTS AN INCREASED RISK OF LOW LIVER VITAMIN A STORES IN WOMEN

[1]Amy L. Rice, [1]Rebecca J. Stoltzfus, [2]Andres de Francisco, [1]Chris L. Kjolhede
[1]*Center for Human Nutrition, Johns Hopkins University, Baltimore, MD* [2]*ICDDR,B: Centre for Health and Population Research, Dhaka, Bangladesh*

Key words: breast milk, vitamin A, liver stores, MRDR test

1. INTRODUCTION

Women in developing countries generally have lower dietary vitamin A intakes and produce breast milk with less vitamin A as compared to women in developed countries[1]. Women with low dietary vitamin A intakes are probably also more likely to have low liver vitamin A stores. However, few studies have assessed liver vitamin A stores and breast milk vitamin A concentrations in the same women.

2. OBJECTIVE

We used data from an individually randomized, placebo-controlled trial of vitamin A and β-carotene supplementation in lactating women in Matlab, Bangladesh[2] to 1) Describe the relationship between liver vitamin A stores (assessed using the modified relative dose response [MRDR] test) and breast milk vitamin A concentrations, and 2) Determine if low breast milk vitamin A could be used as a proxy indicator of risk of low liver vitamin A stores.

Short and Long Term Effects of Breast Feeding on Child Health
Edited by Berthold Koletzko *et al.*, Kluwer Academic/Plenum Publishers, 2000

3.   METHODS

At 2 wk postpartum women were randomized to receive either vitamin A (200,000 IU) [n=74], daily β-carotene (7.8 mg) [n=73], or daily placebo capsules [n=73] until 9 mo postpartum. At each visit (2 wk, 3, 6 and 9 mo), 50% of the women completed an MRDR test and provided a full milk sample (the entire contents of one breast that had not been used to feed an infant for ≥2 h). The following cutoffs were applied to the resulting data: Low liver vitamin A stores = MRDR ratio ≥0.06; low milk vitamin A = <1.05 µmol/L or <8 µg/g milk fat; low serum retinol = <1.05 µmol/L.

4.   RESULTS

At each time point, mean milk vitamin A and serum retinol concentrations were significantly lower (P<0.01) among women with low as compared to adequate liver vitamin A stores. The prevalence of low milk vitamin A ranged from ~40% at 2 wk to nearly 80% at 9 mo. Low milk vitamin A was almost twice as prevalent as low liver stores. Nearly all women with low liver vitamin A stores also had low milk vitamin A, but not all women with low milk vitamin A had low liver stores. The relationship between these two indicators was strongest prior to six months postpartum and stronger when milk vitamin A was measured per gram of fat.

5.   CONCLUSIONS

Breast milk vitamin A concentrations are highly influenced by liver vitamin A stores and milk vitamin A levels decline before liver stores become severely depleted. Although not highly predictive at the individual level, an assessment of milk vitamin A content can be used to identify communities at risk of maternal vitamin A deficiency.

REFERENCES

1. Newman V. Vitamin A and breastfeeding: A comparison of data from develeped and developing countries. Wellstart, San Diego, CA, 1993.
2. Rice AL, Stoltzfus RJ, de Francisco A, Chakraborty J, Kjolhede C, Wahed MA. Maternal vitamin A or β-carotene supplementation in lactating Bangladeshi women benefits mothers and infants but does not prevent subclinical deficiency. Am J Clin Nutr 1999; 129:356-365.

35

VITAMIN A IN MILK CAN POTENTIALLY REDUCE THE REPLICATION OF ENVELOPED VIRUSES IN INFANTS

Isaacs, C.E.[1], Xu, W.[1], Kascsak, R.[2], Pullarkat, R.[1]

[1]*Department of Developmental Biochemistry,* [2]*Department of Virology, New York State Institute for Basic Research in Developmental Disabilities, Staten Island, NY 10314, USA*

Vitamin A (retinol and its derivatives) and provitamin A carotenoids are fat soluble compounds which play a role in maintenance and restoration of epithelial barriers, stimulation of immune function and provide increased resistance to gastrointestinal and respiratory infections[1]. Diarrhea, measles and in some studies respiratory infections are common in vitamin A deficient children[2]. Although most studies indicate that vitamin A status does not reduce the incidence of infectious disease, the severity of some infections, especially those related to diarrhea can be reduced with vitamin A supplementation. Vitamin A present in human milk may help to reduce the severity of viral infections since these infections appear to alter the normal transport and metabolism of retinol. The results presented in this and previous studies[3] show that vitamin A can reduce the production of infectious enveloped virus particles in cultured cells and suggest a direct antiviral effect of vitamin A *in vivo* which is not mediated by immune function.

In the present study the application of retinoic acid, the acid form of vitaminA, inhibited the production of a number of different enveloped viruses regardless of whether they were DNA (herpes simplex virus-1 (HSV-1)) or RNA (measles and vesicular stomatitis virus (VSV)) viruses (Table). Decreases in viral titers ranged from 1,000-fold to as much as 100,000-fold. HSV-1 titers were reduced by similar amounts in both monkey kidney cells and in a differentiated human neuroblastoma cell line (SY5Y) which is similar to the neuronal cells that HSV-1 infects in vivo. Retinoic acid treatment did not interfere with the replication of nonenveloped viruses as evidenced by the results with polio1 and polio 3 viruses in both monkey kidney and an epithelial cell line.

Treatment of HSV-1 infected Vero cells with retinoic acid did not reduce the production of viral glycoproteins, even when the production of infectious virus particles was inhibited by 1,000-fold.   Envelope glycoproteins are a constituent of all enveloped viruses and inhibition of their synthesis would have been one possible mechanism for vitamin A dependent reduction in viral infectivity.   Studies done using labeled carbohydrates however, suggest that retinoic acid treatment interferes with the processing of carbohydrates attached to enveloped virus proteins. These studies indicate that the maintenance of adequate vitamin A levels in breast milk could help to reduce the severity of enveloped virus infections in infants when a vaccine is not available.

Table 1. Susceptibility of Enveloped and Nonenveloped Viruses to Inhibition by Retinoic Acid

Virus[1]	Envelope	Cell Type[2]	Control	Retinoic Acid
Measles	Y	Vero	$10^{5.00}$	$10^{1.25}$
HSV-1	Y	Vero	$10^{6.90}$	$10^{1.40}$
HSV-1	Y	SY5Y	$10^{5.50}$	$10^{0.63}$
VSV	Y	Vero	$10^{8.50}$	$10^{2.75}$
Polio 1	N	ME 180	$10^{3.00}$	$10^{3.25}$
Polio 3	N	LLC	$10^{5.50}$	$10^{5.25}$

[1]Herpes simplex virus-1 (HSV-1); VSV (vesicular stomatitis virus).
[2]Vero (monkey kidney); SY5Y (human neuroblastoma); ME 180 (human cervical epithelial carcinoma); LLC (monkey kidney).
[3]Viral titer numbers are tissue culture infectious doses ($\log_{10}$).

REFERENCES

1.   Ross, A.C., 1992, Vitamin A status: Relationship to immunity and the antibody response. *PSEBM* **200:** 303-320.
2.   Ross, A.C., and Stephensen, C.B., 1996, Vitamin A and retinoids in antiviral responses. *FASEB J.* **10:** 979-985.
3.   Isaacs, C.E., Kascsak, R., Pullarkat, R.K., Xu, W., and Schneidman, K., 1997, Inhibition of herpes simplex virus replication by retinoic acid. *Antiviral. Res.* **33:** 117-127.

36

NUCLEOSIDE ANALYSES OF HUMAN MILK AT 4 STAGES OF LACTATION

[1]Gerichhausen MJW, [1]Aeschlimann AD, [1]Baumann HA, [1]Inäbnit M and [2]Infanger E
[1]*Novartis Nutrition Research AG, Switzerland:* [2]*Cantonal Hospital Sursee-Wolhusen, Sursee, Switzerland*

Key words: Nucleosides, Nucleotides, Human Milk

1. INTRODUCTION

Nucleotides are part of the non-protein nitrogen fraction of human milk. It is suggested that nucleotides are semi-essential nutrients for newborn infants and therefore are added to infant formulas by some manufacturers. Nucleosides (nucleotides without phosphate group) are the preferred form for absorption and they occur both in the free and bound form. In this study we quantified the nucleosides most abundantly present in human milk at 4 stages of lactation, after degradation of the different forms into nucleosides and determined the partition of these different nucleoside sources.

2. METHODS

Human milk samples were collected from 8 healthy lactating women who had given birth to term infants. The samples were stored at -75 °C until analysis. After thawing, samples were pooled by stage of lactation and analysed using enzymatic degradation followed by HPLC separation and quantification of the liberated nucleosides[1].

Short and Long Term Effects of Breast Feeding on Child Health
Edited by Berthold Koletzko *et al.*, Kluwer Academic/Plenum Publishers, 2000

3.   RESULTS AND DISCUSSION

Table1. Nucleosides in pooled human milk by stage of lactation (µmol/L)

	Uridine	Cytidine	Guanosine	Adenosine	Total
0-2 days pp	12	22	14	16	64
3-10 days pp	15	26	13	14	68
1 month pp*	24	38	11	18	92
3 months pp#	34	57	13	20	123
Mean (SD)	**21 (10)**	**36 (16)**	**13 (1)**	**17 (3)**	**87 (27)**

pp: postpartum; *: n=6; #: n=7

The total amount of liberated nucleosides increased over lactation from 64 µmol/L to 123 µmol/L. Comparing colostrum (0-2 days postpartum) with late mature milk values (3 months postpartum), the two pyrimidine nucleosides, uridine and cytidine, seem to be responsible for this rise. The two purine nucleosides, guanosine (11-14 µmol/L) and adenosine (14-20 µmol/L) were remained at a rather constant level. The mean value of total liberated nucleosides over 3 months of lactation was 87 µmol/L.

Table 2. Percentage of total liberated nucleosides in pooled human milk as polymeric nucleotides, monomeric nucleotides, nucleosides and adducts (Mean ± SD)

	Uridine	Cytidine	Guanosine	Adenosine	Total
Polymeric nucleotides	27 ± 8	48 ± 2	66 ± 4	57 ± 6	50 ± 2
Monomeric nucleotides	39 ± 25	43 ± 6	34 ± 4	37 ± 4	40 ± 7
Nucleosides	15 ± 18				4 ± 5
Adducts	19 ± 15	9 ± 6		6 ± 9	6 ± 5

It is shown that the total liberated nucleosides were mainly present in the polymeric (50 ± 2%) and monomeric (40 ± 7%) nucleotide form. The latter being the form normally used to supplement infant formulas. The nucleosides derived from adducts contributed for only 6% to the total and the free form of nucleosides for even less (4 ± 5%). Uridine was the only nucleoside found in the free form (15 ± 18%). Guanosine was only found in the polymeric and monomeric nucleoside form and not linked to adducts, as the others were. Inosine was not found in any of the samples analysed in the entire study (<4 µmol/L).

REFERENCES

[1]Leach JL et al. Total potentially available nucleosides of human milk by stage of lactation. Am J Clin Nutr 1995;61: 1224-30.

37

QUANTITATIVE ANALYSIS OF HUMAN MILK OLIGOSACCHARIDES BY CAPILLARY ELECTROPHORESIS

David S. Newburg, Zuojun Shen, and Christopher D. Warren
Program in Glycobiology, Shriver Center, Waltham, MA, and Massachusetts General Hospital, Harvard Medical School, Boston, MA USA

Key words: capillary electrophoresis, oligosaccharides, acidic oligosaccharides, analysis, human milk

Human milk oligosaccharides may have important biological activities.[1] We developed a sensitive, convenient, quantitative method for the routine study of sialylated (acidic, negatively charged) oligosaccharides in large numbers of milk samples. Capillary electrophoresis (CE) with detection at 205 nm was sensitive to the femtomole level and could resolve and quantify nine acidic oligosaccharides in milk, ranging from tri- to nonasaccharides.

Milk samples from Massachusetts, South Carolina, and Mexico were analysed with a Hewlett Packard 3D capillary electrophoresis apparatus (buffer: 376 mM Trizma H [pH 7.9] and 150 mM SDS, plus 6% [v/v] methanol as an organic modifier; approximately one nanoliter loaded onto the column for each analysis). Peaks were identified by coelution with reference oligosaccharides: 3'-sialyllactose (3'-SL), 6'-sialyllactose (6'-SL), disialyltetraose (DST), 3'-sialyl-3-fucosyllactose (3'-S-3-FL), sialyllacto-*N*-tetraose-a (SLNT-a), sialyllacto-*N*-tetraose-b (SLNT-b), sialyllacto-*N*-neotetraose-c (SLNT-c), disialyllacto-*N*-tetraose (DSLNT), and disialomonofucosyllacto-*N*-neohexaose (DSFLNH). The lower limit of detection was approximately 20 to 70 femtomoles. Typical electropherograms of oligosaccharides from pooled samples contained 16 well-defined peaks eluting between 15 and 30 min. Seven major peaks coeluted with reference SLNT-b, SLNT-c, SLNT-a, 3'-S-3-FL, 6'-SL, 3'-SL, and DSLNT, consistent with previous reports.[2-4] Several other peaks, absent from our panel of reference compounds, were eliminated by hydrolysis of sialic acid residues.

Peak areas were directly proportional to oligosaccharide concentrations between 30 and 2,000 mg/L (correlation coefficient [r], 0.998 to 1.000). Ten identical analyses of authentic samples of the seven major oligosaccharides yielded coefficients of variation from 4% to 9%. Quantitation of each compound was unaffected by the presence of others. Oligosaccharide standards were recovered from pooled milk quantitatively (93% to 102%).

Milks of individual donors at various stages of lactation were compared. SLNT pentasaccharides showed the greatest variation: Sometimes SLNT-c was a major peak, with a smaller peak for SLNT-b and a very small peak or shoulder for SLNT-a; sometimes SLNT-c was a very small peak or shoulder, with larger peaks for SLNT-b and SLNT-a. Relative proportions of 6'-SL and 3'-SL also varied, but usually 6'-SL was larger.

CE of underivatised acidic oligosaccharides compares favourably with high-performance anion-exchange chromatography (HPAEC),[5] which requires prior desialylation and longer running times than does CE. CE also offers higher sensitivity and predictable elution position: large molecules and those with a single charge elute early, and small or doubly charged molecules elute late. Kunz and Rudloff[3], using combinations of chromatography and mass-spectrometry, found, as we did, that SLNT isomers of individual milks vary considerably. Both studies also detected sialylated lactoses and DSLNT, but ours found additional variation in the proportions of 6'-SL and 3'-SL. The CE method will facilitate study of the types, preponderances, and possible anti-pathogenic properties of the acidic oligosaccharides.

REFERENCES

1. Newburg, D.S., 1996, Oligosaccharides and glycoconjugates in human milk: Their role in host defense. *J. Mammary Gland Biol. Neoplasia* 1: 271-283.
2. Newburg, D.S., and Neubauer, S.H., 1995, In *Handbook of Milk Composition* (R.G. Jensen, ed.), Academic Press, San Diego, pp. 273-349.
3. Kunz, C., and Rudloff, S., 1993, Biological functions of oligosaccharides in human milk. *Acta Paediatr.* 82: 903-912.
4. Stahl, B., Thurl, S., Zeng, J., Karas, M., Hillenkamp, F., Steup, M., and Sawatzki, G., 1994, Oligosaccharides from human milk as revealed by matrix-assisted laser desorption/ionization mass spectrometry. *Anal. Biochem.* 223: 218-226.
5. Townsend, R.R., Hardy, M.R., Hindsgaul, O., and Lee, Y.C., 1988, High-performance anion-exchange chromatography of oligosaccharides using pellicular resins and pulsed amperometric detection. *Anal. Biochem.* 174: 459-70.

38

ZINC INTAKES AND PLASMA CONCENTRATIONS IN INFANCY

[1]Sievers E, [1]Schleyerbach U, [2]Garbe-Schönberg D, [2]Arpe T, and [1]Schaub J
[1]Dept. Paediatrics, [2]Dept. Geology, University of Kiel, D-24105 Kiel, Germany

Key words: Zinc intake, breast-feeding, infant formula, supplementary feeds

1.   INTRODUCTION, STUDY DESIGN

Optimal supply of the trace element Zn is of special importance for the growing infant. Its concentration in human milk declines during the first months of lactation and a retention superior to Zn from infant formulas has been described [1]. However, data on Zn intake from supplementary foods are scarce and the question arises whether nutritional differences in early infancy affect subsequent Zn intake or plasma Zn concentration.

The Zn intake of 20 breast-fed and 15 formula-fed healthy term infants was investigated by 72 hour weight-based diet protocols at the ages of 4, 8, 16, 24, 32, 42 and 52 weeks. Electronic scales were used for test-weighing of breast-fed infants, the assessment of the body weight and the intakes of formula or supplementary foods. The Zn intake was calculated using the programme Diät 2 000, Soft & Hard Co., Rimbach. A concentration of 5.0 mg Zn/l was given by the manufacturing firm of the infant formula fed (Pre Aptamil®, Milupa Co.). Nutritional counselling was performed according to present recommendations [3] including exclusive breast- or formula-feeding during the first 4 months of life. The families were subsequently supplied with supplementary foods: Vegetables, meat, fruits as ready-to-feed menus (Hipp KG), as well as cereals, follow-up formula (Aptamil II®, Milupa Co.)

Short and Long Term Effects of Breast Feeding on Child Health
Edited by Berthold Koletzko et al., Kluwer Academic/Plenum Publishers, 2000

and mineral water. Zn plasma concentrations were analysed at the ages of 4,16 and 52 weeks by High- resolution ICP-MS at the Dept. of Geology.

2.   RESULTS, CONCLUSIONS

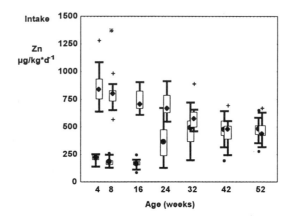

Fig.1: The course of calculated Zn intake; $\perp$ range, 25%-75%, breast-fed: ● median, ● outlier, n=20 (15-16). Formula-fed: ◆ median, + outlier, ＊ extreme value, n = 16 (11-15).

Tab. 1: Plasma Zn concentration in term breast-fed and formula-fed infants.

Age, ± 2 weeks	4	16	52
Group	Plasma Zn concentration (mg/l, median and range)		
Breast-fed	0.65(0.55-0.84); n=10	0.61(0.43-0.71); n=13	0.69(0.55-0.92); n=11
Formula-fed	0.57(0.47-0.69); n=7	0.69(0.55-0.82); n=12	0.68(0.45-0.89); n=8

Zn intake calculations require knowledge of the individual concentration in supplemented formulas. The results suggest that supplementation to the level of 5 mg/l is unnecessary. Zn intake calculation of breast-fed infants should be improved by the use of concentration adjustment according to the stage of lactation. Based on the supply of a choice of infants foods and standardised nutritional counselling, initial nutrition affected neither later Zn intake nor Zn in plasma at the end of the study.

REFERENCES, ACKNOWLEDGMENTS

1. Sievers E, Oldigs HD, Dörner K, Schaub J (1993) Acta Paediatr 1992;81:1-6.
3. Kersting M, Schöch G. Säuglingsernährung 1995. Marseille Verlag GmbH, Munich 1995.

The authors appreciate the co-operation of the families, the support by the DFG (Si 514/1), Bonn, and the supply of infant foods from Milupa Co., Friedrichsdorf, Hipp KG, Pfaffenhofen, and Fürst Bismarck Quelle, Friedrichsruh, Germany.

39

NUTRITIVE SIGNIFICANCE OF ELEMENT SPECIATION IN BREAST MILK
The case of calcium, copper, iron, magnesium, manganese, and zinc

[1]Beatrice Bocca, [1]Alessandro Alimonti, [2]Luciana Giglio, [2]Mauro Di Pasquale, [1]Sergio Caroli, [3]M. Amalia Ambruzzi, [2]Adriana Piccioli Bocca and [2]Ettore Coni
[1] Applied Toxicology Laboratory and [2] Food Laboratory, Istituto Superiore di Sanità, Rome, Italy; [3] Ospedale Pediatrico "Bambino Gesù", Rome, Italy

Key words: Human milk; element speciation

1. INTRODUCTION

Balanced supply of minerals during early childhood allows a good growth of the body tissues and the maturation of several enzymatic systems. The assessment of the total content of the micronutrients in human milk is no longer sufficient to define its nutritional profile. In fact, bioavailability strongly depends on the chemical species of the element when ingested. Speciation analysis provides a suitable tool for achieving data on the element bioavailability. In this study the concentration ranges and binding patterns of Ca, Cu, Fe, Mg, Mn and Zn in milk of 60 lactating Italian mothers (19-40 years aged) were investigated. Size exclusion liquid chromatography with inductively coupled plasma atomic emission spectrometry was used. This approach allows to minimize interactions between the metal protein complexes and the stationary phase as well as to achieve good sensitivity during the multielement quantification.

Short and Long Term Effects of Breast Feeding on Child Health
Edited by Berthold Koletzko *et al.*, Kluwer Academic/Plenum Publishers, 2000

2.   RESULTS AND DISCUSSION

Table 1 reports the statistics of the total concentration of the elements in human milk. The mean concentrations obtained in this study resulted to fall inside the ranges observed in the literature.

Table 1. Elements total content in 60 human milk samples (in $\mu g \ ml^{-1}$)

Element	Mean	SD [a]	Median	25-75 %		Literature range[b]	
Ca	306.6	11.76	224.20	134.11 -	324.44	220.0 - 300.0	
Cu	0.37	0.03	0.26	0.09 -	0.44	0.18 -	0.75
Fe	0.65	0.04	0.33	0.18 -	0.59	0.20 -	1.71
Mg	23.0	0.51	4.11	2.26 -	37.26	9.50 -	62.5
Mn	0.03	0.002	0.01	0.007-	0.03	0.003-	0.04
Zn	2.72	0.07	0.65	0.28 -	2.42	0.70 -	4.00

(a): Standard Deviation; **(b):** from WHO/IAEA 1989 and Caroli *et al* 1994.

Only the Ca mean content exceeds the literature value, i.e., 306.6 ± 11.76 vs. 220.0- 300.0 $\mu g \ ml^{-1}$. A typical milk chromatogram shows five resulting fractions. The first of these was due to the species with molecular weights (MW) > 2000 kDa and presumably accounted for caseins (α_s, β and k) aggregates. The second peak (MW, 500 - 2000 kDa) could be ascribed to immunoglobulins (Igs). The third one (MW, 100 - 500 kDa) could be traced back to human serum albumin (HSA) and lactoferrin (LF). The fourth fraction (MW, 2 - 100 kDa) included the α-lactalbumin (α-La). Finally, the fifth peak represented substances with MW < 2 kDa (non-proteic fractions). Elements such as Cu and Fe were homogeneously spread over all the fractions, from high to low MWs. Calcium and Mg bound preferably to low MW components (48 % and 56 %, respectively). Manganese, in turn, was found in the third (28 %) and fifth (30 %) peaks (i.e., HSA, LF and low MW compounds). Finally, Zn was bound for *ca.* 44 % to the fraction of the α-La, but also citrates, caseins, HSA and LF presented substantial binding percentages. The speciation analysis, thus, highlighted peculiar binding behaviour of the elements investigated. This confirms the important role of some chemical ligands in affecting the bioavailablity of these elements and, consequently, the nutritional potential of human milk.

REFERENCES

WHO/IAEA, 1989, *Minor and trace elements in breast milk.* WHO, Geneva.
Caroli, S., Alimonti, A., Coni, E., Petrucci, F., Senofonte, O., and Violante, N., 1994, *Crit. Rev. Anal. Chem.* **24**: 363-98.

40

HUMAN MILK MERCURY (Hg) AND LEAD (Pb) LEVELS IN VIENNA

[1]Claudia Gundacker, [2]Beate Pietschnig, [1]Karl J. Wittmann and [2]Andreas Lischka

[1]Department of Medical Biology, Schwarzspanierstr. 17, A-1090 Wien, University of Vienna; [2]Kinderklinik Glanzing der Stadt Wien, Wilhelminenspital, A-1160 Wien, Austria

Key words: Pb, Hg, trace metals, heavy metals, human milk

1.   INTRODUCTION

Lead and mercury are potentially toxic. The infant is especially susceptible. Austrian data are sparse [1,2]. Pb concentrations decreased in the last years. Hg concentration in human milk was below the limit of detection[2].

2.   GOALS OF THE STUDY

(1) Measurement of Pb and Hg in human milk (2) Comparison to infant formula and international data [3,4,5].

3.   MATERIALS AND METHODS

5-10 ml individual samples of human milk, voluntarily provided, cow's milk and infant formula samples. Questionnaire: maternal living circumstances and nutrition. Samples were lyophilized, wet ashed and analysed with AAS.

Statistics: Single-criterion ANOVA. The study was approved by the ethical committee. Written informed consent was obtained from the mothers.

4.   RESULTS

Mean maternal age 31 yr, 45 % multipara, mean 27 days p.p. 34.5% LBW.

Table 1. Mercury and lead contents (µg/l) of human milk, cow's milk, formulas

The results of Hg and Pb contents of human milk, cow's milk and infant

		N	mean ± S.D.	min.	max.
Hg	human milk	23	4.1 ± 4.0	0.63	16.8
	infant formula*	2	0.23 ± 0.06	0.18	0.29
	cow's milk	2	not detectable		
Pb	human milk	22	1.5 ± 2.5	0.02	11.17
	infant formula*	2	1.8 ± 1.04	0.88	4.1
	cow's milk	1	0.45		

*: infant formula was prepared with tap water

Hg concentrations of Austrian human milk were within the European range. Austrian Pb values declined sharply during the last 20 years and are now extremely low. Nutritional habits seem to influence Hg levels in milk.

5.   DISCUSSION

For Hg we found significantly higher levels in human milk than in infant formulas, depending on maternal nutrition. For Pb, the human milk and infant formula concentrations are in the same range. Austrian levels decreased since 1981. Thus, there is no risk for the baby of a healthy mother.

Acknowledgements: Study is supported by the Austrian National Bank.

REFERENCES

1) Haschke, F., and Steffan, I., 1981, Die Bleibelastung des jungen Säuglings mit der Nahrung in den Jahren 1980/81. *Wr. Klin. Wochenschr.* **93**: 613-616.
2) Plöckinger, B., Dadak, C., and Meisinger V., 1993, Lead, mercury and cadmium in newborn infants andtheir mothers. *Z. Geburtshilfe Perinatol.* **197(2)**: 104-107.
3) Jensen, A.A., and Slorach, S.A., (eds.), 1991, Chemical Contaminants in Human Milk. CRC Press.
4) Hallen, I.P., Jorhem, L., *et. al.*, 1995, Lead and cadmium levels in human milk and blood. *Sci. Total.Environ.* **166**: 149-155.
5) Sternowsky, H.J., and Wessolowski, R., 1985, Lead and cadmium in breast milk. *Arch. Toxicol.* **57**: 41-45.

41

BREASTFEEDING AND ATOPIC SENSITISATION

Marko Kalliomäki and Erika Isolauri
Department of Paediatrics, Turku University Hospital, 20520 Turku, Finland

1.   INTRODUCTION

Atopic disease may manifest itself even during exclusive breastfeeding[1]. This early sensitisation has been explained by the presence in breastmilk of maternal dietary antigens in low amounts[2,3]. However, the concentrations of dietary antigens in breastmilk do not differ between the mothers feeding atopic and normal infants[3] which apparently explains why the effects of maternal elimination diets during lactation on the development of atopic sensitisation have been controversial[4]. Moreover, these diets may entail nutritional risks for both the mother and the infant[5]. Consequently, maternal dietary restrictions during lactation for primary allergy prevention are not recommended. The data imply that atopic sensitisation during exclusive breastfeeding may depend more on immunological factors than the presence of dietary antigens in breastmilk.

2.   MECHANISMS OF ORAL TOLERANCE

Oral tolerance is a systemic unresponsiveness to orally administered non-pathogenic antigen. Immunological mechanism of oral tolerance is dependent on the dose of antigen[6]. High doses of antigen result the clonal anergy and/or deletion whereas low-dose antigen feeding is characterised by the induction of regulatory T cells producing suppressor cytokines such as transforming growth factor beta (TGF-β). A recent study clues that the latter

Short and Long Term Effects of Breast Feeding on Child Health
Edited by Berthold Koletzko *et al.*, Kluwer Academic/Plenum Publishers, 2000

mechanism may occur in breastfed infants receiving dietary peptides present in breastmilk[7].

3.   TGF-β IN BREASTMILK

Human milk contains TGF-β1 and TGF-β2[8]. In addition to oral tolerance, TGF-β has been shown to have an important impact on the other essential part of the mucosal immune system, namely IgA production[9]. Both the number of IgA-containing cells and the production of TGF-β in intestinal mucosa increase with age[10,11]. Therefore, the impact of TGF-β in breastmilk may culminate at an early age, when new antigens are first encountered by the enteral route and the production of endogenous TGF-β and IgA in the gut are minimal. In a recent study we showed that the concentrations of both TGF-β1 and TGF-β2 were higher in colostrum of mothers whose infants developed atopic disease after weaning compared with those with a preweaning onset atopic disease[12]. Moreover, high TGF-β in maternal colostrum was associated with the infant's ability to produce specific IgA in response to betalactoglobulin, casein, ovalbumin and gliadin, the dietary antigens most frequently responsible for sensitising the infant.

4.   CONCLUSION

The results suggest that TGF-β in colostrum may prevent the development of atopic disease during exclusive breastfeeding and promote specific IgA production in man.

REFERENCES

1.   Isolauri E, et al. (1999) J Pediatr 134:27-32.
2.   Kilshaw PJ, et al. (1984) Int Arch Allergy Appl Immunol 75:8-15.
3.   Cant A, et al. (1985) BMJ 291:932-935.
4.   Zeiger RS (1999) Immunol Allergy Clin North Am 19:619-646.
5.   Arvola T, et al. (1999) Ann Med 31:293-298.
6.   Strober W, et al. (1998) J Clin Immunol 18:1-30.
7.   Pecquet S, et al. (1999) Immunology 96:278-285.
8.   Saito S, et al. (1993) Clin Exp Immunol 94:220-224.
9.   Stavnezer J (1995) J Immunol 155:1647-1651.
10. Perkkiö M, et al. (1980) Pediatr Res 14:953-955.
11. Penttilä IA, et al. (1998) Pediatr Res 44:524-531.
12. Kalliomäki M, et al. (1999) J Allergy Clin Immunol 1999;104:x-y (in press).

42

CYTOKINE PRODUCTION BY LEUKOCYTES FROM HUMAN MILK

Joanna S. Hawkes, Dani-Louise Bryan and Robert A. Gibson
*Child Health Research Institute, Flinders Medical Centre and Flinders University, Bedford Park
SA 5042 and Women's and Children's Hospital, North Adelaide SA 5006 Australia*

1.   INTRODUCTION

Breast milk not only contains factors that provide passive protection, but also bioactive agents that may influence the immunologic development of the recipient infant. Among the many components with immunomodulatory potential that have been identified in human milk are cytokines [1,2] and leukocytes [3]. The aim of this study was to investigate the capacity of breast milk leukocytes to produce cytokines *in vitro*.

2.   MATERIALS AND METHODS

At 2 weeks postpartum breast milk samples (20-30mL) were collected by manual expression from 10 mothers of healthy term infants. Cells were isolated from the whole milk samples by centrifugation at 680xg for 20min. After removing the fat and aqueous fractions the cells were washed and resuspended in RPMI/5%FCS. Cells were cultured ($5x10^6$cells/mL) at 37°C with or without lipopolysaccharide (LPS) (500ng/mL). After 24h, cells were subjected to two freeze-thaw cycles and the supernatants collected for determination of total (secreted + intracellular) cytokine production (IL-1β, IL-6 and TNF-α) by ELISA. ELISAs were established using matched antibody pairs as described previously [1]. The minimum detectable level for each ELISA was 15pg/mL.

Short and Long Term Effects of Breast Feeding on Child Health
Edited by Berthold Koletzko *et al.*, Kluwer Academic/Plenum Publishers, 2000

3. RESULTS

Unstimulated breast milk cells from all donors produced IL-1β, IL-6 and TNF-α. Stimulation with LPS significantly increased cytokine production.

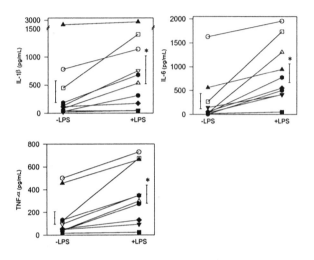

Figure 1. Cytokine production by breast milk cells cultured in vitro with (+LPS) or without (-LPS) LPS. Vertical bars represent the mean±SEM of 10 samples. *p<0.01, t test

4. DISCUSSION

Our data support existing evidence that human milk leukocytes have the capacity to produce cytokines in significant amounts following stimulation with LPS. This type of stimulus may be responsible for activation of milk cells in the gastrointestinal tract of breastfed infants. The presence of immunomodulatory agents such as cytokines in the aqueous phase of breast milk and the capability of breast milk cells to produce these cytokines after stimulation may contribute to the mucosal defence mechanisms of breastfed infants.

REFERENCES

1. Hawkes JS *et al*. Pediatr Res 46(2):194-199, 1999
2. Bryan D-L *et al*. Pediatr Res 45(6):858-859, 1999
3. Goldman AS & Goldblum RM. Curr Top Microbiol Immunol 222:205-213, 1997

BREASTFEEDING AND ASTHMA IN CHILDREN
A Prospective Cohort Study

Wendy H. Oddy
TVW Telethon Institute for Child Health Research, Department of Paediatrics, University of Western Australia, Perth, Western Australia

Key words: asthma, breastfeeding, children

1. INTRODUCTION

Asthma is the leading cause of hospitalisation in Australian children and its prevalence is increasing.[1] Susceptibility to asthma may be heightened by early cessation of exclusive breastfeeding[2] perhaps because breastfeeding may be an important determinant of the immune response.[3] However, whether breastfeeding protects against asthma and/or atopy is controversial.[4]

2. METHODS

The Western Australian Pregnancy Cohort Study is a prospective birth cohort established from 1989 to 1992 in Perth, Western Australia. At age six, 2,602 (91%) children were available for follow-up.

Outcomes and Exposures

Childhood asthma was defined as doctor diagnosed asthma, wheeze in the last year, sleep disturbance due to wheeze in the last year and objective atopy defined by skin prick test. Breast-feeding was measured as the duration of breastfeeding, and the duration of exclusive breastfeeding.

Short and Long Term Effects of Breast Feeding on Child Health
Edited by Berthold Koletzko *et al.*, Kluwer Academic/Plenum Publishers, 2000

3.   RESULTS

Having adjusted for the potential confounders, the introduction of milk other than breastmilk before four months of age was positively associated with all primary end-points of asthma at six years (table 1).

Table 1. Multivariate logistic regression model between asthma and atopy in children at six years and the risk of other milk at less than four months of age (n=2023)*

	Doctor diagnosed asthma	Current wheeze in the last year	Sleep disturbance due to wheeze	Positive skin prick test
OR 95% CI	1.25 (1.02-1.51)	1.32 (1.06-1.64)	1.43 (1.08-1.90)	1.30 (1.05-1.61)
p-value	.028	.014	.013	.016

*Each estimated odds ratio (OR) is adjusted for gender, gestational age & parental smoking.

4.   CONCLUSION

This study provides evidence consistent with others, of a protective effect of exclusive breastfeeding against a range of end-points reflecting asthma and atopy. Delaying the introduction of other milk until at least four months of age may reduce the risk of asthma and atopy later in childhood.

ACKNOWLEDGMENTS

WH Oddy was supported by a Western Australian Health Promotion Foundation Research Award.

REFERENCES

1. Peat JK, Li J. Reversing the trend: Reducing the prevalence of asthma. The Journal of Allergy and Clinical Immunology 1999;103(1):1-10.
2.   Saarinen UM, Kajosaari M. Breastfeeding as prophylaxis against atopic disease: prospective follow-up study until 17 years old. Lancet 1995;346:1065-9.
3.   Hanson LA. Breastfeeding provides passive and likely longlasting active immunity. Annals of Allergy, Asthma and Immunology 1998;81:523-537.
4. Golding J, Emmett PM, Rogers IS. Eczema, asthma and allergy. Early Human Development 1997;49 (Suppl):S121-S130.

44

DOCOSAHEXAENOIC ACID (DHA) STATUS OF BREASTFED MALNOURISHED INFANTS AND THEIR MOTHERS IN NORTH PAKISTAN
An association between DHA in breastmilk and infants red blood cells

[1]Smit EN, [2]Muskiet FAJ, [1]Boersma ER
[1]Departments of Obstetrics/Pediatrics, Perinatal Nutrition and Development Unit, Groningen University Hospital; [2]Pathology and Laboratory Medicine, University Hospital Groningen.

1. INTRODUCTION

The importance of the postnatal docosahexaenoic acid (DHA; $22:6\omega3$) status for neurological and cognitive development is well established. In the North of Pakistan the general diet contains a low content of essential fatty acids (EFA) of the $\omega3$ series. Consequently, we hypothesised that the low erythrocyte (RBC) DHA content of malnourished, breastfed, children living in the North of Pakistan is to a great extent caused by marginal $\omega3$ FA intake from their mothers milk.

2. SUBJECTS AND METHODS

The study population consisted of eight mothers feeding a malnourished child. EDTA anti-coagulated blood (2 ml) was taken from the children. Breastmilk samples (5 ml) were collected by manual expression. Fatty acids were determined as their methyl esters by capillary gas chromatography with flame ionisation detection. The milk fatty acid composition of Pakistani mothers was compared with that of mature milk of 25 Dutch mothers. Between-group differences were analysed with Mann Whitney-U test at

Short and Long Term Effects of Breast Feeding on Child Health
Edited by Berthold Koletzko *et al.*, Kluwer Academic/Plenum Publishers, 2000

395

$p<0.05$. Correlations of the different polyunsaturated fatty acids (PUFA) between breastmilk and infant RBC were tested with the Spearman test at $p<0.05$.

3. RESULTS

Median (range) duration of lactation of Pakistani and Dutch mothers was 12.5 (4.5-21) and 3 (2.5-3.5) months, respectively. The milk of the Pakistani mothers contained significantly lower amounts of all FA of the ω3 series and the main ω6-fatty acids LA, and AA (Table 1). Breastmilk DHA and eicosapentaenoic acid (20:5ω3; EPA) were correlated with infant RBC DHA (r=0.8571, p=0.007; r=0.7186, p=0.045).

Table 1. Fatty acids in mature human milk of Pakistani mothers breast-feeding malnourished children as compared with Dutch controls

	Pakistani (n=8)		Dutch (n=25)	
18:3ω3	0.34	(0.28-0.51)[a]	1.12	(0.64-2.19)
20:5ω3	0.02	(0.01-0.09)[c]	0.05	(0.00-0.29)
22:6ω3	0.06	(0.04-0.14)[b]	0.14	(0.10-0.65)
18:2ω6	8.73	(7.45-10.61)[b]	13.84	(6.44-27.69)
20:4ω6	0.26	(0.20-0.44)[c]	0.33	(0.24-0.43)

Data represent median (range), and are expressed in mol% (mol/100 mol).
[a] $p<0.0001$, [b] $p<0.005$, [c] $p<0.05$

4. DISCUSSION

Under the prevailing conditions in North Pakistan breast-fed malnourished children and their mothers have a poor EFA status. Their ω3 status is more severely affected, than their ω6 status. The low maternal milk LCPUFAω3 content is presumably caused by low fish consumption in the North of Pakistan. The low LCPUFAω3 status of malnourished breastfed children in North Pakistan is most probably caused by the low LCPUFAω3 content of their mother's milk. Improvement of the EFA status of both mother and child may be accomplished by EFA supplementation of the mother.

45

LONG TERM EFFECT OF BREAST FEEDING ON ESSENTIAL FATTY ACID STATUS IN HEALTHY, FULL-TERM INFANTS

Tamás Decsi, Barbara Kelemen, Hajnalka Minda and István Burus
Department of Paediatrics, UniversityMedical School of Pécs, József A. u. 7., H-7623 Pécs, Hungary

Key words: arachidonic acid, docosahexaenoic acid, infant feeding

1.   INTRODUCTION

Human milk contains not only the essential fatty acids linoleic (C18:2ω-6) and α-linolenic (C18:3ω-3) acids but also their long-chain polyunsaturated fatty acid derivatives arachidonic (C20:4ω-6) and docosahexaenoic (C22:6ω-3) acids.[1] In contrast, infant formulae with traditional fat blends contain only the essential fatty acids but are devoid of long-chain polyunsaturates.[2] Here we report data obtained at investigating the fatty acid composition of plasma phospholipids in 6- to 12-month old, healthy, full-term infants fed either human milk or formula.

2.   SUBJECTS AND METHODS

The infants were enrolled into the study if interview with the parents allowed unequivocal characterisation of feeding history to exclusive breast feeding (no breast milk substitute formula) or exclusive formula feeding (no human milk feeding after the age of 1 month). Fatty acid composition of plasma phosphoplipids was analysed by high-resolution capillary gas liquid chromatography. The analytical procedure has been recently described in detail elsewhere[3].

3.   RESULTS

In the breast-fed group, the mean duration of breast feeding was 26 ± 8 weeks, one infant was still exclusively breast-fed, three infants were weaned, and eight infants received partial breast feeding. In the formula fed group, seven infants still received breast milk substitute formula, four infants were given follow-on formula, and one infant was fed diluted cow's milk. Contribution of the essential fatty acids C18:2ω-6 and C18:3ω-3 to the fatty acid composition of plasma phospholipids did not differ between the two groups (Table 1). In contrast, plasma phospholipid C20:4ω6 and C22:6ω-3 values were significantly higher in breast-fed than in formula fed infants (Table 1).

Table 1. Major polyunsaturated fatty acids in plasma phospholipids of 6 to 12-month-old, healthy, full-term infants fed human milk or formula. Data are % weight/weight expressed as mean±SD. * = P < 0.001, ** = P < 0.0001.

Fatty acid	Breast-fed (n=12)	Formula fed (n=12)
Linoleic	18.32±4.11	20.91±2.69
Arachidonic	9.79±1.97*	6.74±1.45
α-Linolenic	0.06±0.03	0.12±0.13
Docosahexaenoic	1.96±0.36**	1.00±0.25

4.   DISCUSSION

In the present study feeding formula without long-chain polyunsaturated fatty acids was found to be associated with significantly lower plasma phospholipid C20:4ω-6 and C22:6ω-3 values in formula fed than in breast-fed infants. The data obtained in the present study support the concept that the type of infant feeding exerts relatively long term effect on the fatty acid composition of infantile lipids.

REFERENCES

1. B. Koletzko et al. *J. Pediatr.* **120:** S62-S70, 1992
2. B. Koletzko et al. *Acta Paediatr. Scand.* **78:** 513-521, 1989
3. T. Decsi et al. *Acta Paediatr.* **88:** 500-504, 1999

46

HUMAN MILK FATTY ACID PROFILES FROM AUSTRALIA, CANADA, JAPAN, AND THE PHILIPPINES

Rebecca Yuhas, Charles Kuhlman, Joan Jackson, Kathryn Pramuk and Eric Lien
Wyeth Nutritional International, Philadelphia, PA, USA

Key words: long chain polyunsaturated fatty acids, human milk

1.   INTRODUCTION

Human milk (HM) fatty acids (FAs) are derived from both dietary sources and from mammary gland synthesis. Dietary sources of essential FAs, linoleic acid (LA) and α-linolenic acid (ALA)[1], as well as some long chain polyunsaturated FAs, such as docosahexaenoic acid (DHA), are a reflection of maternal diet. Mammary gland synthesis of saturated FAs, particularly up to a chain length of 14 carbons, is the predominant source of these FAs.[2] However, dietary considerations also enter into the HM levels of saturated FAs, since low fat, high carbohydrate diets lead to elevated HM levels of lauric acid. The present study evaluates HM FA profiles from four countries, with approximately 50 samples evaluated per site.

2.   MATERIALS AND METHODS

HM samples were full breast expressions stored in polypropylene bottles at -70°C until analyzed. Samples were extracted using a modified Roese

Gottlieb mixed ethers method and analyzed by GC with an Omegawax™ capillary column and FID.

3.   RESULTS AND DISCUSSION

Table 1. FATTY ACID COMPOSITION OF HUMAN MILK (wt % ± SEM)

FA	Australia (A)	Canada (C)	Philippines (P)	Japan (J)
12:0	$5.49\pm0.22^{a*}$	5.25 ± 0.23^a	13.82 ± 0.47^b	5.89 ± 0.24^a
16:0	22.26 ± 0.31^c	18.67 ± 0.32^a	23.02 ± 0.28^c	20.21 ± 0.26^b
18:2n-6	10.66 ± 0.35^b	11.48 ± 0.43^b	7.90 ± 0.24^a	12.63 ± 0.25^c
18:3n-3	0.90 ± 0.04^b	1.22 ± 0.05^c	0.43 ± 0.02^a	1.32 ± 0.05^c
20:4n-6	0.38 ± 0.01	0.37 ± 0.01	0.39 ± 0.01	0.39 ± 0.01
22:6n-3	0.23 ± 0.03^a	0.17 ± 0.01^a	0.74 ± 0.05^b	0.98 ± 0.09^c

*Means sharing a common superscript are not significantly different (P<0.05)

Saturated FAs. Although the lauric acid content was similar among A, C, and J (between five and six weight percent), the level in P is exceptionally high, 13.8%.

Polyunsaturated FAs. LA was lowest in P, suggesting a diet low in FAs, and particularly polyunsaturated FAs. Arachidonic acid (AA) levels were similar among all countries demonstrating the highly protected nature of this FA. DHA varied greatly, ranging from 0.17% in C (samples collected in Edmonton, Alberta) to almost 1% in J. Due to relatively constant AA levels and large differences in DHA levels, the AA/DHA ratio varied seven-fold.

4.   CONCLUSION

The results of this study demonstrate the substantial variability of HM FA profiles. Consideration of optimal neonatal intake of specific FAs and suggestions for supplementation of maternal diets and infant formula should take this variability into consideration.

REFERENCES

1.   Jensen, R.G.,1989, The lipids of human milk, CRC Press., Boca Raton, Pp 93-151.
2.   Thompson, B.J., and Smith, S., 1985, Biosynthesis of fatty acids by lactating human breast epithelial cells: An evaluation of the contribution to the overall composition of human milk fat. Pediatr. Res. **19**:139-143.

47

SHORT-AND LONG TERM VARIATION IN THE PRODUCTION, CONTENT, AND COMPOSITION OF HUMAN MILK FAT

[1]Leon R. Mitoulas, [2]Jill L. Sherriff and [1]Peter E. Hartmann
[1]*Department of Biochemistry, The University of Western Australia, Nedlands, WA, 6907*
[2]*The School of Public Health, Curtin University, GPO Box U1987, Perth, WA, 6845*

Key words: Milk fat content, fatty acid composition, infant intake

1.   INTRODUCTION

Many studies have manipulated maternal diet to increase the proportion of specific fatty acids (FA) in human milk. However, few have investigated short- and long-term variations of milk fat content and FA composition and the implications these have on infant intake. We determined milk fat content (spectrophotometrically[1]) and FA composition (using gas chromatography[2]) in fore- and hind-milk samples from each feed, from each breast over 24 h periods at 1, 2, 4, 6, 9 and 12 months of lactation in 5 women.

2.   SHORT-TERM VARIATION

Fat content varied over the day with a mean (±SD) daily coefficient of variation (CV) of 44.7 ± 2.1 %. Fatty acid composition also varied over the day with a mean (±SD) daily CV of 14.3 ± 7.7 % for all FA. However, there was no consistent circadian rhythm for either fat content or the proportion of individual FA between women or with stage of lactation.

Short and Long Term Effects of Breast Feeding on Child Health
Edited by Berthold Koletzko *et al.*, Kluwer Academic/Plenum Publishers, 2000

3.   LONG-TERM VARIATION

Mean (±SD) milk production (376±154 mL/breast) differed between breasts, between women and with stage of lactation (p<0.05). Milk fat content (35.5±7.86 g/L) and the percentage composition of 18:1n9 (32.24±3.3), 18:2n6 (9.18±2.66), 18:3n3 (0.76±0.21), 20:4n6 (0.37±0.07), 22:5n3 (0.17±0.04) and 22:6n3 (0.2±0.07) differed only between women and with stage of lactation (p<0.05). In contrast, the amount delivered to the infant differed (p<0.05) between women only for 18:3n3, 22:5n3 and 22:6n3 and no differences in amounts delivered were observed for any of the FA from 1 to 12 months of lactation. Each child received a mean (±SD) of 8.27±2.84 g 18:1n9; 2.38±0.98 g 18:2n6; 194±73 mg 18:3n3; 92±31 mg 20:4n6; 43±14 mg 22:5n3 and 49±21 mg 22:6n3 every 24 h from breastmilk over the first year of life.

4.   CONCLUSIONS

Short-term patterns of variation for milk fat content are largely determined by infant feeding pattern and are therefore different between women. These results, when combined with the short-term variability in FA composition, emphasise the importance of appropriate sampling protocols. In addition, they suggest that the average fat content and FA composition of human milk quoted in the literature are of little value when assessing energy and FA intakes of individual breastfed infants. Furthermore, changes in milk production, fat content and composition over the long-term have highlighted that variation in the percentage composition of individual FA may not always translate to variation in the amount delivered to the infant and that milk production and fat content have to be taken into account.

REFERENCES

1. Atwood, C.S. and Hartmann, P.E. 1992. Changes in the composition of fore- and hind–milk from the sow. *J. Dairy Res.,* **59**:287:298.
2. Makrides, M., Neumann, M.A., Byards, R.W., Simmer, K. and Gibson, R.A. 1994. Fatty acid composition of brain, retina, and erythrocytes in breast and formula-fed infants. *Am. J. Clin. Nutr.,* **60**:189-194.

†   This study was supported by the Grains Research and Development Corporation of Australia, Meadow Lea Foods Ltd. and the Lotteries Commission of Western Australia

48

DIETARY FISH AND THE DOCOSAHEXAENOIC ACID (DHA) CONTENT OF HUMAN MILK

Lotte Lauritzen; Marianne H. Jørgensen; Kim F. Michaelsen
Research Department of Human Nutrition and LMC Centre for Advanced Food Studies, The Royal Veterinary and Agricultural University, Rolighedsvej 30, 1958 Frederiksberg C, Denmark

Key words: DHA, fatty acids, human milk, fish

1.   INTRODUCTION

DHA is ubiquitous in human milk, although in varying concentrations from 0.1% in some western societies to 1.4% in Inuit populations. It is possible that the neurologic development of breast fed infants could be affected by the level of maternal milk DHA. In order to investigate whether DHA is essential for term infants, and if it is, what the optimal level is, we need to understand the variations in milk DHA and influencing factors. The richest dietary source of DHA is marine organisms. Thus, in the studies described here our aim has been to describe the fluctuations in milk DHA and the effect of fish and fish oil intake on milk DHA levels.

2.   RESULTS AND DISCUSSION

The mean DHA-content in milk from Danish mothers is 0.41±0.36% range (0.12% to 1.98%)[1]. This variation probably reflect the variation in fish intake. 25% of Danish fertile women never eat fish, whereas the intake in the upper decile is >39 g/day[2]. I one of our studies 55% of the variation in milk DHA could be explained by differences in maternal fish intake[1,3]. In another study women, who reported never to eat fish, had a milk DHA content of

Short and Long Term Effects of Breast Feeding on Child Health
Edited by Berthold Koletzko *et al.*, Kluwer Academic/Plenum Publishers, 2000   403

$0.26\pm0.11\%$[1]. In a group of women, who did eat fish, those who had fish 2.1 ± 1.2 times a week had a mean DHA content of $0.47\pm0.39\%$ (n=10) and those who ate fish 4.2 ± 1.6 times/week 0.57 ± 0.28 %[4].

Mothers who ate fish on the day before they delivered a morning milk sample had a 50% higher DHA concentration than those who did not[1]. Those who had fat fish had milk DHA levels $82\pm17\%$ higher, whereas lean fish only gave rise to an insignificant increase of $32\pm35\%$[4]. Fish oil test meals (2-8 g) resulted in an acute increase in milk DHA, which started after a few hours, peaked after 8-10 hours at 150-300% of morning level, and lasted for approximately 24 hours[4].

In a cross sectional study of 4 mo old infants we found a positive association between visual acuity (SWEEP-VEP), and the DHA content of their mother's milk controlled for fish intake the day before milk sampling[3]. However, this association between milk DHA and visual acuity were not confirmed neither in a cross-sectional study of American/Canadian infants nor in an Australian intervention study[5]. Therefore, we cannot from this limited data make any conclusions about functional effects of different levels of DHA in breast milk.

In conclusion, consumption of fish and marine oils have a pronounced and immediate effect on the concentration of DHA in human milk. The increase in milk DHA peaks after approximately 10 h. In mothers with a high BMI the increase was less (unpublished data). Because of this pronounced effect of fish meals and consequently large fluctuations in milk DHA it is difficult to asses the exact DHA intake of breast fed infant if the mother eats fish. The assessment would be better if it is based on an average of several milk samples taken at different times of the day and not on a single morning milk sample. Another approach would be to indirectly assess the DHA intake of the infant through an assessment of the DHA status of the mother. This is normally done by measuring the fatty acid composition of her erythrocytes or adipose tissue. We found that the fatty acid composition of erythrocytes in the mother is a better bio-marker for milk DHA than the composition of adipose tissues (unpublished data).

3.   REFERENCES

1. Lauritzen, L., Jørgensen, M.H., and Michaelsen, K.F. FASEB Journal 1998;12(4):A201.
2. Levnedsmiddelstyrelsen. Dietary habits in the Danish Population 1995. Main Results (in Danish), Levnedsmiddelstyrelsen, Copenhagen, 1996.
3. Jørgensen, M.H. et al. FASEB Journal 1998;12(5):A970.
4. Lauritzen, L. et al. Pediatric Research 1999;45(6):916.
5. Jørgensen, M.H., Lauritzen, L., and Michaelsen, K.F. Journal of Human Lactation 1999; 15(1):3-6.

49

FATTY ACID COMPOSITION OF MATURE BREAST MILK ACCORDING TO THE MOTHERS DIET DURING PREGNANCY

M. Moya; M. Juste; E. Cortés; F. Carratalá

Pediatric Department Hospital Universitario San Juan. Universidad Miguel Hernández. Alicante. Spain

Key words: Breast milk. Fatty acids, mother diet

1.   INTRODUCTION

Breast milk fats (98% TG) reflect not only the mothers nutritional condition but also their diet. We studied wether a diet containing small amounts of fish during whole gestation increases the content of DHA and eicosapentaenoic acid (EPA, 20:5n-3) in breast milk.

2.   METHODS

102 healthy mothers were interviewed twice filling a questionnaire assessing the usual habits over the past year (Black G et al. J Am Epidemiol 1986;124:453-69). That enabled us to identify a group of 86 mothers having at least a portion of fish (200 g) per week ($\geq$ 28 g/day, fish group) and another group of 16 mothers eating fish never or less than once per week

A sample of mature (> 15 days) breast milk was obtained for measuring total fat, FA pattern (mass spectrometry) vitamin D and 25 D (HPLC and binding protein).

3.   RESULTS

Maternal and newborn nutritional status was normal in all cases. In the table are the values for fatty acids and total fat in both groups.

BREAST MILK COMPOSITION ACCORDING FISH INTAKE; < 200 g/week (n=16); ≥200 g/week (n=86)					
FA wt/wt	<200 g/wk	>200 g/wk	FA %wt/wt	<200 g/wk	>200 g/wk
10:0	1.67(1.32)	1.28(1.03)	20:3n-6	.55(.28)	.52(.25)
12:0	5.18(3.23)	4.49(3.12)	20:4n-6	.63(.27)	.60(.25)
14:0	7.03(3.22)	6.31(2.58)	20:5n-3	.09(.10)	.07(.07)
14:1n-5	.15(.14)	.30(1.87)	22:00	.37(.52)	.27(.41)
16:0	21.6(4.66)	22.3(5.06)	22:1n-9	.18(.22)	.19(.14)
16:1n-7	1.43(.79)	1.34(.58)	22:2n-6	.14(.17)	.12(.10)
18:0	7.44(2.79)	7.57(2.57)	22:3n-3	.16(.19)	.18(.22)
18:1n-7*	1.99(.10)	2.21(.29)	22:4n-6	.13(.17)	.11(.17)
18:1n-9	27.8(9.48)	32.9(6.96)	22:5n-3**	.20(.12)	. 29(.12)
18:2n-6	17.9(8.80)	16.1(4.08)	22:5n-6	.21(.34)	.17(.17)
18:3n-3	.63(.42)	.54(.25)	22:6n-3	.36(.19)	.46(.23)
20:0	.19(.07)	.21(.06)	24:0	.11(.13)	.18(.13)
20:1n-9	.48(.21)	.55(.24)	24:1n-9**	.14(.14)	.20(.14)
20:2n-6	.68(.37)	.70(.40)	Total fat g/dl	3.04(1.38)	2.69(1.44)

Mean (sd) ; * p<.05; ** p<.01

Vitamin D content showed no differences (.57± .32 ng/ml, vs .51 ± .26 ng/ml) conversely 25 hydroxyvitamin D was significantly (P< .05) higher in the group taking fish (.62 ± .43 ng/ml vs .98 ± .60 ng/ml).

4.   SUMMARY

Mothers taking 200 g of fish per week, showed a greater content in mature breast milk of n-3 fatty acids, particularly DHA. AA was not decreased.

Vitamin D content was low despite mothers were living in a sunny and template area. The content of 25 hydroxyvitamin D is increased in the group on fish intake, probably pointing out its marine source.

REFERENCES

1. Ackman R.G. Docosahexaenoic acid in the infant and its mother. Letter. Lipids 1999;34:125-8.
3.   Genzel-Boroviczény O. et al. Fatty acid composition of human milk during the 1st month after term and preterm delivery. Eur J Pediatr 1997;156:142-7.

50

CONTRIBUTION OF DIETARY AND NEWLY FORMED ARACHIDONIC ACID TO MILK SECRETION IN WOMEN ON LOW FAT DIETS

Martha Del Prado[1], Salvador Villalpando[1], Alejandra Lance[1], Eunice Alfonso[1], Hans Demmelmair[2] and Berthold Koletzko[2].

1 Unidad de Investigación Médica en Nutrición. Instituto Mexicano del Seguro Social México, D.F.; 2 Klinderklinik and Kinderpoliklinik, Dr. von Haunersches Kinderspital, Ludwig-Maximilians University, Munich, Germany.

1. INTRODUCTION

Long chain polyunsaturated fatty acids in breast milk are derived from dietary intake, from endogenous conversion and from maternal body stores. The diet of rural Mexico is low in fat (17% of energy) and although the arachidonic acid (AA) intake in women from these regions is low, the amount of AA in the milk is similar to values reported for women from developed countries.[1,2] The aim of this study was to estimate the contribution of dietary and endogenously synthesised AA to milk in this women .

2. METHODS

An oral bolus of U-^{13}C-linoleic acid (LA, 2.5 mg/kg) was given to 10 lactating women.. Milk and breath samples were collected before and until 72h after tracer administration. The ^{13}C enrichment in CO_2 and milk fatty acids was measured by isotope-ratio mass spectrometry, while milk fatty acids were quantified by gas chromatography. Breast milk intake was measured for 48 h by test weighing of the infant.[2] The total amounts of LA and AA transferred directly from diet into milk fat were calculated by multiplying the 24 h intakes of LA and AA times the % of ^{13}C-LA recovered in milk . We assumed a similar transfer rate into milk for dietary AA and LA based on the observations by Sauerwald who showed a similar transference for palmitic, oleic and docosahexaenoic acid.[3]

3.   RESULTS

Within 72 h after administering the dose, about 16% of the labelled LA was recovered in milk as LA, 0.01% as AA and 16% as breath CO_2 (Table I). The calculated transfer of LA and AA from the diet into milk contributed with about 33 and 12% of the total LA and AA secreted into milk, respectively. The detectable endogenous conversion of ^{13}C-LA to milk AA was low and contributed 1.1% of the total AA secreted into milk.

Table I Calculated contribution of LA and AA from diet and AA from endogenous synthesis to the LA and AA secretion in milk.

Transfer into milk		Linoleic acid	Arachidonic acid
from diet	(g/d)	1.8 ± 0.8	0.011 ± 0.007
	(% of total)	32.8 ± 18.0	11.8 ± 6.6
from endogenous synthesis	(g/d)		0.0008 ± 0.0004
	(% total)		1.14 ± 0.80

4.   CONCLUSIONS

About 70% of the LA and 80% of the AA secreted into milk were not derived directly from the diet. Only a minor fraction of milk AA stems from direct conversion of dietary LA. Maternal body stores, with low turnover, are the major source for milk LA and AA in woman on low fat diets.

REFERENCES

1. Villalpando, S., Butte, N., Flores-Huerta, S., and Thotathuchery, M. 1998, Qualitative analysis of human milk produced by women consuming a maize-predominant diet typical of rural Mexico. *Ann Nutr Metab* 42:23-32

2. Demmelmair, H., Baumheuer, M., Koletzko, B., Dokoupil, K., and Kratl, G. 1998, Metabolism of U^{13}C- labelled linoleic acid in lactating women. *J. Lipid Res.* 39: 1389-1396.

3. Sauerwald, T., Fidler, N., Pohl, A., Demmelmair, H., Koletzko, B 1998, Docosahexaenoic acid recovery in human milk after dietary supplementation. *Ped Res.* 43: 268A.

This work was supported by grants from the Consejo Nacional de Ciencia y Tecnología, México and from the Deutsche Forschungsgemeinschaft, Bonn, Germany (Ko912/5-2).

51

[13]C-LINOLEIC ACID OXIDATION AND TRANSFER INTO MILK IN LACTATING WOMEN WITH CONTRASTING BODY MASS INDEX

Alejandra Lance[1] , Salvador Villalpando[1] , Martha Del Prado[1], Eunice Alfonso[1],
Hans Demmelmair[2] and Berthold Koletzko[2]
*1 Unidad de Investigación Médica en Nutrición. Instituto Mexicano del Seguro Social México,
D.F.; 2 Klinderklinik and Kinderpoliklinik, Dr. von Haunersches Kinderspital, Ludwig-
Maximilians University, Munich, Germany*

1. INTRODUCTION

The diet of the rural community of San Mateo Capulhuac Mexico, is marginal in energy (45 kcal/kg body weight/day) and protein (0.8 g/kg body weight/day) and low in fat (17% of total energy). The milk lipid concentration in women from this community was positively correlated with maternal weight, body mass index (BMI) and body fat.[1] The aim of this study was to investigate differences in the metabolic distribution of dietary lipids between women with a low or a high BMI by following the metabolism of an oral dose of ^{13}C-linoleic acid (LA).

2. METHODS

Ten lactating women from San Mateo Capulhuac, Mexico with a BMI<22.5 (n=5) or BMI>23.5 were recruited. The first day of the study they received orally 2.5 mg/kg body weight of U-^{13}C-linoleic acid. Milk samples were collected at 0, 6, 9, 12, 15, 24, 36, 48 and 72h after the tracer dose. Breath samples were taken at 0, 1-12h, 24, 48 and 72h after the dose. The [13]C

Short and Long Term Effects of Breast Feeding on Child Health
Edited by Berthold Koletzko *et al.*, Kluwer Academic/Plenum Publishers, 2000

enrichment in CO_2 was measured by isotope-ratio mass spectrometry (IRMS). Breast milk intake was measured for 48 h by test weighing of the infant. The fatty acid composition of milk samples was measured by gas chromatography and ^{13}C enrichment by IRMS.

3.   RESULTS

Women in the high BMI (HBMI) group had a body weight 10 kg higher than those of the low BMI (LBMI) group (45.7 ± 3.8 Vs 54.3 ± 5.1, p= 0.019). The energy and fat intakes were not different between groups (2216.6 ± 395.1 vs 2328.2 ± 356.0 Kcal/d and 43.05 ± 6.15 vs 50.99 ± 14.26 g/d). Milk volume was higher and milk lipid concentration was lower in the LBMI than in the HBMI group (763 ± 93 vs 676 ± 149 g/d and 2.66 ± 0.61 vs 3.58 ± 1.24 g/dL, p= 0.03). HBMI women had a higher 72h cumulated $^{13}CO_2$ production, cumulated ^{13}C-LA recovered in milk LA at 72h was not different between groups (Table I).

Table I Cumulative recovery of orally applied ^{13}C-linoleic acid in lactating women

	% dose		
	BMI <22.5	BMI>23.5	P
Breath CO2	8.6 ± 3.5	22.8 ± 9.4	0.01
Milk 18:2 n-6	17.70 ± 6.68	14.82 ± 6.49	n.s.
Total recovered	26.3 ± 10.7	37.6 ± 14.4	n.s.

4.   CONCLUSIONS

Our results showed that lactating women with BMI <22.5 had a lower oxidation of dietary fat in comparison to women with BMI >23.5 from the same community, eating a similar low fat diet. The percentage of a dose of ^{13}C-LA transferred to milk was similar between groups. An important portion of the dose may be taken up by a maternal compartment with a low turnover rate, such as the adipose tissue.

REFERENCES

1. Barbosa, L., Butte, N.F., Villalpando, S., Wong, W.W., Smith, E.O. 1997, Maternal energy balance and lactation performance of Mesoamerindians as a function of BMI. *Am J Clin Nutr.* 66: 575-583.
This work was supported by grants from the Consejo Nacional de Ciencia y Tecnología, México and from the Deutsche Forschungsgemeinschaft, Bonn, Germany (Ko912/5-2).

52

ARACHIDONIC (AA) AND DOCOSAHEXAENOIC (DHA) ACID CONTENT IN HEALTHY INFANTS FED WITH AN HA MILK FORMULA SUPPLEMENTED WITH LCPUFA AND IN BREAST FED INFANTS

Francesco Savino, Paola Serraino, Alessandra Prino, Roberto Oggero, Roberta Bretto and Michael Mostert
Department of Paediatrics, University of Turin, P.zza Polonia 94, Torino 10126 Italy.

Key words: Lcpufa, Supplementation, ha milk formula

1. INTRODUCTION

In infants fed with supplemented formulas plasma and erythrocyte membrane phospholipid composition in AA and DHA is comparable to that of breast fed infants. In addition to their role in development, LCPUFA may also play a role in atopic disease [1,2]. Reports describe disorders of essential fatty acids metabolism, specifically of impaired conversion of 18 carbon precursors to their LCPUFA products, that lead to modified fatty acids profiles in atopic children[3]. Therefore, the supplementation of HA formulas with LCPUFA should be useful.

2. AIM

To examine composition in AA and DHA of *plasma phospholipids* and *erythrocyte membrane phospholipids* in infants fed a HA formula supplemented with LCPUFA (HA) and in breast fed (BM) infants.

3. METHODS

Forty six term, AGA infants with a family history for atopic disease fed from birth with a HA formula supplemented with LCPUFA (Aptamil HA 1, Milupa) and twenty five exclusively breast fed infants, constituted the case series. At three months of age the composition in AA and DHA of plasma and erythrocyte membrane phospholipids was determined on venous blood samples, after 3 hours fasting, by means of gaschromatography. Differences between means for the two groups were analyzed. Statistical analysis was performed using Student's t-test. A value of $p < 0.05$ was used for statistical significance.

4. RESULTS

No significant differences between breast fed infants and infants fed Aptamil HA 1 milk formula were observed.
The table below reports the mean values and (standard deviation)of AA and DHA in plasma (Table 1) and erythrocite membrane phospholipids (Table 2) in %wt/wt .

Table 1	BREAST MILK	HA+LCPUFA	Statistical Analysis
AA (C20:4n6)	11.68 (2.31)	9.96 (2.23)	NS
DHA (C22:6n3)	4.28 (0.90)	3.75 (1.07)	NS
Table 2	BREAST MILK	HA+LCPUFA	Statistical Analysis
AA (C20:4n6)	12.42 (2.61)	12.05 (2.21)	NS
DHA (C22:6n3)	4.95 (1.43)	4.39 (2.19)	NS

5. CONCLUSIONS

AA and DHA content of plasma and erythrocyte membrane phospholipids in infants fed the examined HA formula supplemented with long chain polyunsaturated fatty acids and breast fed infants is similar suggesting that the supplementation is useful.

REFERENCES

1. Gibson, R.A., and Makrides, M., 1998, The role of long chain polyusaturated fatty acids (LCPUFA) in neonatal nutrition. *Acta Paediatr.* 87: 1017-1022.
2. Hamosh, M., 1998, Atopic disease and milk fatty acid composition. *Acta Paediatr.* 87: 719-720.
3. Yu, G., Kjellman, N-I.M., and Bjorksten, B., 1996, Phospholipid fatty acids in cord blood: family history and development of allergy. *Acta Paediatr.* 85: 679-683.

53

LOW CONTRIBUTION OF DOCOSAHEXAENOIC ACID TO THE FATTY ACID COMPOSITION OF MATURE HUMAN MILK IN HUNGARY

Tamás Decsi, Szilvia Oláh, Szilárd Molnár and István Burus
Department of Paediatrics, UniversityMedical School of Pécs, József A. u. 7., H-7623 Pécs, Hungary

Key words: arachidonic acid, docosahexaenoic acid, human milk

1.   INTRODUCTION

Contribution of the long-chain polyunsaturated fatty acids to the fatty acid composition of human milk exhibits considerable variability among populations.[1] More than a decade ago, an obstetrical study comparing the influence of steroidal contraceptives on milk lipids and fatty acids in Hungary and Thailand showed unexpectedly low docosahexaenoic acid (C22:6w-3) values in the Hungarian milk samples.[2]

2.   SUBJECTS AND METHODS

Human milk samples of 10 ml volume from 24-hour collections were obtained from 15 lactating women twice with 2 weeks of intervals. The mean duration of lactation was 4 months (ranges: 1 to 14 months) at the first sample collection. Technical details of fatty acid analysis have been recently described.[3]

Short and Long Term Effects of Breast Feeding on Child Health
Edited by Berthold Koletzko *et al.*, Kluwer Academic/Plenum Publishers, 2000

3. RESULTS

Values of the ω-6 essential fatty acid, linoleic acid (C18:2ω-6) were considerably higher, whereas those of the ω-3 essential fatty acid, α-linolenic acid (C18:3ω-3) were considerably lower in mature human milk in Hungary in 1998 than in 1986 (Table 1). In spite of the very similar contribution of C18:3ω-3 to the fatty acid composition of mature human milk in Hungary in 1998 to that reported from other five European countries[4-8] in the 1990ies, the C22:6ω-3 values in the Hungarian milk samples were considerably lower than the values reported for other European populations (Table 1).

Table 1. Major polyunsaturated fatty acids in mature human milk in Hungary in 1986[2] and in 1998. The Hungarian data are compared to the mean of values recently reported in five studies[4-8]. Data are % weight/weight, mean (SD).

Fatty acid	Hungary 1986	Hungary 1998	Europe 1993-1998
Linoleic	11.0	15.72 (4.39)	11.6
Arachidonic	0.5	0.52 (0.10)	0.5
α-Linolenic	1.2	0.71 (0.25)	0.7
Docosahexaenoic	0.1	0.17 (0.05)	0.3

4. DISCUSSION

The low contribution of C22:6ω-3 to the fatty acid composition of milk lipids in Hungary may be the consequence of low dietary intake of preformed C22:6ω-3 in the form of fish and fish products. It is to be emphasised, however, that neither the present study nor the aforementioned previous report[2] found any indication of low dietary intake of the C22:6ω-3 precursor essential fatty acid, C18:3ω-3.

REFERENCES

1. B. Koletzko et al. *J. Pediatr.* **120:** S62-S70, 1992
2. M. Sas et al. *Contraception* **33:** 159-178, 1986
3. T. Decsi et al. *Acta Paediatr.* **88:** 500-504, 1999
4. G. Serra et al. *Biol. Neonate* **72:** 1-8, 1997
5. S. Presa-Owens et al. *J. Pediatr. Gastroenterol. Nutr.* **22:** 180-185, 1996
6. O. Genzel-Boroviczény et al. *Eur. J. Pediatr.* **156:** 142-147, 1997
7. P. Guesnet et al. *Eur. J. Clin. Nutr.* **47:** 700-710, 1993
8. I.B. Helland et al. *Eur. J. Clin. Nutr.* **52:** 839-845, 1998

54

MALNOURISHED MOTHERS MAINTAIN THEIR WEIGHT THROUGH OUT PREGNANCY AND LACTATION

Results From Guatemala

[1]Anna Winkvist, Ph.D., [2]Jean-Pierre Habicht, M.D., Ph.D., [2]Kathleen M. Rasmussen. Ph.D. and [2]Edward A. Frongillo Jr., Ph.D.
[1]Epidemiology, Dept. of Public Health and Clinical Medicine, Umeå University, Umeå, Sweden: [2]Div. of Nutritional Sciences, Cornell University, Ithaca, NY, USA

Key words: pregnancy, lactation, weight, Guatemala, malnutrition

1. INTRODUCTION

We have shown that moderately malnourished Pakistani and Guatemalan women lose weight over a reproductive cycle without compromising the birthweight of their second compared to their prior infant. Surprisingly, malnourished women did not lose weight over the reproductive cycle, but their second was smaller than their prior infant. These findings were consistent with results among Indonesian women and with our work in animals.

2. OBJECTIVE

Here we again use data from a supplementation trial of pregnant and lactating women by Institute of Nutrition in Central America and Panama in Guatemala 1969-1977, to estimate the thresholds in maternal body weight at which the trade-offs between maternal and fetal health occur. Impact of maternal experiences of periods of non-pregnancy/non-lactation (NPNL) or overlap of lactation with the next pregnancy also are evaluated.

3.   METHODS

Information on two consecutive deliveries were available for 176 women. Change in maternal weight (3 mo postpartum) over the reproductive cycle (ΔW) and difference between the two birthweights (within 24 h of delivery; ΔBW) were calculated. Women with supplement intake in the top two tertiles were contrasted with the others. The relationships of ΔW and ΔBW to initial maternal weight were investigated for both supplement groups, using piece-wise regression analyses.

4.   RESULTS

The threshold below which lower initial maternal weight in Low Supplement predicted lower ΔBW was 48.4 kg (± 2.7). High levels of maternal supplement eliminated this association. Above this threshold, ΔBW was independent of initial maternal weight in both supplement groups. On the maternal side, the threshold below which ΔW was higher the lower the initial maternal weight, was 49.6 kg (± 1.6). High levels of maternal supplement eliminated this association. The threshold above which ΔW was unrelated to initial maternal weight for Low Supplement was 55.3 kg (± 1.3). Between 49.6 kg and 55.3 kg, lower initial maternal weight was associated with lower ΔW for women in Low Supplement. High levels of supplement eliminated this association. Separate analyses for women with NPNL vs. overlap yielded similar results.

5.   CONCLUSIONS

We identified a threshold in initial maternal weight below which the nutritional flow during reproduction benefits the infant more than the mother, and an even lower threshold where the nutritional flow benefits the mother at the expense of the infant. The benefits of a maternal nutritional supplement are partitioned to counteract these dynamics. Whether the mother had experienced periods of non-pregnancy/non-lactation or overlap of lactation with the next pregnancy, had no impact on these results.

55

EFFECT OF EXERCISE AND ENERGY RESTRICTION ON LEPTIN DURING LACTATION

Ratna Mukherjea [1], Phylis Moser-Veillon [1] and Cheryl Lovelady [2]
[1] *Dept of Nutrition and Food Science, University of Maryland, College Park;* [2] *Dept of Nutrition and Food Service Systems, University of North Carolina, Greensboro.*

1.   INTRODUCTION

Leptin, a hormone originally thought to play a role only in control of food intake, energy expenditure and regulation of body weight, may have a role in energy utilisation during lactation. The objectives of the present study were to determine the effect of exercise and energy restriction on leptin and examine the relationship between leptin, prolactin and insulin during lactation.

2.   METHODS

Four to five week exclusively breast feeding women with BMI >25<30 were recruited for the study. The subjects were assigned to a treatment group (n=8) and a control group (n=6). The treatment group was put on an energy restriction and aerobic exercise program. Data collection was done at 4-5 weeks postpartum and 10 weeks after intervention. Fasting plasma was analysed for leptin, prolactin and insulin. BMI, fat mass and % body fat were determined. Three-day diet records were kept prior to each visit. ANOVA was used to determine differences between groups. Correlation and regression were done to determine the relationship between leptin, prolactin and insulin.

Short and Long Term Effects of Breast Feeding on Child Health
Edited by Berthold Koletzko *et al.*, Kluwer Academic/Plenum Publishers, 2000

3.   RESULTS

Pre-pregnancy BMI was not significantly different between the treatment (24.9 ± 2.27) and control (26.4 ± 3.19) group. There was no significant effect of intervention on leptin, prolactin or insulin concentrations. A significant decrease ($p<0.05$) in body weight (4.3 ± 1.08 kg) and fat mass (3.8 ± 1.15 kg) was observed only in the treatment group after intervention. Further there was no treatment effect on leptin even when analyses were done with % body fat as a covariate. Hence the groups were combined for further analyses. There was a significant correlation between leptin and BMI ($r = 0.5$, $p<0.05$), leptin and fat mass ($r = 0.6$, $p<0.05$) and leptin and % body fat ($r = 0.7$, $p<0.05$). There was a significant correlation only between change in leptin and change in energy intake ($r = 0.6$, $p<0.05$). BMI, % body fat, and prolactin ($p <0.05$) independently predicted leptin. Leptin concentrations were also predicted by BMI and insulin ($R^2 = 0.6$, $p<0.05$), prolactin and insulin ($R^2 = 0.53$, $p<0.05$) and by % body fat, insulin and the interaction between % body fat and insulin ($R^2 = 0.77$, $p<0.05$).

4.   DISCUSSION

Fat mass is correlated with BMR and 74% of the change in BMR during pregnancy can be explained by leptin[1]. Another study observed a 66% increase in leptin early in pregnancy prior to significant changes in body fat[2]. We have previously shown that leptin is elevated in lactating women when compared to never pregnant controls. In the present study although change in leptin did not correlate with changes in body composition, there was a significant correlation between change in leptin and change in energy intake. A relationship between leptin, prolactin and insulin was also demonstrated. Thus, in addition to adiposity, change in energy intake and hormones such as prolactin and insulin affect leptin concentrations during lactation.

REFERENCES

[1] Lang, K.E., Bonnel, E.L., Havel, P.J., Gale, B., Reilly, J., Van Loan, M., King, J.C. 1999, Changes in leptin and body fat mass relate to the rise in BMR during pregnancy. FASEB J. Abs # 760.2

[2] Catalano, P.M. 1999, Pregnancy and lactation in relation to range of acceptable carbohydrate and fat intake. Eur. J. clin. Nutr. 53 : 1 : s124-131

56

FOOD INTAKES IN A GROUP OF BREAST-FEEDING AND NOT BREAST-FEEDING MOTHERS

Francesco Savino, Giuseppina Bonfante, Maria Cristina Muratore, Amalia Peltran, Francesco Cresi, Michael Mostert and Roberto Oggero.
Department of Paediatrics, University of Turin, P.zza Polonia 94, Torino 10126, Italy

Key words: food intakes, breast-feeding mothers.

1. ABSTRACT: INTRODUCTION

The relation between mother's diet and breast milk composition is still an open question. An important issue is whether mothers who are breast feeding modify, respect to before lactation,food intake to satisfy the increased requirements.

2. AIM

To compare food intakes in a group of breast-feeding and not breast-feeding mothers with the respective LARN values [1].

3. MATERIALS AND METHODS

In the period February - May 1998 the healthy mothers of 48, singleton, term infants, aged 25-35 days and seen at the Infants' Department of our institution for a routine medical visit were enrolled. Twenty five infants were breast fed and the rest were exclusively fed on formula milk. Mothers filled

Short and Long Term Effects of Breast Feeding on Child Health
Edited by Berthold Koletzko *et al.*, Kluwer Academic/Plenum Publishers, 2000

in a detailed questionnaire concerning dietary habits over two days. Italian recommended daily assumption levels of nutrients (LARN) values for breast-feeding (LA) and not breast-feeding (LB) mothers were used for the purpose of comparisons. The data collected were processed by Dietosystem software to obtain the daily nutrient intakes.

4. RESULTS

Breast-feeding mothers' diet is hyperproteic and hypocaloric and intake is inadequate for vitamins B1, B2, PP, B6, B12, E and folic acid, and for Fe, Ca, Mg and Zn.

Not breast-feeding mothers diet is hyperproteic, isocaloric, inadequate for vitamins B6 and E and for Fe and Mg.

Intake of nutrients in not breast-feeding and breast-feeding mothers is closer to the respective LARN values in the former.

Table 1. Breast-feeding (A) and not breast-feeding (B) mothers' intakes (mean of 2 days) compared with Recommended Daily Assumption Levels of Nutrients (LA) (LB) respectively.

	Cal Kcal	Prot G	B1 mg	B2 mg	B6 mg	fol µg	B12 µg	C Mg	A µg	D3 µg	E µg	Fe mg	Ca mg	P mg	Mg mg	Zn mg
A	1765	116	0.81	1.27	1.16	158	2.3	119	1407	13.6	4.3	11.6	689	1134	221	10.1
SD	495	25	0.29	0.3	0.42	51.2	0.88	90.5	982	4.3	1.9	3.4	260	303	75.5	4.4
B	2164	96	1.03	1.4	0.9	229	2.4	130	1207	15	5.2	13	889	1121	270	10.9
SD	600	30	0.33	0.5	0.39	49.2	0.81	99.1	973	5.2	2	2.8	199	289	74.8	3.8
LA	2650	70	1.1	1.7	1.3	350	2.6	90	950	10	8	18	1200	1200	475	12
LB	2150	53	0.9	1.3	1.1	200	2	60	600	10	8	18	800	800	325	7

5. DISCUSSION

It is necessary to improve nutrients intake in breast-feeding mothers and not breast-feeding mothers, but more so in the former.

It is important that pediatricians inform breast-feeding mothers on the advantages of improving quality of intake of nutrients.

REFERENCES

1.   LARN- Livelli di assunzione raccomandati di energia e nutrienti per la popolazione italiana. Società Italiana di Nutrizione Umana-Revisione 1996.

57

ILLNESS-INDUCED ANOREXIA IN THE BREAST-FED INFANTS. ROLE OF IL-1β AND TNF-α

Mardya Lopez-Alarcon, M.D, M.Sci*., Salvador Villalpando, M.D., PhD., Cutberto Garza, M.D., PhD*.
*Unidad de Investigación Médica en Nutrición, Instituto Mexicano del Seguro Social and *Cornell University*

Key words: Illness-induced anorexia, breast-fed infants, TNF, IL-1

1.   BACKGROUND

Infants are reported to eat less than normal amounts during infections [1,2]. Some have reported that breast-fed infants are less prone to anorexia during infectious illnesses [1,2]. In animals, illness-induced anorexia (IIA) is associated with the release of interleukin-1 and tumor necrosis factor whose main mediators are the prostaglandins [3]. Prostaglandins, cytokines, anti-inflammatory factors and the PUFAs docosahexaenoic (DHA) and arachidonic (AA) are among the substances present in human milk that likely modulate an infant's immune system and may account for the putative dampening of anorectic responses during illnesses of breastfed infants. It also is noteworthy that DHA and AA are prostaglandin precursors. AA derived prostaglandins are more potent than those derived from DHA. This study's aims were to assess energy intakes of breast- and formula-fed infants during and after an infectious episode and to assess possible relationships between circulating concentrations of IL-1 and TNF, and DHA and AA tissue levels to anorectic responses in both groups. This study was approved by the Research Committee of the Mexican Institute of Social Security and by the Human Use Committee of Cornell University.

Short and Long Term Effects of Breast Feeding on Child Health
Edited by Berthold Koletzko *et al.*, Kluwer Academic/Plenum Publishers, 2000   421

2.   SUBJECTS AND METHODS

Twenty-eight infants hospitalized with pneumonia in 2 hospitals of Mexico City were enrolled. Daily energy intake (test-weighing procedure) was estimated and peripheral venous blood was collected at hospitalization for the determination of IL-1β and TNF-α (ELISA), and erythrocytes fatty acid profiles (gas chromatography). To compare energy intakes during illness (the day of hospitalization), convalescence (the day of discharge), and post convalescence (three weeks after discharge), infants were readmitted for three days three weeks after discharge. Paired t-Test, Wilcoxon, Student t-Test and regression analyses were performed as appropriate.

3.   RESULTS

Of the 28 selected infants, 13 returned for reevaluation. Formula-fed infants (FFI) were older (5.9 ± 0.9 Vs 4.2 ± 0.9 mo) and had higher body temperature (37.6 ± 0.2 Vs 36.8 ± 0.3 °C) and cardiac rate (150 ± 4.6 Vs 140 ± 3.7) than breast-fed infants (BFI). Energy intakes were reduced in both groups during illness period (64.25 ± 43 and 62.59 ± 6.6 kcal/kg/day) compared to intakes observed in the convalescent (82.98 ± 9.2 and 86.36 ± 7.2 kcal/kg/day) and post-convalescent periods (84.02 ± 7.7 and 111.15 ± 6.7 kcal/kg/day). However, the relative reduction in intake was significantly lower in BF than in FFI (23.5 Vs 43.7%). BFI also recovered the appetites sooner. The mean proportion of DHA in the erythrocyte membranes was higher in BFI as compared to FFI (3.9 ± 0.2 Vs 2.4 ± 0.3). The increase of IL-1β was similar in both groups (36 and 37%), but the increase of TNF-α was significantly higher in FFI (164%) than in BFI (89%). Reduction in energy intake was related positively to IL-1β and TNF-α levels, and negatively to the proportion of DHA in the tissues (p< 0.05, R = 0.64).

REFERENCES

1. Hoyle B Y, Chen LC. Breast-feeding and food intake among children with acute diarrheal disease. Am J Clin Nutr 1980; 33:2365-2371.
2. Brown KH and Perez F. Determinants of dietary intake during childhood diarrhea and implications for appropriate nutritional therapy. Acta Paediatr 1992; 381(Suppl):127-32.
3. McCarthy DO, Kluger MJ, Vander AJ. The effect of peripheral and intracerebroventricular administration of interleukin-1 on food intake of rats. In: The physiologic, metabolic, and immunologic actions of interleukin-1. Alan R. Liss, Inc., New York. USA 1985, pp 171-179.

58

MATERNAL PERCEPTION OF THE ONSET OF LACTATION: A VALID INDICATOR OF LACTOGENESIS STAGE II?

Donna Chapman M.S, R.D. and Rafael Pérez-Escamilla, Ph.D.
Department of Nutritional Sciences, University of Connecticut, Storrs, CT USA, 06269-4017

Key words: lactogenesis stage II, onset of lactation

1. INTRODUCTION

The measurement of milk transfer (MT) by test weighing is the „gold standard" for documenting the onset of lactogenesis stage II (OL)[1]; however, test weighing is impractical for routine use. From a public health perspective, maternal perception (MP) of the timing of OL may be a useful proxy for OL, as it describes when women actually feel their milk „came in." This study compares the determinants and consequences of delayed OL, as measured by both MT and MP.

2. METHODS

Study data were obtained from a previously described randomized clinical trial [2]. Following Cesarean delivery in a USA hospital, 57 subjects were randomly assigned to study group (breast pumping or control) and were interviewed 3 times daily regarding MP.   Test weights were obtained 3 times daily between 24 and 72 hours pp to generate individual MT/feeding curves.   MP and OL were categorized as early or late, using cutoffs of 72 hours pp for MP and 9.2 g/feeding for MT at 60 hr pp. Multivariate logistic regression analyses were used to identify the determinants of delayed OL. Multivariate survival analyses examined the association between OL and breastfeeding (BF) duration.

3.   RESULTS

The determinants common to both low MT and delayed MP included: delayed BF initiation (MT: OR=7.5; MP: OR=9.5), milk transfer at 30 hr pp (MT: OR=0.81; MP: OR=0.83); breast pumping*parity (MT: $p<0.05$; MP: $p<0.01$); and maternal obesity*BF frequency (MT:$p=0.03$; MP:$p=0.06$).   Intended BF duration interacted with both MT ($p<0.001$) and MP ($p<0.001$) to determine the duration of any BF.

4.   DISCUSSION AND CONCLUSIONS

Our findings strongly suggest that MP is a useful, non-invasive, public health marker of OL.   This conclusion is based on the striking consistency observed between the determinants and consequences of low MT and delayed MP in our population.   Our data replicate our previous finding that among women planning to breastfeed for at least six months, those with delayed perception of the onset of lactation are more likely to discontinue BF sooner than their counterparts with early perception of OL [3].   Future studies are needed in different cultures and settings to conclusively validate MP as a marker of OL.

REFERENCES

1. Daly S, Hartmann P. Infant demand and milk supply. Part 2: The short-term control of milk synthesis in lactating women. J Hum Lact 1995;11:27-37.

2. Chapman D. Impact of breast pumping on the onset of lactogenesis stage II following Cesarean delivery: A randomzied clinical trial.   Doctoral dissertation, University of Connecticut, Department of Nutritional Sciences, Storrs, CT, 1999.

3. Chapman D, Pérez-Escamilla R. Does delayed perception of the onset of lactation shorten   breastfeeding   duration?   J   Hum   Lact   1999;15:107-111.

59

THE ONSET OF LACTATION: IMPLICATIONS FOR BREAST-FEEDING PROMOTION PROGRAMS

Rafael Pérez-Escamilla, Ph.D. and Donna Chapman, M.S., R.D.
Department of Nutritional Sciences, University of Connecticut, Storrs, CT USA, 06269-4017

Key words: breast-feeding promotion, lactogenesis stage II, onset of lactation

1.   INTRODUCTION

A delay in the onset of lactation (OL), defined herein as the maternal perception of the initiation of copious amounts of breast milk production, may lead to an early introduction of infant formula and an early termination of breast-feeding (BF) even after controlling for maternal original BF intentions[1]. Women perceive OL between 12 hours and 5 days after delivery[1-4]. The objective of this study is to examine the implications of OL for infant feeding decisions.

2.   RESULTS

Mutivariate analyses performed on samples from different countries consistently indicate that a 'delayed' OL is a risk factor for poor BF outcomes. A longitudinal study conducted in urban Mexico[1] found that OL, expressed as a continuous variable in days post-partum (pp), was inversely associated with the likelihood of BF at 2 months pp (Odds Ratio (OR)=0.60, N=124, p=0.02). A cross-sectional survey conducted in Honduras[2] among women with children $\leq$ 2 y old indicated that OL > 72 h pp was positively

Short and Long Term Effects of Breast Feeding on Child Health
Edited by Berthold Koletzko *et al.*, Kluwer Academic/Plenum Publishers, 2000   425

associated with the use of milk-based prelacteal feeds (OR=1.89, N=2116, p<0.05) which in turn was associated with a lower likelihood of BF (OR=0.21, P<0.05). A longitudinal study conducted in Hartford, Connecticut, USA[3] found, among women planning to breastfeed for at least six months, that the median BF duration among women with OL < 72 h pp was longer than among women with OL ≥ 72 h pp (11.7 mo vs. 3.4 mo, N=56, p<0.001).

3.   DISCUSSION

Empirical data suggest that the longer it takes for women to perceive OL the more likely it is that they will become stressed and begin using breast milk substitutes. This may further delay OL leading to an early termination of BF. The sharp drop in progesterone subsequent to the removal of the placenta is considered a major trigger of OL. Delayed BF initiation, lack of rooming-in, stress during labor and delivery, emergency Cesarean deliveries, maternal obesity, and IDDM are risk factors for a delayed OL[4]. Further understanding of the determinants of OL should be a priority for BF promotion programs.

4.   CONCLUSIONS

International studies are needed to describe the epidemiology of OL. It is important to provide sound lactation management and psycho-social support to women who experience a 'delayed' OL. Future studies should emphasize the relationship between biological and psychosocial stress with OL and subsequent infant feeding outcomes.

REFERENCES

1. Pérez-Escamilla R, Segura-Millan S, Pollitt E, Dewey K. Determinants of lactation performance across time in an urban population from Mexico. Soc Sci & Med 1993;37:1069-1078.

2. Pérez-Escamilla R, Segura-Millan S, Canahuati J, Allen H. Prelacteal feeds are negatively associated with breast-feeding outcomes in Honduras. J. Nutr. 1996;126:2765-2773.

3. Chapman D, Pérez-Escamilla R. Does delayed perception of the onset of lactation shorten breast-feeding duration? J Hum Lact 1999;15:107-111.

4. Chapman D, Pérez-Escamilla R. Identification of risk factors for delayed onset of lactation. J Am Diet Assoc 1999;99:450-454.

60

PRE-TERM DELIVERY AND BREAST EXPRESSION: CONSEQUENCES FOR INITIATING LACTATION

Mark D. Cregan, Thalles R. de Mello, and Peter E. Hartmann
Department of Biochemistry, The University of Western Australia, Nedlands, Australia, 6907.

Key words: Lactogenesis II, pre-term expressing women, prolactin

1.   INTRODUCTION

Lactogenesis II (initiation of copious milk secretion) occurs 30-40 hours after birth in breastfeeding women[1] and is associated with changes in milk composition that stabilise by day 5 post-partum. Milk components which change from day 1 to day 5 include citrate (1.0 to 5.0 mM), lactose (90 to 160 mM)[1], sodium (60 to 10 mM) and total protein (40 to 10 g/L)[2], making them ideal lactogenesis II markers. We have demonstrated that pre-term expressing women produce lower volumes of milk at day 10 post-partum than both breastfeeding and full-term expressing women[3]. Thus the aim of this study is to determine the success of lactogenesis II in women expressing milk for their pre-term (31-35 weeks gestation) infants (expressing women), by measuring milk citrate, lactose, sodium, and total protein on day 5 post-partum, and comparing them to women breastfeeding full-term infants.

2.   INITIATION IN PRE-TERM EXPRESSING WOMEN

No significant differences were seen between the means ($\pm$ SD) of the lactogenesis II markers (citrate, lactose, sodium, and total protein) for expressing (3.4 ± 1.4 mM; 126 ± 17 mM; 30 ± 13mM; 15.3 ± 2.5 g/L respectively) and breastfeeding (4.3 ± 0.7 mM; 147 ± 10 mM; 12 ± 6 mM; 14.0 ± 1.5 g/L respectively) women. There was however a greater variation about the mean in expressing women (coefficient of variation in expressing women of 40% for citrate, lactose 14%, sodium 42%, and total protein 17%) when compared to breastfeeding women (17%, 7%, 33%, and 10% respectively). Thus implying there is variation in the success of initiation of lactation in these expressing women. Further statistical analysis[1] showed that 80% of expressing women had at least one lactogenesis II marker at pre-initiation concentrations, but none had all four (data not shown).

Whilst participating in our study the lactogenesis II markers of one expressing women changed from those indicating a failed initiation to a successful initiation over the course of day 5 (data not shown). Thus suggesting that a delay in lactogenesis II may, in part, be responsible for the compromised initiation observed in pre-term expressing women. In addition, the prolactin concentration (mean ± SD) of the milk did not differ significantly between expressing (54 ± 14 mM) and breastfeeding (60 ± 17 mM) women, nor was there a greater variation about the mean (coefficient of variation of 27% and 28% respectively). This finding suggests that prolactin deficiency was not responsible for the compromised initiation observed in pre-term expressing women.

3.   CONCLUSIONS

It was concluded that many pre-term expressing women undergo a compromised lactogenesis II, such that at day 5 of lactation some, but not all, lactogenesis II markers indicate a failure to initiate. Although the cause for a compromised initiation of lactation in pre-term expressing women has yet to be elucidated, it may be related to drug treatment for high risk pregnancy, complications arising from pre-term delivery and/or incomplete milk removal due to the failure of the milk ejection reflex.

4.   REFERENCES

1. P.G. Arthur, M. Smith, and P.E. Hartmann, Milk lactose, citrate and glucose as markers of lactogenesis in normal and diabetic women. *J. Pediatr.Gastroenterol. Nutr.* 9:488 (1989).
2. J.K. Kulski, and P.E. Hartmann, Changes in human milk composition during the initiation of lactation. *Aust. J. Exp. Biol. Med. Sci.* 59:101 (1981).
3. M.D. Cregan, and P.E. Hartmann, Computerized breast measurement from conception to weaning: Clinical Implications. *J. Hum. Lact.* 15:89 (1999).
This project was funded by MEDELA^{TM} Inc.

61

BREASTFEEDING RATES OF VLBW INFANTS—
Influence of Professional Breastfeeding Support

Pietschnig B, IBCLC, Siklossy H., Göttling A., Posch M, Käfer A., Lischka A.
Kinderklinik der Stadt Wien, Glanzing im Wilhelminenspital, Montleartstr. 37, 1171 WIEN

Key words: premature infant, neonatology, breastfeeding, human milk

1.   INTRODUCTION

Breastfeeding rates for VLBW- infants are by far lower than for term babies, however, nutritional and psychological advantages of mother's milk or breastfeeding for VLBW - infants are well documented.[1]

2.   OBJECTIVE

Is to document the difference between breastfeeding outcomes before (1994/95) and after (1997/8) introduction of professional support (IBCLC*) and staff training in helping mothers to initiate and maintain lactation.

3.   SUBJECTS AND METHODS

266 patients < 1500g, admitted to the NICU 1994/95 and 1997/98. Retrospective data from records. Statistics: Chi-squared test and analysis of variance. Before 1995, no specific lactation management measures were

Short and Long Term Effects of Breast Feeding on Child Health
Edited by Berthold Koletzko *et al.*, Kluwer Academic/Plenum Publishers, 2000

taken. Since 1995, individual mothers were counselled, during 1997 we offered intensive staff training by an IBCLC and improved the infrastructure for the mothers.[2,3,4.]

4.   RESULTS

	Number	Multiplet	<29week	Cesarian	Died	Transfer
1994/95	134	28	26	75	37	13
1997/98	137	34	13	5	8	1
P	n.s.	n.s.	n.sn	0.001	0.001	0.001

	Dismissed	Breastfed	Totally bf	Part.bf	Formula
1994/95	84	17	9	8	67
Ind.95	14	13	5	8	1
1997/98	127	81	44	37	46
94/95vs97/98 + ind95		0.001	0.001	0.001	0.001

Ind.95 Individual mothers counselled 1995 by IBCLC.

5.   DISCUSSION

Our study proves the influence of good lactation counselling on the breastfeeding rates of VLBW- infants. Retrospective maternal interviews reveal better bonding and contentedness, if the mother breastfeeds.

6.   CONCLUSION

Professional may support significantly increases breastfeeding in VLBW-infants. (* IBCLC- International Board Certified Lactation Consultant)[5]

REFERENCES

1. Lawrence: Breastfeeding, a Guide for the medical profession, Mosby 1994
2. Meier J., Engstrom et. Al: Breastfeeding support Services in the Neonatal Intensive care Unit, JOGGN, 1993,Vol22/4,33-347
3. Meier P, Brown L, Strategies to assist Breastfeeding in Preterm Infants, Recent Advances in Pediatrics, 137-150,1998
4. Furmann L, Minich NM et al: Breastfeeding VLBW-infants, JHL 14, 1, 29-34, 1998
5. Schanler R., Shulman R-J-: Feeding Strategies for premature infants, Randomised trial of gastrointestinal priming and tube feeding, Pediatrics 103, 2, 434-4-1997

62

BREASTFEEDING IN GENT, BELGIUM
A cohort study on breastfeeding rate and duration

Myriam Van Winckel, Nathalie Van De Keere, Sylvie Deblaere, Veerle Van Put, Eddy Robberecht
Department of Paediatrics, University Hospital, De Pintelaan 185, B 9000 Gent

Key words: breastfeeding habits

1.   INTRODUCTION

Little is known about infant feeding practices in Flanders, Belgium, beyond the neonatal period. This study describes breastfeeding rate and duration in Gent.

2.   METHOD

All 538 healthy term infants born between may 20 and august 19 in 1997, living in Gent and followed at well-baby clinics (Kind en Gezin) were eligible for the study. Privacy law prohibits direct contact with the parents, nurses of "Kind en Gezin" asked 324 (60%) parents permission for an interview regarding infant feeding habits. Of these, 27 (8%) refused.. Thus 297 (125 boys, 172 girls) infants were included. The study population was comparable to the population of Flanders regarding age, ,parity and degree of employment of the parents. 39% of the mothers had a full-time job, 16,5% worked part-time. Compared to the general population however, parents in the study population were more highly educated. 51% of the mothers and 45% of the fathers had attended high school or university, compared to 28% of women and 20,8% of men in Flanders. At the age of 5 months, a structured interview was performed at home.

Short and Long Term Effects of Breast Feeding on Child Health
Edited by Berthold Koletzko *et al.*, Kluwer Academic/Plenum Publishers, 2000   431

3.   RESULTS

206 (67%) infants received breastfeeding at birth. Parents had made the decision to breastfeed before pregnancy (93%). Breastfeeding rate was positively correlated with the educational level of the parents. Breastfeeding rate declines steadily during the first 5 months of life. It is stopped before the age of 2 weeks in 18/206 (9%) infants, between 2 and 6 weeks in 33 (16%), between 6 and 12 weeks in 62 (30%) and between 12 and 20 weeks in 47 (23%). Weaning foods were started before the age of 12 weeks in 25 (12%), between 14 and 16 weeks in 94 (45%), between 16 and 20 weeks in 50 (24%) infants. At the age of 5 months 98% of the infants received weaning foods, 17 (8%) received breastfeeding as the only milk source, 29 (14%) were partially breastfed and partially bottle-fed. Return to the workplace was the most frequent reason to stop breastfeeding (31%), followed by insufficient milk supply (20%), fatigue of the mother (17%), regurgitations and crying of the baby (11%), breast-problems (9%).and other reasons (12%). Parents said they took the decision to stop breastfeeding themselves (86%).. Introduction of weaning foods was advised by nurses of "Kind en Gezin" (49%) or by a paediatrician (10%). In 35% introduction of weaning foods was the parent's own decision.

4.   DISCUSSION AND CONCLUSION

In Belgium, reality differs greatly from the ideal situation where every infant receives exclusive breastfeeding during the first 4 to 6 months of life. In this study, 67% of the infants receive breastfeeding at birth. According to the parents, the decision to breastfeed is made before pregnancy. So, strategies to enhance breastfeeding rate should be targeted at adolescents. Breastfeeding rate declines rapidly and continuously during the first 5 months of life. Strategies aimed at increasing breastfeeding duration include better lactational support and lobbying for increasing maternity leave for working mothers and/or creating more opportunities to combine work and lactation successfully. Weaning foods were introduced before 4 months in 57% of the infants, whereas current guidelines advice to introduce them between 4 and 6 months of life. As parents introduced weaning foods most frequently as advised by health-care workers, these health-care workers obviously need better up to date information and education on infant nutrition.

63

BREAST-FEEDING PATTERN AND INFLUENCING FACTORS IN LITHUANIA

J. Vingraite[1]; A. Raugale[1]; K. Kadziauskine[2], K.F. Michaelsen[3]

[1]*Clinic of Children Diseases, Vilnius University, Lithuania,* [2]*National Nutrition Centre Vilnius, Lithuania and Research Department of Human Nutrition and LMC Centre for Advanced Food Studies,* [3]*The Royal Veterinary and Agricultural University, Rolighedsvej 30, 1958 Frederiksberg C, Denmark*

Key words: infant feeding, breast-feeding, influencing factors

1.   INTRODUCTION

Breast-feeding rates in Lithuania during the Soviet times were low, and exclusive breast-feeding was very rare. However, there are no well-collected and systemised data on infant feeding from that time. It was recommended to introduce juices and complementary feeding during the first months, as it was believed that the breast-fed infant needed extra water, vitamins, minerals and protein.

The aim of the present publication is to present preliminary data on duration of breast-feeding and influencing factors from an ongoing prospective study of infant nutrition in Lithuania, and to compare the results with data from a cross-sectional study performed in 1991/1992.

2.   METHODS , RESULTS AND DISCUSSION

In the first study a nation wide random sample of 702 mothers with a child between 6 and 36 years of age were interviewed about duration of breast-feeding, current feeding practices, and factors which potentially could influence breast-feeding duration.

The ongoing study is carried out in the capital Vilnius. Infants are followed from birth to 12 months with home visits at 3, 6, 9 and 12 months. At each visit the mother is asked about breast-feeding and when complementary foods were introduced. We present data for the first 165 infants who turned 6 months old before September 1999.

Breast-feeding rates in 1991/92 and 1998/99 are compared in the figure. The rates are not very different except for some longer duration of almost exclusive breast-feeding (i.e. infants drinking water/tea/juice in addition to breast-milk) during the first 3 months in 1991/92. No data are available on exclusive breast-feeding in 1991/92.

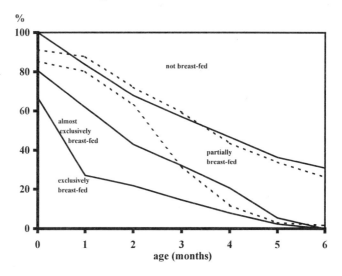

Figure 1. Breast-feeding rates in 1991/92 and 1998/99. (The three solid lines (the 1998/99 study) divide the infants into exclusively, almost exclusively, partially and not breast-fed. The two dashed lines (the 1991/92 study) divide the infants into almost exclusively, partially or not breast-fed.)

In the 1991/1992-year-study duration of breast-feeding was strongly associated with mother's age (≤ 20 y, mean 2.3 months; ≥ 31 y, 4.8 months; p=0.009), and duration of mother's education (p<0.00001) and negatively with smoking (p=0.05). There was no association with parity, time span since the last delivery and mother's employment status.

Breast-feeding rates are still low and there is no sign of an increasing trend. Exclusive breast-feeding is rare. The results suggest that support of breast-feeding is not sufficient, and that it is especially the youngest mothers and those having the lowest education who need more information and support.

64

FACTORS INFLUENCING A MOTHER'S DECISION TO BREASTFEED

Carol L. Wagner, M.D., Mark T. Wagner, Ph.D., and Thomas C. Hulsey, Sc.D.

Div. of Neonatology and Epidemiology, Dept. of Pediatrics and the Depts. of Psychiatry and Behaviorial Sciences & Neurology, Medical University of South Carolina, Charleston, SC

Key words: breastfeeding, personality traits, maternal attitudes

1.   INTRODUCTION

Mothers choose to breastfeed for a variety of reasons; however, little is known to what extent environmental and intrapsychic factors may influence that decision, if at all. We conducted a survey of mothers delivering at a university hospital to test whether infant-feeding choice was associated with personality traits.

2.   METHODS

Any mother delivering at an inner city, University hospital on postpartum days 1-4 during 2 periods (June-August 1996 & June-August 1997) was eligible for enrollment into the study. Based on observed/self-reported behavior, women were classified either as (1) initiators of breastfeeding only or as (2) initiators of formula feeding only. Combination breast/formula feeders were excluded from the study (n = 16).

A structured interview and a 264-question Revised NEO Personality Inventory were used to objectively determine attitudinal, cultural and personality traits. A Hollingshead score was calculated for each subject based on occupation and educational level. Following the interview, the subjects were asked to complete the personality inventory.

Short and Long Term Effects of Breast Feeding on Child Health
Edited by Berthold Koletzko *et al.*, Kluwer Academic/Plenum Publishers, 2000   435

3.   RESULTS

There were significant socio-economic differences between initiators of breastfeeding and formula feeding. Mothers who had chosen breastfeeding were older, of higher socio-economic status as defined by the Hollingshead score, and were married. The independent association between socio-economic status and personality on breastfeeding was determined by logistic regression. Compared to unskilled workers, professional mothers were 5.1 times as likely to initiate breastfeeding (95% CI: 1.1-23.4; p=0.04).

Maternal life experiences were associated with a mother's decision to initiate breastfeeding in the first four days after delivery. Of those women who were themselves breastfed, 74% chose to breastfeed compared with 40% who chose to breastfeed when they themselves were not breastfed (p<0.03). A similar relationship was found if father had been breastfed.

In the final group of 209 subjects, 73 returned the NEO (43 BF and 30 FF). While compliance was a major factor in completed NEO inventories, the respondents were similar to the non-respondents in terms of sociodemographic characteristics. Significant group differences were found on 3 major Personality Factor Domain group mean T-scores. After controlling for socio-economic status in a logistic regression analysis, the personality factor traits Extraversion and Openness remained the dimensions significantly associated with breastfeeding.

4.   SUMMARY OF STUDY FINDINGS

(1) Socioeconomic factors were strongly associated with feeding type decision. Breastfeeding women in this cohort were older, more educated, of higher socioeconomic status, and married.

(2) Prior maternal and paternal experiences with breastfeeding influenced a mother's decision to initiate breastfeeding.

(3) Of the 73 responders, certain personality characteristics of mothers were associated with a mother's infant feeding decision.

(a) When socioeconomic status was controlled, breastfeeding mothers' personality traits contrasted with formula-feeders as being more affectionate, friendly, active, optimistic, receptive to emotional experience, and willing to try new activities.

(b) Formula feeding mothers contrasted with breastfeeders as being more reserved, less likely to try new activities, less exuberant, less likely to acknowledge feeling states as important, and more skeptical.

65

USE OF SOFT LASER IN THE THERAPY OF SORE NIPPLES IN BREASTFEEDING WOMEN

Pietschnig Beate IBCLC, Pani Michael, Käfer Astrid, Bauer Wais Elisabeth and Lischka Andreas.
Wilhelminenspital der Stadt WIEN, Kinderklinik Glanzing, Austria

Key words: Low level laser therapy, sore nipples, cracked nipples, breastfeeding

1. INTRODUCTION

AAP, WHO/UNICEF and the Austrian Pediatric Society recommend exclusive breastfeeding or the first 4-6 months. Sore nipples are responsible for early weaning[1,2.] The main reasons are wrong positioning, candida albicans and bacterial infection [3].

Low level laser irradiation ("softlaser") improves the microcirculation and proliferation of keratinocytes.[4,5,6,7] however, the therapy of sore nipples with softlaser has never been published.

2. GOAL OF THE STUDY

The main aim was to report the causes and therapies of a group of mothers with sore and cracked nipples.

3.   PATIENTS / METHODS / STUDYDESIGN

31 mothers with sore nipples (1998), who came for an "ultimate ratio".
All mothers were counselled for proper lactation management, medicated
as necessary and used pure lanolin. Softlaser was started at the first visit. We
used a 5mW / 780nm laser for 2 minutes at a distance of 5 cm every other
day. All mothers reported pain - intensity on a 0-10 scale[8].

4.   RESULTS

The mean number of treatment sessions was 6.92 (SD 3.72). The mean
painvalue was 9.17 (SD 0.89) in the beginning and 1.95 (SD0.76) at the last
visit. Antimycotics were used in 16 mothers topically, 3 systemic, antibiotics
in 6 and 4 mothers, resp. No nipples shields were used. 28 mothers went on
breastfeeding, 2 were not sure, 1 mother quit.

5.   DISCUSSION

Sore represent a severe problem. Low level laser therapy may be a
valuable adjuvant therapy, together with counselling and medication.

REFERENCES

1) Haschke F, Schilling R, Thun- Hohenstein L, Schuster E (1985): Säuglingsernährung in
    Österreich, eine Studie im Auftrag des BMUG
2) Bronneberg G, Frank W: (1998): Stillen in Österreich, BMUG
3) Livingstone VH, Willis CE, Berkowitz J: (1996): Staphylococcus aureus and sore nipples.
    Can. Fam. Physician Apr.42 654-9
4) Yu W, Naim JO, Lanzafame RJ: (1997): Effects of photostimulation on wound healing in
    diabetic mice. Lasers Surg Med 20(1): 56-63
5) Landau Z: (1998): Topical hyperbaric oxygen and low energy laser for the treatment of
    diabetic foot ulcers. Arch. Orthop. Trauma Surg 117(3): 156-8
6) Grossmann N, Schneid N., Reuveni H, Halevy R, Lubart R: (1998): 780 nm low power
    laser irradiation stimulates proliferation of keratinocyte cultures: involvement of reqactive
    oxygen species. Lasers Surg Med 22(4): 212-8
7) Schindl A, Schindl M, Schon H, Knobler R, Havelec L, Schindl L⊗ 1998) Low- intensity
    laser irradiation improves skin circulation in patients with diabetic microangiopathy.
    Diabetes Care Apr., 21(4): 580-4
8) Carey SJ, Turpin C, Whatley J, Haddox D: (1997): Improving pain management in an
    acute care setting. The Crawford Long Hospital of Emory University experience. Orthop.
    Nurs Jul-Aug 16(4): 29-36

66

NATURAL FEEDING OF PREMATURE INFANTS

Magdalena Salamon[1] , Anna Sendecka[2]
[1]Obstetrics Ward of the Independent Public Health Service in Nowy Sacz. Poland .
Head of Department: Dr. Andrzej Bieniasz M.D., Ph.D. [2]The Chair and Department of
Clinical Nursing , Nursing Faculty of the Medical Academy in Lublin. Poland. Chief of
Department: Prof. Krzysztof Turowski M.D., Ph. D.

Key words: natural feeding, premature infants, breast feeding

1.   INTRODUCTION

The Breast-feeding Promotional Program in Poland (begun in 1992) establishes that by the year 1997, 50,0% of all newborns shall be exclusively breast-feed to the end of their fourth month of life. For this reason a retrospective study was performed to answer the following question : by which method were pre-mature infants feed during the years 1993-1996 at the Regional Hospital in Nowy Sącz .

2.   MATERIALS AND METHODS

Research questionnaires polled 99 mothers and 110 pre-mature infants during the years 1993-1996.The number and percentage of pre-mature infants depending on pregnancy duration is presented in table 1.

Table 1.Number and percentage of pre-mature infants born depending on pregnancy duration.

Pregnancy Duration (weeks)	Children born in 1993-1994 y.(**Gr.I**)		Children born in 1993-1994 y.(**Gr.II**)		Total	
	N	%	N	%	N	%
To end 33	9	17,0	12	21,2	21	19,1
34 –36	44	83,0	45	78,8	89	80,9
Total	53	100,0	57	100,0	110	100,0

3.   RESULTS

According to the literature, newborns delivered at the end of the 33rd week of gestation do not have a fully mature sucking reflex, whereas newborns delivered after the 33rd week of gestation have a mature sucking reflex. Among the studied groups, almost 84,0% of pre-mature infants had a developed sucking reflex, while 86,0% of pre-mature babies in both group possessed a developed swallowing reflex. Worth noting is that 67,9% of infants from group I and 82,5% from group II were born in good state according to the Apgar Scale, which may explain their ability to be breast-fed. Nevertheless none of the pre-mature infants, possessing developed sucking and swallowing reflexes, were breast-feed in the delivery room. During hospitalization, 68,0% of infants from group I and 72,0% of infants from group II undertook breast-feeding. In both groups 82,0% of the pre-mature infants born after the 33rd week of pregnancy were breast-feed in obstetric department. Almost all children born before the 33 week of pregnancy were artificially fed.

4.   CONCLUSION

The Polish Program Promoting Breastfeeding set the goal that by the year 1997, 50,0% of all infants would be exclusively breastfed during the first four months of life. In group I 43,4% infants were breastfed at home, where among these infants 35,8% were exclusively breastfed until the end of the 4th month of life. In group II 50,9% infants were breastfed at home, where among these baby 33,3% were naturally fed until the 4th month of life.

WHO recommends feeding exclusively with breast milk until 4th – 6th month of infant life. In group I 17,0% of premature infants and 29,8% in group II (almost 13,0% more) were fed with breast milk for at least 4 to 6 months.

67

NEWS ABOUT HUMAN MILK BANKING IN GERMANY

Skadi Springer, M.D., IBCLC
Dept. Neonatology, Children's Hospital, University of Leipzig, Germany

Key words: human milk banking, donor milk, guidelines, screening, distribution

1.   HISTORY

Germany has a longstanding tradition of donor human milk banking. The first human milk bank was founded in 1919. While human milk banking was widespread during the 1950s, by 1972 it reached its lowest level (52.000 l/year). By the end of the 80's it had climbed to its highest level before reunification of the two parts of Germany: About 200.000 l/year were collected in the 60 milk banks of the eastern part of Germany. The need for donor milk throughout this region was more than adequately met. After the reunification of Germany, a lot of milk banks were closed.

Position Statement of the Nutrition Commission of the German Pediatric Society, (July 1991):

Donor milk is needed as an important option for the care and treatment of premature and sick newborns and babies. Its use in pediatrics has a primarily preventive and therapeutic character particularly in immature newborns and in cases of serious intestinal illness in infancy such as Necrotizing Enterocolitis (NEC), Morbus Hirschsprung, intractable diarrhea and cow's milk protein intolerance.

2.   HUMAN MILK BANKS IN GERMANY

In 1998, the 15 remaining milk banks were able to supply about 8000 liters of donor milk from more than 500 nursing mothers. The collection capacity varies widely from 50 up to 3000 l/year. Nine of the 15 milk banks meet the demand of donor milk in their region.

3.   GUIDELINES

Strict collection and storage procedures are necessary to provide safe, high quality donor milk to those infants who need it. The guidelines for German milk banks are comparable with the ones in the United States and the United Kingdom. It is important that the milk is uncontaminated and that the donors are selected and screened carefully like blood donors. Samples of each bottle of milk are collected and screened for bactaria. None of the donor milk is pooled to further reduce the risk of contamination.

The donor milk is offered as:

1. — frozen human milk (–18°C/6 months)
2. — pasteurized human milk (+4°C/48 hours or –18°C/6 months)
3. — untreated human milk (+4°C/72 hours)
4. — freeze-dried human milk (room temperature/1 year)

If a preterm mother is able to provide a surplus of breast milk above the needs of her own infant this milk is preferred for the early feedings of an other preterm baby because of the special needs of the premiees. Half of the human milk banks carry out the collection on a daily basis. This make it possible to provide fresh milk with its clear advantages, especially immunological and infectological ones. Necrotising enterocolitis, for example, is extremely rare in the neonatal unit of our hospital. The interest in feeding of very low birth weight newborns with human milk is steadily increasing in other countries. Along with this interest there is the need to learn more about management of human milk banks in the modern world. Therefore we want to get in contact with the staff of milk banks in Europe and worldwide.

REFERENCES:

1. Balmer SE, Williams AF 1995 Guidelines for the establishment and operation of human milk banks in UK. Midwifery 5(3): 342-342

Contributors

Bengt Björksten
Dept. of Pediatrics
University Hospital
S-58185 Lingköping
Sweden
Benbj@ped.liu.se

Rudy Boersma
Pediatrician
NL-9728 NH Groningen
Netherlands
e.r.boersma@med.rug.nl

Ana Maria Calderón
CIAD
883000 Hermosillo, Sonora
Mexico
Amc@cascabel.ciad.mx

Donna Chapman
University of Connecticut
Cept. Nutritional Sciences
Storrs, CT 06269
USA
Dic95005@uconnvm.uconn.edu

Mark Cregan
University of Western Australia
Dept. of Biochemistry
Perth 6907
Australia
Mdcregan@cyllene.uwa.edu.au

Tamás Decsi
University of Medical Sciences
Dept. of Paediatrics
H-7623 Pécs
Hungary
Decsi@apacs.pote.hu

Martha Del Prado
Unidad de Investigación en Nutrición
México D.F. 06700
Mexico
Svnutri@data.net.mx

Suzanne Filteau
Institute of Child Health
GB-London WC1N 1EH
England
Sfiltreau@ich.ucl.ac.uk

Monique Gerichhausen
Novartis Nutrition Research
CH-3176 Neuenegg
Switzerland
Monique-gerichhausen@ch.novartis.com

Jean-Pierre Habicht
Cornell University
Ithaca, NY 14853
USA
Jh48@cornell.edu

C. N. Hales
Dept. of Clinical Biochemistry
University of Cambridge
Addenbrooke's Hospital
Cambridge CB2 2QR
England
Cnh1000@cam.ac.uk

Klaus Hamprecht
Hygiene-Institut der Universität Tübingen
Abt. f. Med. Virologie und Epidemiologie
der Viruskrankheiten
72076 Tübingen
Germany
Klaus.hamprecht@uni-tuebingen.de

Lars Ake Hanson
University of Göteborg
Dept. of Clinical Immunology
S-41346 Göteborg
Sweden
Lars.a.hanson@immuno.gu.se

Joanna Hawkes
Child Nutrition Research Centre
Women's & Children's Hospital
CNRC, Level I Rieger Building
North Adelaide 5006
Australia
Jo.hawkes@flinders.edu.au

Olle Hernell
Dept. of Pediatrics
Umeå University
S-90185 Umeå
Sweden
Olle.hernell@pediatri.umu.se

Tadashi Iizuka
Kihoku Hospital
Wakayama Medical College
649-7113 Wakayama
Japan
Taiizuka@wakayama-med.ac.jp

Charles E. Isaacs
Institute for Basic Research
Staten Island, NY 10314
USA
Chisi@cuny.edu

Alan Jackson
Institute of Human Nutrition
University of Southhampton
UK
a.jackson@ihnsoton.easynet.co.uk

Christian Kind
Ostschweizer Kinderspital
CH-9006 St. Gallen
Switzerland
Christian.kind@gd-kispi.sg.ch

Nigel Klein
Great Ormond Street Hospital for
Children Trust and Institute of Child
Health
30 Guilford Street
London WC1N 1EH
England
n.klein@ich.ucl.ac.uk

Berthold Koletzko
University of Munich
Dept. of Pediatrics
80337 München
Germany
Berthold.koletzko@kk-i.med.uni-
muenchen.de

Michael Kramer
McGill University
Montreal H3A 1A2
Canada
Mikek@epid.lan.mcgill.ca

Clemens Kunz
Institute of Nutrition
University of Giessen
Wilhelmstr. 20
35392 Giessen
Germany
Clemens.kunz@ernaehrung.uni-giessen.de

Alejandra Lance
Unidad de Investigación en Nutrición
México D.F. 14490
Mexico
Lance@datasys.com.mx

Frauke Lehner
Kinderklinik & Kinderpoliklinik
Universität München
80337 München
Germany
Frauke-Lehner@pk-i.med.uni-
muenchen.de

Bernhard Liebl
Landesuntersuchungsamt of the State of
Bavaria
D-85762 Oberschleißheim
München
Germany
Liebl_lua@compuserve.com

Eric L. Lien
Wyeth Nutritionals International
Philadelphia, PA 19101
USA
Liene@war.wyeth.com

Mardya Lopez-Alarcon
Tlalnepantla 54090
Mexico
Saumar2@dfl.telmex.net.mx

Chessa Lutter
Pan American Health Organization
Washington, DC 20037
USA
Lutterch@paho.org

Grace S. Marquis
Iowa State University
Dept. of Food Science and Human
Nutrition
Ames, IA 50011-1061
USA
Gmarquis@iastate.edu

Kim Fleischer Michaelsen
Research Dept. of Human Nutrition
The Royal Veterinary and Agricultural
University
DK-1958 Frederiksberg C
Denmark
Kim.F.Michaelsen@fhe.kvl.dk

Leon Mitoulas
University of Western Australia
Dept. of Biochemistry
Perth 6907
Australia
Lrobert@cyllene.uwa.edu.au

Manuel Moya
Hospital U. San Juan
E-03550 San Juan, Alicante
Spain
Manuel.moya@umh.es

Ruth Nduati
University of Nairobi
P.O. Box 19676
Nairobi
Kenya
Rnduati@iconnect.co.ke

David S. Newburg
Shriver Center
Waltham, MA 02452
USA
DNewburg@shriver.org

Wendy Oddy
Institute for Child Health Research
The University of Western Australia
Perth 6872
Australia
Wendyo@ichr.uwa.edu.au

Adelheid Onyango
World Health Organization
Nutrition for Health & Development
CH-1211 Geneva 27
Switzerland
Onyango@who.ch

Rafael Peréz-Escamilla
University of Connecticut
Dept. of Nutritional Sciences (U-17)
Storrs, CT 06269-4017
USA
Rperez@canrl.cag.uconn.edu

Beate Pietschnig
Wilhelminenspital der Stadt Wien
Montleartstr. 37
A-1171 Wien
Austria
Pietschnig@Eunet.at

Hildegard Przyrembel
Federal Health Office
BgVV
14195 Berlin
Germany
h.przyrembel@bgvv.de

Amy Rice
The Johns Hopkins University
School of Public Health
Baltimore, MD 21205
USA
Arice@jhsph.edu

Kristiina Saarinen
Hospital for Children and Adolescents
University of Helsinki
00029 Helsinki
Finland
Kristiina.saarinen@huch.fi

Francesco Savino
Via Reymond 7
I-10126 Torino
Italy
Savino@pediatria.unito.it

Magdalena Salamon
Spzoz Nowy Sacz
PL-33 300 Nowy Sacz
Poland
Magdasa@mp.pl

Thorsten Sauerwald
Kinderklinik & Kinderpoliklinik
Universität München
80337 München
Germany
Thorsten.sauerwald@kk-i.med.uni-
muenchen.de

Felicity Savage
World Health Organization
Dept. of Child and Adolescent Health
Development
CH-1211 Geneva 27
Switzerland
Savagekingf@who.int

Horst Schroten
University Children's Hospital
Heinrich Heine Universität
Düsseldorf
Germany
Schroten@uni-dusseldorf.de

Kirsten Simondon
Research Institute for Development
F-34032 Montpellier
France
Kirsten.simondon@mpl.ird.fr

Ella N. Smit
% Th. Hiemstra
71000 Sarajevo
Bosnia and Herzegovina
Pip@bib.net.ba

Otmar Tönz
Schlösslihalde
CH-6006 Luzern
Switzerland
o.toenz@bluewin.ch

Myriam van Winckel
Univeristy Hospital Gent
UZG 5K6
B-9000 Gent
Belgium
Myriam.vanwinckel@rug.ac.be

Jovile Vingraite
2050 Vilnius
Lithuania
Jovi@ktl.mii.lt

Rüdiger von Kries
Institut uur Soziale Pädiatrie und
Jugendmedizin
Kinderzentrum München
81377 München
Germany
Ag.epi@lrz.uni-muenchen.de

Carol Wagner
Medical University of S.C.
Dept. of Pediatrics
Division of Neonatology
Charleston, SC 29425
USA
Wagnercl.@musc.edu

Agnes Wold
University of Göteborg
Dept. of Clinical Immunology
Guldhedsgatan 10, SE-41346
Göteborg
Sweden
Agnes.wold@immuno.gu.se

Anne L. Wright
Tucson, AZ 85704
USA
Awright@resp-sci.arizona.edu

INDEX

1